NUTRACEUTICALS IN CANCER PREVENTION, MANAGEMENT, AND TREATMENT

AAP Advances in Nutraceuticals

NUTRACEUTICALS IN CANCER PREVENTION, MANAGEMENT, AND TREATMENT

Edited by

Raj K. Keservani, MPharm

Bui Thanh Tung, PhD

Sippy Singh, DPhil

Rajesh K. Kesharwani, PhD

AAP | APPLE ACADEMIC PRESS

First edition published 2024

Apple Academic Press Inc.
1265 Goldenrod Circle, NE,
Palm Bay, FL 32905 USA

760 Laurentian Drive, Unit 19,
Burlington, ON L7N 0A4, CANADA

CRC Press
2385 NW Executive Center Drive,
Suite 320, Boca Raton FL 33431

4 Park Square, Milton Park,
Abingdon, Oxon, OX14 4RN UK

Library and Archives Canada Cataloguing in Publication

CIP data on file with Canada Library and Archives

Library of Congress Cataloging-in-Publication Data

CIP data on file with US Library of Congress

ISBN: 978-1-77491-327-7 (hbk)
ISBN: 978-1-77491-328-4 (pbk)
ISBN: 978-1-00339-255-2 (ebk)

ABOUT THE BOOK SERIES: AAP ADVANCES IN NUTRACEUTICALS

Series Editor:
Raj K. Keservani, MPharm
Faculty of B. Pharmacy, CSM Group of Institutions, Allahabad, India
Telephone: +91-7897803904 / Email: rajksops@gmail.com

Rajesh K. Kesharwani, PhD
Nehru Gram Bharati (Deemed to be University), Prayagraj, India

Anil K. Sharma, PhD, MPharm
Department of Pharmacy, School of Medical and Allied Sciences,
GD Goenka University, Gurugram, India

In the modern era, mankind has witnessed a paradigm shift with respect to fundamental eating behavior. The lack of physical workouts and busy schedules at offices and in households have promoted the consumption of junk foods, which eventually results in numerous diseases and disorders since the nutritional content from fast food is inadequate. Plumpness and obesity have become a global health threat. The leading causes of death from most developing nations are noncommunicable diseases such as cardiovascular diseases, cancer, arthritis, osteoporosis, and liver toxicity. Patients suffering from such lifestyle ailments are a bit apprehensive towards prolonged use of costly modern therapeutics, which encourages instead the use of alternative approaches for management of such diseases and disorders.

The emerging sector of the nutraceutical industry encompasses products derived from nature, dietary supplements, and functional foods. Nutraceuticals are used for treatment and prevention of a broad range of diseases, such as the common cold, arthritis, sleep-related disorders, cancers, cardiovascular complications, metabolic disorders, and others.

The research on nutraceuticals is increasing day by day, considering the beneficial effects of food or food supplements in the management of diverse diseases. The issue of paramount concern is standardization and establishment of clinical efficacy of nutraceuticals, which is in fact a challenge for researchers around the globe.

This book series aims at realizing the significance of the variety of nutraceuticals for human well-being. The books in the series will also emphasize the role of dieticians and nutritionists for the prescription of judicious eating habits. The key food components such as carbohydrates, proteins, and lipids as well as micronutrients (vitamins, minerals) are demonstrated to maintain good health, obviating the need for medicines. Thus, nutraceuticals that are indeed derived from food ingredients are believed to be potential alternative therapeutics.

Asymptomatic diseases/disorders necessitate proper diagnosis. Stressed circumstances have been reported to cause weight loss. Workplace stress is a key variable in the genesis and propagation of metabolic disorders. The nuances of the underlying mechanisms are still to be deciphered. Poor lifestyle trends have been attributed along with the consumption of junk foods in several such instances. Sugar-rich carbonated beverages, the use of contraband drugs, and the consumption of liquor in excess are assigned as risk factors. This book series will cover advances and applications in addition to providing the basics of nutraceuticals.

The books in this series may be valuable resources for industry professionals to design and develop quality products for end users. In addition, the book series will be fortified by ideas of innovation, concept building, manufacturing aspects, quality control, and regulatory status of nutraceuticals.

Ostensibly, business has seen a rise in the nutraceutical consumption in recent years. Pure, safe, efficacious products are the need of the hour globally. There are a number of books on nutraceuticals in the market, yet these are only a few books presenting certain aspects of nutraceuticals therein. This book series aims to offer a holistic view of this promising strategy, which is picking up pace with time. This book series will be a unique endeavor to bring manufacturing, research and development, and marketing strategies under a single umbrella.

CURRENT BOOKS IN THE SERIES

- **Micronutrients and Macronutrients as Nutraceuticals**
  Editors: Prakash Chandra Gupta, PhD, Sayan Bhattacharyya, MBBS, MD, Nisha Sharma, PhD, MPharm, Rajesh K. Kesharwani, PhD, and Raj K. Keservani, MPharm

- **Formulations, Regulations, and Challenges of Nutraceuticals**
  Editors: Tingirikari Jagan Mohan Rao, PhD, Rajesh K. Kesharwani, PhD, Raj. K. Keservani, MPharm, and Anil K. Sharma, PhD
- **Food Supplements and Dietary Fibers in Health and Disease**
  Editors: Bhushan R. Rane, PhD, MPharm, Raj K. Keservani, M Pharm, Durgesh Singh, DPhil, Nayan A. Gujarathi, PhD, and Ashish S. Jain, PhD
- **Nutraceuticals in Cancer Prevention, Management, and Treatment**
  Editors: Raj K. Keservani, MPharm, Bui Thanh Tung, PhD, Sippy Singh, DPhil, and Rajesh K. Kesharwani, PhD
- **Advances in Flavonoids for Human Health and Prevention of Diseases**
  Editors: Nisha Sharma, PhD, Deepika Saini, PhD, Rajesh K. Kesharwani, PhD, Prakash Chandra Gupta, and Raj. K. Keservani, MPharm
- **The Flavonoids: Extraction and Applications**
  Editors: Deepika Saini, PhD, Rajesh K. Kesharwani, PhD, and Raj K. Keservani, MPharm
- **Immune-Boosting Nutraceuticals for Better Human Health: Novel Applications**
  Editors: Urmila Jarouliya, PhD, Raj K. Keservani, MPharm, Rajesh K. Kesharwani, PhD, Virendra K. Patel, PhD, and Adi D. Bharti
- **Applications of Functional Foods in Disease Prevention**
  Editors: Raj K. Keservani, MPharm, and Eknath D. Ahire, MSPharm
- **Plant Metabolites and Vegetables as Nutraceuticals**
  Editors: Raj K. Keservani, MPharm, Bui Thanh Tung, PhD, Rajesh K. Kesharwani, PhD, MPharm, and Eknath D. Ahire
- **Preventive and Therapeutic Role of Vitamins as Nutraceuticals**
  Editors: Khemchand R. Surana, Eknath D. Ahire, Raj K. Keservani, MPharm, and Rajesh K. Kesharwani, PhD
- **Nutraceuticals and Bone Health**
  Editors: Deepak Sharma, PhD, Madan Mohan Gupta, PhD, Anil K. Sharma, PhD, MPharm, Raj K. Keservani, MPharm, and Rajesh K. Kesharwani, PhD
- **Flavonoids as Nutraceuticals**
  Editors: Rajesh K. Kesharwani, PhD, MTech, Deepika Saini, PhD, Raj K. Keservani, MPharm, and Anil Kumar Sharma, PhD, MPharm

- **Herbals as Nutraceuticals: Their Role in Healthcare**
  Editors: Raj K. Keservani, MPharm, Rajeshwar Kamal Kant Arya, PhD, MPharm, and Rajesh K. Kesharwani, PhD, MTech
- **Nutraceutical Fruits: Overview and Disease Prevention**
  Editors: Raj K. Keservani, MPharm

ABOUT THE EDITORS

Raj K. Keservani, MPharm
Associate Professor, Faculty of B. Pharmacy, CSM Group of Institutions, Prayagraj, India

Raj K. Keservani, MPharm, is currently working as an Associate Professor, faculty of B. Pharmacy, CSM Group of Institutions, Prayagraj, India. He has more than 12 years of academic (teaching) experience from various institutes in India in pharmaceutical education. He has supervised more than 25 UG students for their research work, has published 31 peer-reviewed papers in the field of pharmaceutical sciences in national and international journals, has one patent, 43 book chapters, three co-authored books, and 19 edited books. He is also active as a reviewer for several international scientific journals. Mr. Keservani graduated with a pharmacy degree from the Department of Pharmacy, Kumaun University, Nainital (Uttarakhand), India. He received his Master of Pharmacy (MPharm) (specialization in pharmaceutics) from the School of Pharmaceutical Sciences, Rajiv Gandhi Proudyogiki Vishwavidyalaya, Bhopal, India. Mr. Keservani is a life member of the Society of Pharmaceutical Education and Research (SPER). His research interests include nutraceutical and functional foods, novel drug delivery systems (NDDS), transdermal drug delivery/drug delivery, health science, cancer biology, and neurobiology.

Bui Thanh Tung, PhD
Faculty of VNU School of Medicine and Pharmacy, Vietnam National University, Hanoi, Vietnam

Bui Thanh Tung, PhD, is the Faculty of VNU School of Medicine and Pharmacy at Vietnam National University, Hanoi, Vietnam. Bui Thanh Tung received his PhD in Pharmacology from Seville University, Spain, in 2014. Then, he worked as a Lecturer in the School of Medicine and Pharmacy, at Vietnam National University Ha Noi. In 2018, he was appointed as an Associate Professor. His main research focuses on medicinal plants for the treatment of various diseases such as diabetes, Alzheimer, cancer, etc. His special interest is in the development of new drugs from Vietnamese natural resources. He writes and presents widely on issues of natural products, bioactive compounds, and their pharmacological activities.

Sippy Singh, DPhil
Assistant Professor, Department of Zoology, S.S. Khanna Girls' Degree College, Prayagraj (A Constituent College of University of Allahabad, Prayagraj), India

Sippy Singh, DPhil, is an Assistant Professor in the Department of Zoology at S.S. Khanna Girls' Degree College, Prayagraj (A Constituent College of the University of Allahabad, Prayagraj). She has more than seven years of academic experience in various institutes in India. Dr. Singh has completed her DPhil in Zoology with a specialization in Neurobiology from the University of Allahabad. She has also served as Project Co-coordinator of the Societal Research Fellowship (SoRF) Scheme of the Department of Science and Technology, GoI at NASI, Prayagraj (The Oldest Science Academy). Dr. Singh has edited one book and has 20 publications in the form of research papers, book chapters, and popular articles in international and national journals of high repute. She is a life member of scientific bodies: ISCA, IAN, ISCB, ABRF, and IFEE. Dr. Singh is a member of IQAC. She is the recipient of two international awards: the S.S. Parmar Foundation Award" of IAN and the "Young Scientist Award 2019 of IFEE, and three national awards. Her research interest includes neurobiology and cell biology.

Rajesh K. Kesharwani, PhD
Associate Professor, Department of Computer Application, Nehru Gram Bharati (Deemed to be University), Prayagraj, India

Rajesh K. Kesharwani, PhD, MTech, is currently working as an Associate Professor in the Department of Computer Application at Nehru Gram Bharati (Deemed to be University), Prayagraj, India. He has more than 11 years of research and nine years of teaching experience in various institutes in India, imparting bioinformatics and biotechnology education. He has received several awards, including the NASI-Swarna Jayanti Puruskar by The National Academy of Sciences of India. He has supervised one PhD, and more than 20 UG, and PG students for their research work, and has authored over 49 peer-reviewed articles, 20 book chapters, and 14 edited Books with international publishers (e.g., Springer Nature, IGI Global, Taylor & Francis, etc.). He has been a member of many scientific communities as well as a reviewer for many international journals. He has presented many papers at various national and international conferences. Dr. Kesharwani received his PhD from the Indian Institute of Information Technology, Allahabad, and worked at NIT Warangal for two-semester. He has been a recipient of the Ministry of Human Resource Development (India) Fellowship and a Senior Research Fellowship from the Indian Council of Medical Research, India. His research fields of interest are medical informatics, protein structure and function prediction, computer-aided drug designing, structural biology, drug delivery, cancer biology, nano-biotechnology, and biomedical sciences.

CONTENTS

CONTRIBUTORS

Raghu Ram Achar
Division of Biochemistry, School of Life Sciences, JSS Academy of Higher Education and Research, Mysuru, Karnataka, India

Tushar B. Agam
Shri D. D. Vispute College of Pharmacy and Research Center, Panvel, Maharashtra, India

Bhavana Ahire
Department of Quality Assurance Techniques, NDMVP's, College of Pharmacy, Nashik, India

Eknath D. Ahire
Department of Pharmaceutics, MET's Institute of Pharmacy, Adgaon Nashik, India

Rabia Shabir Ahmad
Department of Food Science, Government College University Faisalabad, Faisalabad, Pakistan

Aliashraf Bagheri
Department of Nuclear Engineering, Faculty of Sciences and Modern Technologies, Graduate University of Advanced Technology, Kerman, Iran

Atun Roy Choudhury
Manager (HoD), Fecal Sludge Management Division, Banka BioLoo Limited, India; Scholar, Department of Biological Sciences, BITS Pilani Hyderabad Campus, India

Ozan E. Eyupoglu
Department of Biochemistry, School of Pharmacy, Istanbul Medipol University, Istanbul, Turkey

Prakash Chandra Gupta
School of Pharmaceutical Sciences, Chhatrapati Sahu Ji Maharaj University, Kanpur, India

Zeinab Haghi
Department of Plant Protection, School of Agriculture, Shiraz University, Shiraz, Iran

Sadia Hassan
Department of Nutritional Sciences, Faculty of Science and Technology, Government College Women University Faisalabad, Faisalabad, Pakistan
Department of Dietetics and Nutritional Sciences, The University of Faisalabad, Faisalabad, Pakistan

Muhammad Bilal Hussain
Department of Food Science, Government College University Faisalabad, Faisalabad, Pakistan

Shaista Jabeen
Department of Zoology, Vellore, Tamil Nadu, India

Anil G. Jadhav
Department of Pharmacognosy, Sandip Institute of Pharmaceutical Sciences, Savitribai Phule Pune University, Nashik, Maharashtra, India

Emad Jafarzadeh
Department of Toxicology and Pharmacology, Faculty of Pharmacy, Tehran University of Medical Sciences (TUMS), Tehran, Iran

Ashish S. Jain
Shri D. D. Vispute College of Pharmacy and Research Center, Panvel, Maharashtra, India

Amna Javed
Department of Food Science, Government College University Faisalabad, Faisalabad, Pakistan

Ashish A. Karle
Shri D. D. Vispute College of Pharmacy and Research Center, Panvel, Maharashtra, India

Raj K. Keservani
Faculty of B. Pharmacy, CSM Group of Institutions, Prayagraj, Uttar Pradesh, India

Ritesh Khairnar
Department of Pharmaceutical Chemistry, St. John Institute of Pharmacy & Research, Palghar, Maharashtra, India

V. Kiruthiga
Assistant Professor, PG & Research Department of Zoology,
D.K.M. College for Women (Autonomous), Tamil Nadu, India

Sanjay Kshirsagar
Department of Pharmaceutics, MET's Institute of Pharmacy, Adgaon Nashik, India

Sunil Mahajan
Department of Pharmaceutical Chemistry, MGV's Pharmacy College, Panchvati, Nashik, India

Arezoo Matin
Public Health School, Bam University of Medical Sciences, Bam, Iran

Mohammad Mehdizadeh
Department of Agronomy and Plant Breeding, Faculty of Agriculture and Natural Resources, University of Mohaghegh Ardabili, Ardabil, Iran; Ilam Science and Technology Park, Ilam, Iran

Zoleikha Mehdizadeh
Department of Biology, Payame Noor University, Tehran, Iran

Dang Kim Ngan
VNU University of Medicine and Pharmacy, Vietnam National University, Hanoi, Vietnam

Anahita Omidi
Department of GIS and Remote Sensing, Faculty of Geography, University of Tehran, Tehran, Iran

Ritesh Pawar
Department of Pharmaceutical Chemistry, Poona College of Pharmacy, Pune, Maharashtra, India

Ramsaneh Raghuwanshi
Professor, Department of Pharmaceutical Chemistry, Corporate Institute of Pharmacy,
Bhopal, Madhya Pradesh, India

Bhushan R. Rane
Shri D. D. Vispute College of Pharmacy and Research Center, Panvel, Maharashtra, India

Kalsoom Saleem
Department of Pharmaceuticals Sciences, Riphah Institute of Pharmaceutical Sciences, Islamabad, Pakistan

Nisha Sharma
School of Pharmaceutical Sciences, Chhatrapati Sahu Ji Maharaj University, Kanpur, India

Ashwini V. Shelke
Department of Pharmaceutical Chemistry, Sandip Institute of Pharmaceutical Sciences, Savitribai Phule Pune University, Nashik, Maharashtra, India

K. C. Sumukha
Division of Biochemistry, School of Life Sciences, JSS Academy of Higher Education and Research, Mysuru, Karnataka, India

Khemchand Surana
Department of Pharmaceutical Chemistry, Shreeshakti Shaikshanik Sanstha, Divine College of Pharmacy, Satana, Nashik, India

Swati G. Talele
Department of Pharmaceutics, Sandip Institute of Pharmaceutical Sciences, Savitribai Phule Pune University, Nashik, Maharashtra, India

Bui Thanh Tung
VNU University of Medicine and Pharmacy, Vietnam National University, Hanoi, Vietnam

Madhuri Verma
Naraina Group of Institutions of Pharmacy, Kanpur, Dr. APJ. Abdul Kalam Technical University, India

A. Vinodhini
Assistant Professor, PG & Research Department of Zoology, D.K.M. College for Women (Autonomous), Tamil Nadu, India

Marwa Waheed
Department of Food Science, Government College University Faisalabad, Faisalabad, Pakistan

ABBREVIATIONS

5-DMN	5-demethylonobiletin
AA	arachidonic acid
AB23A	alisol B 23-acetate
AGNPs	silver nanoparticles
AICR	American Institute of Cancer Research
ALA	acid a-linolenic acid
ALA	α-linolenic acid
AUC	area under curve
AuNPs	gold nanoparticles
BALF	bronchoalveolar lavage fluid
BBR	berberine
BCRP	breast cancer resistance proteins
BC-SLNs	beta-carotene-loaded solid lipid nanoparticles
BPA	bisphenol A
BPA	phthalates and bisphenol A
BSA	bovine serum albumin
CAA	Consumer Affairs Agency
CCL2	CC chemokine ligand 2
CDC	center for disease control
CDK2	cyclin-dependent kinase 2
CH	chitin
CIMP	CpG island methylator phenotype
CIN	chromosomal instability
CMC	critical micelle concentration
CME	C. alata flower methanol extract
CNS	central nervous system
CNTs	carbon nanotubes
COX-2	cyclooxygenase 2
CPP	casein phosphopeptides
CRC	colorectal cancer
CS	chitosan
DADS	diallyl disulfide
DAPI	4,6-diamidino-2-phenylindole
DAPK1	death-associated protein kinase 1

DAS	diallyl sulfide
DATS	diallyl trisulfide
DDR	DNA damage response
DHA	docosahexaenoic acid
DPPH	2,2-diphenyl-1-picryldrazyl
DT	dihydroisotanshinone I
EGCG	epigallocatechin-3-gallate
EGFR	epidermal growth factor receptor
ENA	European Nutraceutical Association
EPA	eicosapentaenoic acid
ER	estrogen receptor
ESPEN	European Society for Clinical Nutrition and Metabolism
FA	ferulic acid
FA-CLAP	folate-functionalized PEG cross-linked acrylic polymer
FIM	Foundation for Innovation in Medicine
GA	gallic acid
GDP	gross domestic product
GIT	gastrointestinal tract
GO	garlic oil
GSE	grape seed extract
GSH	glutathione
H2O2	hydrogen peroxide
HER2	human epidermal growth factor receptor 2
HGPIN	high-grade prostatic intraepithelial neoplasia
HIF-1	hypoxia-inducible factor-1
HK	honokiol
HMG-CoA	hydroxy β-methylglutaryl-CoA
HO-1	heme oxygenase-1
HPS	harmonized polysaccharide
I3C	indole-3-carbinol
IARC	International Agency for Research Cancer
IBD	inflammatory bowel disease
ICDS	integrated child development services
IGF	insulin-like growth factor
JNK	c-Jun N-terminal kinase
LOOH	lipid hydroperoxide
MAPK	mitogen-activated protein kinases
MCRC	metastatic colorectal cancer
MDR	multi-drug resistance

MMP	mitochondrial membrane potential
mPEG-PCL	methoxy-poly(ethylene glycol)-block-poly(ε-caprolactone)
MSI	microsatellite instability
MTT	3-(4,5-dimethylthiazol-2-YL)-2,5-diphenyltetrazolium
NAC	N-acetylcysteine
NAC	N-acetylcysteine
NCI	National Cancer Institute
NF-κB	nuclear factor κB
NIR	near infrared
NK	natural killer
NO	nitric oxide
NOB	nobiletin
Nrf	nuclear factor
Nrf2	nuclear factor (erythroid-derived 2)-like 2
NSAID	nonsteroidal anti-inflammatory drugs
NSCLC	non-small cell lung cancer
OP	organophosphate
OPP	oxygen partial pressure
OSCs	organic sulfur compounds
PA	palmitic acid
PAHs	polycyclic aromatic hydrocarbons
PAMAM	polyamidoamine
PARP	poly(ADP-ribose) polymerase
PCa	prostate cancer
PCL	poly ε-caprolactone
PEG	polyethylene glycol
PGE2	prostaglandin E2
P-gp	P-glycoproteins
PI	propidium iodide
PIA	proliferative inflammatory atrophy
PLA	polylactic acid
PLGA	poly lactic-co-glycolic acid
PMA	phorbol 12-myristate 13-acetate
PMF	polymethoxyflavone
PR	progesterone receptor
PSA	prostate-specific antigen
PUFAs	polyunsaturated fatty acids
PVC	polyvinyl chloride

QDs	quantum dots
RB	rinoxia B
RNS	reactive nitrogen species
ROS	reactive oxygen species
RT-PCR	polymerase chain reaction
SCLC	small cell lung cancer
SEDDs	self-emulsifying drug delivery system
SENDDS	self-nanoemulsifying drug delivery system
SFN	sulforaphane
SKP	S-phase kinase-associated protein 2
SLNs	solid lipid nanoparticles
SMEDDS	self-micro-emulsifying drug delivery systems
T2DM	type 2 diabetes mellitus
three-MA	three-methyladenine
TNF	tumor necrosis factor
Topo-I	topoisomerase-I
TUNEL	terminal deoxynucleotidyl dutp nick-end-labeling
UPR	unfolded protein response
UV	ultraviolet light
VDR	vitamin D receptor
VEGF ELISA	vascular endothelial growth factor-ELISA
XTT	XML tunneling technology
ω-3 PUFA	omega-3 polyunsaturated fatty acid

PREFACE

Nutraceuticals are natural and bioactive products with nutritional value to help maintain energy balance in the body and promise significant therapeutic value in various diseases. They may have chemopreventive effects, as suggested by traditional medicine. Nutraceuticals are now part of dietary supplements over-the-counter, and self-prescribing is increasing on a large scale. This book illustrates the role of multiple nutraceuticals in the avoidance and/or management of human malignancies that are known to be mediated through alteration at numerous molecular targets. The book begins with a chronological viewpoint on the value of natural agents in the prevention of human malignancies, followed by a series of present topics on various nutraceuticals targeting several cancers.

The present book strives to provide requisite information to its readers relevant to nutraceuticals in cancer. The text of this book is written by highly skilled, experienced, and renowned scientists and researchers around the globe with up-to-date information to offer insights on herbal medicines to readers, researchers, academicians, scientists, and industrialists worldwide.

This book, *Nutraceuticals in Cancer Prevention, Management, and Treatment,* comprises 10 chapters that describe the use of medicinal plants for the prevention and treatment of cancer and its mechanism. The details of history and the latest trends in nutraceuticals and cancer have been presented in Chapter 1, "Nutraceuticals and Cancer: Past, Present, and Future," written by Bhushan R. Rane and colleagues. The authors have given an introduction to the history of nutraceuticals for cancer treatment and its future.

Chapter 2, "Nutritional Strategies for the Prevention of Cancer," written by Eknath D. Ahire and associates, provides an overview of nutritional strategies for the prevention of cancer.

Chapter 3, "Phytochemicals in Cancer Treatment," written by Shaista Jabeen and colleagues, gives a general introduction to phytochemicals proven to be potential in the treatment of various cancers. Further, it illustrates bioactive components like thymoquinone, curcumin, gingerol, cumin aldehyde, and allicin, etc., played a promising role in multiple types of cancers.

Chapter 4, "Nanotechnology in Nutraceuticals Delivery for the Prevention and Treatment of Cancer," written by Ozan E. Eyupoglu and Kalsoom Saleem, focuses on nutraceuticals delivery through nanotechnology. They show that nanotechnology-based formulations can be explored to enhance the bioavailability and anti-cancer potential of nutraceuticals. There have been multiple implications and advancements in the use of nanotechnology in delivering nutraceuticals to prevent and treat cancer.

Chapter 5, “Oxidative Stress in Cancer,” written by Muhammad Bilal Hussain, illustrates how oxidative stress induces cancer and how to counteract it. Free radicals have secured immense importance in biological studies owing to their role in cancer.

Breast cancer, the leading cancer in women, is one of the three most common cancers worldwide. Chapter 6, “Breast Cancer Prevention by Nutraceuticals,” written by Dang Kim Ngan and associates, provides the potential of nutrition for breast cancer prevention and treatment. The chapter reviews diverse nutraceuticals that are used to prevent breast cancer.

Chapter 7, “Prostate Cancer Prevention by Nutraceuticals,” written by Swati G. Talele, discusses the benefit of major promising nutraceutical-based agents such as Vitamin D, Vitamin E, green tea, and green tea polyphenols, zinc, silibinin, grape seed extract (GSE), grape skin extract and resveratrol, fish oil, omega-3-fatty acid, and cruciferous vegetables.

Prebiotics, probiotics, fiber, polyunsaturated fats, antioxidants, and other plants/natural foods are examples of food products utilized as nutraceuticals. Chapter 8, “Lung Cancer Prevention by Nutraceuticals,” written by Eknath D. Ahire and associates presents medicinal plants used for lung cancer.

Colon cancer develops as a result of factors like gender, age, genetic predisposition, lifestyle, diet, or as a complication of inflammatory bowel disease. Chapter 9, “Colon Cancer Prevention by Medicinal Plant,” written by Madhuri Verma discusses phytochemical, preclinical, and clinical studies of medicinal plants for colon cancer.

Chapter 10, “Skin Cancer Prevention by Nutraceuticals,” written by Mohammad Mehdizadeh and colleagues, gives information on nutraceuticals and herbal medicines for skin cancer treatment. In this regard, the main classes of nutraceutical compounds with powerful anti-cancer potential are discussed in this chapter including phenolic acids, flavonoids, carotenoids, vitamins, and terpenes.

CHAPTER 1

NUTRACEUTICALS AND CANCER: PAST, PRESENT, AND FUTURE

BHUSHAN R. RANE,[1] RAJ K. KESERVANI,[2] TUSHAR B. AGAM,[1] ASHISH A. KARLE,[1] RAMSANEH RAGHUWANSHI,[3] and ASHISH S. JAIN[1]

[1]Shri D. D. Vispute College of Pharmacy and Research Center, Panvel, Maharashtra, India

[2]Faculty of B. Pharmacy, CSM Group of Institutions, Prayagraj, Uttar Pradesh, India

[3]Professor, Department of Pharmaceutical Chemistry, Corporate Institute of Pharmacy, Bhopal Madhya Pradesh, India

ABSTRACT

Since ancient times, humans have recognized natural products as the primary source of high nutritional value. Dietary requirements were important long before the concept of "nutrition" was developed. In fact, the subject has always been a source of fascination as well as an important area of research. Many numbers of advanced scientific studies have been demonstrated to observe all probable effects of various dietary active and inactive ingredients on the development and spreading of cancer. One particular topic of interest is the impact of food contaminants. Human food contains a wide range of carcinogenic and mutagenic chemicals. Some of these chemicals are naturally present in food ingredients, while others are the consequence of pesticide residues, pollution, food additives, food preparation, food processing techniques, and fungal infection. Cancer has become one of the prominent consequential community health issues. According to World

Nutraceuticals in Cancer Prevention, Management, and Treatment. Raj K. Keservani, Bui Thanh Tung, Sippy Singh, & Rajesh K. Kesharwani, PhD (Eds.)

Health Organization, cancer is an enormous group of diseases that can begin in any tissue or organ of the human body, when affected cells grow disorderly and surpass their usual limits to pierce neighboring parts of the body and/or spread to various other organs. This further process is known as metastasizing and is a primary cause of death from cancer. A malignant tumor and neoplasm are other synonyms names for cancer. Nutraceuticals which contain carotenoids have anti-oxidant properties and can help prevent cancer. Indian and Chinese medicines have used the anticancer effects of different plant and animal-derived compounds since ancient times. Many historical civilizations, including ancient Egypt, Greece, and Rome, employed herbal remedies and plants to heal and prevent disease. Nutraceuticals with nano-delivery methods have been progressively favored in recent years for the curing of neoplasms.

1.1 HISTORY

Natural products have long been acknowledged by mankind as the principal source of high nutritional value. Dietary needs were significant even before the term "nutrition" was used. In actuality, the topic has always fascinated people and has been a crucial focus of study. When it comes to biomedical research, the last two decades have revealed the importance of diet in maintaining overall health. Many ancient civilizations, including the Indians, Chinese, Egyptians, and Sumerians, were among the first to recognize food as a source of nutrition or medicine. The origins of nutraceuticals can be traced back three thousand years. To predict the connection between suitable food for health, fitness, and therapeutic effects, Hippocrates (460–377 BC), the well-known father of modern medicine, said, "Let food be the medicine, and medicine be my food." Nutraceuticals are not a new concept; however, they have progressed significantly over time. In the United States, during the early period of the 1900s, the first thrive at generating a functional component through fortification was made when a food company started to install iodine to salt for the prevention of avoid goiter (Andlaur et al., 2002; Kingsley et al., 2020).

1.2 INTRODUCTION

Dr. Stephen L. DeFelice, who is Founder and Chairman of Foundation of Innovation Medicine (FIM) located in Crawford, New Jersey, gave the phrase "nutraceutical." In 1989, "nutraceutical" was coined from the words "nutrition" and "pharmaceutical." The word nutraceutical is frequently used in the market, but yet it is not defined by legislation. Nutraceuticals are natural bio-active or chemical compounds that have health-promoting, disease-curing, or preventive measures in comparison to their dietary amount. Lipids, carbohydrates (Singh et al., 2017b), proteins (Keservani et al., 2015), minerals, vitamins (Singh et al., 2017a), and other essential nutrients are found in nutraceuticals. Nutraceuticals have been found to be potential agents in the treatment of a variety of disease, including cardiovascular disease, atherosclerosis, cancer, diabetes, and neurological disorders, according to research. Isolated nutrients, dietary supplements, herbal items (Rane et al., 2020a; Rane et al., 2020ab; Rane et al., 2020ac), and treated foods such as cereals, drinks, and soup are all examples of nutraceuticals (Sachdeva et al., 2020). Nutraceuticals' principal underlying mechanism is to give functional benefits by strengthening the supply of natural building blocks in the body. Nutraceuticals is a broad term used to refer to any food-derived product that provides additional health advantages beyond the fundamental nutritional quality present in foods. Most of the dietary substances, functional foods, and natural origin substances have been investigated and found to be extremely active, have a significant effect on cell metabolism, and have few negative consequences. It's only natural that people focus is switching to positive approaches to disease prevention in order to remain healthy. Nutraceuticals are useful in improving our overall health. There are many types of nutraceuticals, which truly useful to increase our energy, like all the vitamins, mainly from the Vitamin B family, which prevents chronic diseases, improves sleeping patterns, and relieves anxiety. Nutraceuticals are also herbal products with a variety of disadvantages and limits. Nutraceuticals may be limited by inadequate targeting, low solubility, low permeability, rapid metabolism, and other factors. As a result of these shortcomings, researchers have been motivated to seek and develop innovative methods to enhance the concentration in blood, absorption, distribution metabolism, and effectiveness of these products (Chakrabarty et al., 2021).

1.3 CLASSIFICATION OF NUTRACEUTICALS

Nutraceuticals can be categorized on the criteria of their origin: natural or traditional and unnatural or nontraditional. Nutraceuticals that are obtained or produced from living organisms or they are derived from plants, animals, minerals, or microorganisms come under natural sources. This refers to traditional nutraceuticals. The nutraceuticals which are produced with the help of biotechnology are referred to as nontraditional nutraceuticals, or Unnatural in short, which are synthesized in the laboratory.

1.3.1 DEFINITION

Stephan DeFelice has coined the word "nutraceuticals" for nearly three decades, yet there is still no precise definition for the products or ingredients that fall under this area. It is well known that the word is derived from nutrients and pharmaceuticals, but they are more than nutrients because of their proven health/medicinal benefits. In various diseases like anemia, nutraceuticals serve as a functional food that helps in restricting and treatment of diseases (Keservani et al., 2010, 2020). Even though nutraceuticals are mostly referred as pharmafoods, there are no official definitions or accepted statements from governing bodies. Nutraceuticals are preferred over drugs, and conventional therapy to cure pathological conditions in patients who may not be eligible for conventional drug therapy. As a result, it is critical to establish a clear and specific definition of nutraceuticals as well as agreed regulations (Souyoul et al., 2017).

In the United States of America, nutraceutical products are regulated as "dietary supplements, food ingredients, and drugs" as not have a specific definition (Santini et al., 2017).

"A food or parts of food that provide medical or health benefits, including the prevention and/or treatment of disease" is considered as nutraceuticals as defined by Defelice and backed by Dietary Supplement Health and Education Act 1994 (DSHEA), Food and Drug Administration (FDA), and Dietary Supplement Health and Education Act of 1994 (DSHEA) (Santini et al., 2017).

Nutraceuticals, as per European Nutraceutical Association (ENA), are nutritional products that provide health and medical benefits, including the prevention and treatment of disease (Santini et al., 2017).

As per the new notification from FSSAI dated in 2020 states that "a nutraceutical is a food or food-related component that intends for health benefits even in treatment and prevention of aliments." In India, are considered as nutraceutical (Santini et al., 2017).

According to the United States Government Office, 1994, food supplements means "any product excluding tobacco in the form of a powder, capsule softgel, and gelcap are considered as supplement in the diet to enhance health that includes more than one of the following dietary ingredients: a dietary substance, mineral, botanical, amino acid, or other botanical or vitamin" (Santini et al., 2017).

1.4 DAILY DIET INCLUDE

1.4.1 CONTAMINANT

Contaminants are disease-causing organisms and substances such as parasites, bacteria, and viruses that are spread by inappropriate handling of raw or cooked food. Toxins are produced by these organisms, which lead to food poisoning. Improper food handling, preparation, storage, inadequate sanitization, cleaning, and infestation by pests and insects such as cockroaches and flies are all potential sources of contamination.

Numerous scientific studies have been performed on the possible effects of various dietary (Keservani et al., 2020) components on the development of cancer. One particular topic of interest is the impact of food contaminants. Through the evaluation of hundreds of chemicals, various mixtures, and natural products, the International Agency for Research Cancer (IARC) and the United States Toxicology Program were able to come up with a set of cancer risk assessments. Aflatoxin, alcoholic beverages, and 2,3,7,8-tetracholordibenzo-p-dioxin are among the contaminants having the greatest level of evidence. Acetaldehyde, polycyclic aromatic hydrocarbons, certain nitrosamines, and yerba mate are among the agents with a reasonable degree of evidence. Bracken fern, fumonsin B1, ochratoxin, and other agents have a low level of evidence. It is reported in studies that the four main components are causative factors for cancer. The first are natural compounds that are always present in food. The method of manufacturing salted fish, for example, produces carcinogens that are difficult to avoid. Second, there are natural products that may be prevented, like grain adulterated by the neoplasmic fungal metabolic aflatoxin, which can be decreased or eliminated by implementing optimal grain storage practices. Third, food may contain anthropogenic chemicals. 2,3,7,8-tetracholordibenzo-pdioxin, for example, was generated accidently during the manufacturing of chlorinated hydrocarbons, but it pollutes the surroundings, prevents deprivation, and collects in particular foods. Anthropogenic compounds purposely added to foods, such as artificial sugar or food coloring, represent a fourth type of concern, but they are not covered in this chapter because they are not pollutants because they are introduced intentionally. While a high-energy, low-fiber diet has been connected to an increased risk of cancer, several specific foods have also been identified as having the potential to cause cancer (carcinogenic).

Artificial sweetening agents, such as cyclamate, saccharin, aspartame, and cyclamate, are among them. If laboratory rats are fed massive doses of saccharin or cyclamate, they can develop bladder cancer, however, at levels thousands of times higher than in a typical diet. As animals are affected, humans are not get affected. It is determined on the basis of international studies. Artificial sweeteners are regarded as safe to consume (Abnet et al., 2007).

Cured, pickled, or salty foods (having a chemical called nitrate), which when consumed in excessive amounts, have the potential to cause cancer, specifically colon cancer. To be safe, keep the amount of cured meats in your diet to a minimum, as they are typically excess in lipid content and salt. Stomach cancer risk can be increased due to excessive consumption of salt; thus, it should be used in moderation.

Foods that have been overcooked or burned can form a type of carcinogenic compound described as polycyclic aromatic hydrocarbons (PAHs). Although charred or smoked foods may contain traces of polycyclic aromatic hydrocarbons, scientists believe that the ordinary Australian diet does not include enough. The average human diet is far too low to pretense a severe neoplasm hazard. When cooking, however, it's preferable to utilize low-heat methods wherever feasible and minimize your intake of charcoal-grilled meats and meals. Roasting, baking, microwaving, stewing, casseroling, poaching, braising, microwaving, and steaming boiling are all low-temperature cooking methods.

Eating peanuts contaminated with toxin-producing molds can cause cancer in some test animals. Peanuts sold in most parts of countries are normally uncontaminated, and contamination is constantly checked.

Drinking alcohol raises the risk of oral, pharyngeal, laryngeal, esophageal, breast, bowel, and liver cancers. High risk is observed in those people who smoke. Even small amounts of alcohol can make you more vulnerable. To minimize the risk of disease, males should avoid drinking more than two standardized drinks per day, also for females not more than one standardized drink per day (Dumiterscu et al., 2005).

1.4.2 AIR POLLUTION

Outdoor air pollution is a significant factor in the global illness load. Due to emissions from industry, electricity production, transportation, and residential burning, the majority of the world's population now lives in areas where air pollution levels far surpass the World Health Organization's air-quality guidelines based on human health. Because it is omnipresent and has numerous major negative public health effects, including cancer, outdoor air pollution is an urgent global public health concern. There is currently enough evidence from human and experimental animal research, as well as mechanistic evidence, to indicate a causal association between outdoor (environmental) air pollution, particularly particulate matter in outdoor air, and lung cancer incidence and mortality. Hundreds and thousands of lung cancer fatalities are predicted to occur each year around the world to particulate matter air pollution. There is less epidemiological data on the risk of causing breast cancer and bladder cancer caused by outdoor air pollution (Cao et al., 2011). Outdoor air pollution has also been linked to a lower chance of surviving cancer. Lung cancer is the most prevalent disease diagnosed and the main cause of cancer mortality globally. Through the absorption, metabolism, and distribution of inhaled carcinogens, outdoor air pollution may induce cancer in locations other than the lungs. Multiple forms of cancer have also been linked to other inhalable contaminants. A meta-analysis of home air pollution caused by solid fuel combustion found links to oral, cervical, and esophageal cancer. Occupational exposure to numerous agents, such as diesel and gasoline exhaust, polyaromatic hydrocarbons (PAHs), inhalable dusts (metals, silica), activities in trucking, mining, foundries, or carbon black manufacturing, and work with asphalt, has also been known to cause cancer at different locations (Campanale et al., 2020).

1.4.3 PESTICIDES

Pesticides are chemical or biological agents that are sprayed on crops to protect vegetation from insects, weeds, and pathogens. In the United States, acutely harmful organophosphate (OP) insecticides are commonly utilized. Pesticides are used on non-edible crops such as flowers, grass, and cotton, as well as fruits, vegetables, wheat, rice, olives, and rapeseed pressed into oil. Malathion and chlorpyrifos, major Organophosphate insecticides, are widely used on various wheat, vegetables and fruits. Pesticides are applied to crops that are fed to animals, although pesticide residue is rarely seen in meat or dairy products. Pesticides are most often consumed on; and are present in our food, which exposes most newborns, children, and adults to them. Pesticides are touched and breathed in by workers in farm and occupational settings, exposing them at risk of acute and chronic poisoning. For many years, epidemiological investigations of pesticide exposure in people have been studied across the world. Hemopoietic, prostate, pancreatic, brain, liver, and other body organ cancers have all been linked to insecticides, herbicides, and fungicides. Because of their intrinsic toxicity and widespread application, many of them are also potent immunosuppressors, which indicates they can operate as promoters through immune suppression. A number of epidemiological studies have reported that parental exposure to industrial or non-occupational pesticides increases the relative risk of cancer development in offspring. Furthermore, some researches looking into children's direct exposure to pesticides have established a favorable link. Crops, vegetables, and fruits are exposed to pesticides to protect them against insects, weeds, and fungus. It is dangerous to come into touch with significant concentrations of pesticides. Despite the fact that most produce has some pesticide residue, food testing guarantees that pesticide levels are low enough to pose no harm to human health (George et al., 2011; FAO and WHO, 2020).

1.4.4 PLASTIC

According to a new study, microplastics are plastic particles ranging in size from 1 nanometer to 5 millimeters that are progressively polluting not just aquatic life but also water and food which is consumed. Drinking water contributes to a major portion of microplastic in our diet, which includes bottled water, tap water, ground water, and surface water. According to a 2019 WWF assessment, the average individual intakes around 1,769 microplastic particles on a weekly basis. According to a 2020 research published in Environmental Research, microplastics were discovered in common consumables such as vegetables and fruits. Red and green apples had the maximum microplastic concentration, with 195,500 particles per gram, followed by cauliflower and carrots, all of which contained over one lakh particles per gram. The least contaminated vegetable was lettuce. Sea fish and seafood from plastic-polluted waters have greater levels of microplastic in their digestive and respiratory system. Microplastic deposition was observed in the muscles of marine fishes in a 2020 research. Plastic waste and textile fibers were identified in the intestines of one-third of the marine fish samples collected from California, Indonesia Makassar, US markets, according to a 2015 article. The long-term impacts of plastic ingestion on human body are yet unknown, although research is being conducted. However, studies in fisheries and aquaculture have previously shown that plastic ingestion is hazardous. This toxic chemical emission reached and exposed to fetus in the womb, having a devastating impact on them. Phthalates and bisphenol A (BPA) are two of the most well-known harmful compounds. The two substances are known as endocrine disruptors because they interfere with our body's hormonal system (Wesley et al., 2012).

1.4.4.1 PHTHALATES

Phthalates are a class of compounds used in the production of polyvinyl chloride (PVC), a plastic that is more flexible, plant-based, and difficult to break. These substances act as male reproductive toxicants after being consumed through food. It has an impact on both men and women. These compounds are widely used to soften and bend vinyl polymers, which are incorporated in a variety of products. Humans are at the biggest risk of exposure to these chemicals because they are found everywhere from toys to medical instruments. Adult women, in particular, are at greater risk than males due to the usage of phthalates in cosmetics such as shampoo, soaps, and body washes (Turner et al., 2020; Rillig et al., 2017).

1.4.4.2 BISPHENOL-A

A bisphenol-a (BPA) is an ingredient that is utilized in manufacturing hard plastics such as polycarbonate, which is commonly used in food and beverage storage containers such as water bottles, lunch boxes, and storage cans. Bisphenol-a has recently gained considerable attention because of its negative health consequences in people. The chemical has recently been the subject of debate due to its possible adverse effects on the prostate gland and developing brain of fetuses, babies, and children. In 2011, a research found that pregnant women with high levels of bisphenol-A had a higher risk of anxiety, hyperactivity, and depression in their children.

These two compounds have gotten a lot of attention because of their rizing adverse health effects, but there are a lot of other chemicals in plastics that have comparable effects, such as anti-oxidants and colorants.

Microwaves accelerate the release of chemicals from plastics in food, and they're not the only method that chemicals from plastics contaminate food. Even without microwaves, food and beverages kept in plastic containers discharge toxins into the meal. When plastic is left in a hot climate or exposed to the sun, it releases a lot of compounds. Tomatoes as well as other acidic foods absorb toxins from the can food coating quickly. Apart from food containers, chemicals including phthalates in home decor items emit gases into the air over time, increasing the risk of breathing dangerous compounds. Even if the plastics are not in touch with the food, vapors from them can release toxins. When a plastic spatter cover is used over a microwave dish, vaporized plastic containers discharge their gases into the food.

1.5 TYPES OF CANCER DUE TO BAD QUALITY OF FOOD

Human food contains a wide range of carcinogenic and mutagenic chemicals. Some of these chemicals are naturally present in food ingredients, while others are the consequence of pesticide residues, pollution, food additives, food preparation, food processing techniques, and fungal infection. Natural alkyl benzens found in herbal tea are tannins, edible mushrooms contain hydrazines and safroleare also found in flavorings and spices, are all naturally occurring carcinogens. Flavonoids (Keservani and Sharma, 2014), which are found in a wide range of food plants and fruits, are mutagenic (Lotha et al., 2018). Aflatoxin is a strong carcinogenic mycotoxins produced by fungus infection of preserved food. Aflatoxin contamination of grain has been linked to higher than predicted rates of liver cancer in various African countries. In the human diet, nitrosamines are a substantial source of carcinogens. Nitrosamines are created when nitrite reacts with secondary or tertiary amines. Plants, meats, and dairy products naturally contain a bacterial reproduction product called sodium nitrite. They're also commonly found in smoked pork and salted seafood as preservatives. Nitrosamines are powerful carcinogens, such as dimethyinitrosamine. Consumption of nitrate and nitrite has been linked to an increased risk of stomach and esophageal cancer in epidemiological studies. Because of the increased proportion of esophageal cancer in some areas of Saudi Arabia, this discovery may be of interest (Roudebush et al., 2004). Ascorbic acid and other anti-oxidants can help to minimize the production of nitrosamines in stored food and the stomach. Sugimura has isolated a group of carcinogenic heterocyclic amines that form during the cooking of raw fish and meat due to pyrolosis. Tryptophan, glutamic acid, and soybean pyrrolysates also are carcinogenic. Polyaromatic hydrocarbons can also be discovered in charbroiled beef. Human food contain various diethylstilbestrol which is type of growth enhancer, polychlorinated biphenyls, asbestos, heavy metals, arsenic are some type of industrial pollutants, and chlordane, DDT are insecticides. Cooked proteins include heterocyclic amines, which are strong carcinogens (Wesley et al., 2012). Human food is contaminated with mycotoxins produced by a variety of molds, and some of these toxins are strong carcinogens. Aflatoxin, for example, is found in cereals, peanuts, and other preserved foods and has been established in animal and human epidemiologic investigations to be a human carcinogen. Oral, pharyngeal, esophageal, and stomach cancer have all been linked to alcohol usage, particularly among smokers (Dumiterscu et al., 2005). The extent of the danger posed by these compounds is mainly unclear. There is no confirming link between carbohydrate and cancer. The risk of developing liver cancer with high intake of potato starch has been reported. Diet rich in proteins can be related to an increased risk of breast cancer, colon cancer, pancreatic cancer, prostate cancer, etc. According to epidemiological research. Nevertheless, the strong interrelationship between protein and fat consumption in the Western diet makes data interpretation problematic. Protein seems to have little impact at or below the quantities necessary for optimal development in most cases. The difficulty of getting a reliable history of alcohol usage limits most investigations on the link between ethanol consumption and cancer. According to recent research, excessive alcohol consumption is linked to an increased risk of cancers of the respiratory tract and oral cavity. Smoking is also connected to certain malignancies. A recent prospective study found that high beer consumption is linked to colorectal cancer (Slattery et al., 2004). Moderate drinkers have been linked to an increased risk of breast cancer as compared to nondrinkers, particularly for women who began drinking before the age of 30, independent of later consumption levels. The International Agency for Research on Cancer (IARC) believes the evidence sufficient to categorize alcoholic drinks as carcinogenic based on an examination of epidemiologic research. When alcohol is consumed in conjunction with cigarette smoking, the most convincing research found an increased cancer risk. Multiple ingredients with potential biologic action may be found in beer, wine, distilled spirits, and regionally produced drinks. In fermented preparations, ethanol is not a mutagen, although it is usually associated with mutagenic components. Hepatoxicity, which is frequently linked with ethanol intake, may obstruct the proper metabolism and elimination of potentially carcinogenic substances. (Dumiterscu et al., 2005).

1.6 SOME COMMON CANCERS ASSOCIATED WITH FOOD CONSUMPTION

1.6.1 LUNG CANCER

Across the world death rate due to cancer is high in that lung cancer is one of the major cancer types responsible for death which is mainly due to smoking. It includes few more factors like eating red meat, and smoking processed type meat which can also cause risk of cancer but it required more research on it (Dumiterscu et al., 2005).

1.6.2 BREAST CANCER

Breast cancer is the world's most frequent malignancy among women. Rapid early growth, adult height, and adult weight gain all increases the chances to cause cancer of the breast. There are factors which impact on the estrogen level and are responsible for breast cancer. It includes the age at which starting of the period that is menarche, the number of pregnancies, habits of nursing, late starting of menarche, and late first pregnancy. Breast cancer becomes more common as people get older. Breast cancer risk is more than doubled in postmenopausal women who are overweight, especially around their midsection. Monounsaturated fat-rich foods, such as olive oil, canola oil, certain nuts and seeds, and a high-vegetable diet may lower the risk. Breast cancer may be accelerated by excessive alcohol usage (Aetna et al., 2009).

1.6.3 PROSTATE CANCER

The most frequent malignancy among Australian males is prostate cancer. Males aged above 50 are more vulnerable. It can, however, be noticed in younger males as well. A high-fat diet that consists typically of animal fat sources (such as fatty meats, dairy products, and greasy meals) may reduce the risk, but a high-fat diet that consists primarily of fat vegetable sources (such as soy) may raise the risk. Prostate cancer risk may be reduced by maintaining a healthy body weight. Anti-oxidant like Lycopene which found in tomato and tomato-based food, strawberries, and watermelon may reduce the incidence of prostate cancer. Consuming one to two servings of tomatoes per day (equivalent to 12 cups or 75 grams) has been linked to a lower risk of cancer (Andic et al., 2009).

1.6.4 COLORECTAL CANCER

Colorectal cancer which is commonly known as bowel cancer is 2nd leading cause of cancer death in the world. If followed healthy lifestyle, it can reduce up to 70% of occurrences. Balancing a fit weight, doing physically active exercise, and consuming a diet heavy in vegetables and fiber are protective, however consuming a excessive of red meat, treated meat, and drinking alcohol may raise the risk.

1.6.5 COLON CANCER

It is one of the leading causes of cancer across the world. Cancers of the downward colon and the sigmoid junction, on the other hand, appear to be linked to the kind and amount of fat ingested. This might be unsettled to the fact that cholesterol production and total bile acid flow function as a promoter at this location. Because promoters are extremely dosage-dependent, lowering bile acid concentrations by reducing fat consumption may reduce the risk of colon cancer. A high fiber diet increases stool volume, which decreases the amount of bile acids in the gut and, as a result, lowers the promoter's potential. Some vegetables and fruits include different forms of fiber that may not always enhance stool size in the same way as cereal does. Fecapentaenes, which are direct-acting mutagens, have been found in the feces of 10–20% of persons who eat a normal Western high-fat, low-fiber diet. Fecapentaene synthesis is aided by bile acids and anaerobic storage. Consumption of various types of vegetables and fruits on a regular basis is recommended.

1.6.6 GASTRIC CANCER

Gastric cancer is connected with diet such as smoked fish, dried salted fish, and pickled vegetables. Diet which not includes vitamin A, E and C is also cause gastric cancer. Nitroso indoles or diazonium compounds produced from nitrite and certain substrates might be the active carcinogens. These causative agent inhibited by the vitamin such as vitamin E and vitamin C. (Andic et al., 2009).

1.7 HOW NUTRACEUTICALS ARE IMPORTANT IN CANCER?

Cancer has become one of the most serious public health issues. According to World Health Organization, the neoplasm is a wide group of diseases that begin in any part of tissue, cell or organ. When it starts to mobilize from one specific organ site to another site, this further process is referred to as metastasis. Cancer is the second most common cause of death worldwide, in 2018 accounting for 9.6 million fatalities, or one out of six deaths. Females are more likely to develop breast, thyroid, lung, cervical, and colon cancers. Whereas males are more prone to prostate gland cancer, stomach cancer, liver cancer, and lung cancer. When cancer cells are exposed to chemotherapeutics over an extended period of time, they attempt to evade the drug's harmful effects by up-regulating key survival signals. Increasing the drug's dose could be a method to get over this problem, but the massive negative effects that lie ahead will completely block that option. This is where the importance of looking for fresh lead compounds in nature that can boost the therapeutic efficiency of present medications while being fully non-toxic to normal cells comes into play. The search for active biochemical's medicinal drugs and commercially valuable materials can be obtained from various animal and plant-based origins. And molecular pharmacology researchers have demonstrated that a broad range of nutraceuticals, primarily phytochemicals, might impact cancer cell survival pathways generated by carcinogens. Nutraceuticals, functional foods, and additional micronutrients have been shown to decrease cancer cell proliferation and induce apoptosis in cancer cells. A variety of natural dietary items have been found to have a role in cancer prevention and therapy, and are regarded as a successful technique (Roudebush et al., 2004).

As shown in Figure 1.1, patients with cancer showed various alterations in their body functions.

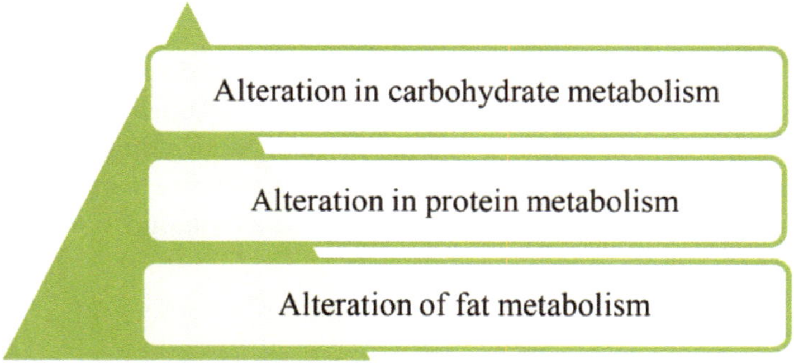

FIGURE 1.1 Patient with cancer shows the following alteration in their body functions.

Nutraceuticals that contain carotenoids have anti-oxidant properties and can help prevent cancer (Linnewiel-Hermoni et al., 2015). Lycopene and other carotenoids, such as beta-carotene, have quite a role in cancer prevention. Lycopene-rich vegetables and fruits possess anticancer properties by reducing oxidative stress and DNA damage. Tomatoes, pink grapefruit, guava, watermelon, and papaya all contain lycopene. Pectin, a soluble fiber present in apples, has been shown to help prevent prostate cancer by preventing cancer cells from connecting to other body cells. Gallic acids, curcumin, ferulic, and caffeic acids are examples of naturally occurring phenolic chemicals that have been demonstrated to have anticancer properties. Curcumin, a polyphenol produced from the Curcuma longa plant, has been shown to be anticarcinogenic, antioxidative, and anti-inflammatory. Consumption of a certain product containing polyphenols lowered cancer risk (Roudebush et al., 2004; Abnet et al., 2007; Rajamanikam et al., 2008). Carbohydrates are good for human physiology and metabolism. It aids in the prevention of a variety of chronic illnesses, including cancer, cardiovascular disease (Keservani et al., 2016a), diabetes, obesity (Jarouliya and Keservani, 2019), and gastrointestinal problems.

Lipids are a broad category of molecules with the feature of being hydrophobic in nature but mostly soluble in organic solvents. Recent technologies, on the other hand, combine the beneficial effects of fatty acids with triacylglycerol molecules to boost lipid nutrition. Seaweed has been found to be a good source of nutraceuticals, according to research. Flaxseed is a high-lipid source that might be used as a nutraceutical, according to recent studies. Flaxseed is thought to lower cancer risk.

Vitamins have a significant role in human health and can be used as nutraceuticals due to their anti-oxidant properties. People on special diets and smokers are particularly vulnerable to vitamin deficiencies and might benefit from these nutraceutical items. Seaweeds are a rich source of vitamins since their nutritional profiles contain adequate concentrations of B complex vitamins (B1, B2, B12), anti-oxidant vitamins (i.e., vitamin C and E), provitamins A, E, and carotenoids. It aids in the decrease of deaths caused by cerebrovascular illnesses and has a beneficial effect on both lung and cervical malignancies. People who consume vitamin C-rich diets have a lower chance of acquiring stomach cancer than patients who consume a typical diet (Nobili et al., 2009).

Polysaccharides (ß-glucans), peptides, mineral elements, unsaturated fatty acids, dietary fibers, terpenes, glycoproteins, alcohols, and anti-oxidants are among the active ingredients found in edible mushrooms. Mushrooms are regarded as great functional foods due to the high bioavailability of ergothioneine, selenium, Vitamin B and D following oral administration. Mushrooms' distinctive biologically active chemicals make them pharmaceutically vital for boosting the immune system in order to cure and prevent life-threatening disorders such as cerebral stroke and cancer (Pandey et al., 2010).

Animals are unable to synthesize carotenoids and must get them from food intake and metabolize them in order to utilize them for physiological purposes. Green leafy veggies include lutein and beta-carotene. Few carotenoids (around 50 out of 600 discovered) have provitamin A activity, with the most significant being a-carotene, ß-carotene, and ß cryptoxanthin. Consumption of these carotenoids may so prevent humans from major eye ailments. Carotenoids boost oxidative stress resistance and function as antioxidants in all species. Carotenoids are also anticancer agents (Sharma et al., 2009).

Flavonoids can be found in nature as glycosides and anti-oxidants. Rutin, a flavonoid derived from Ruta graveolens, is a nutraceutical with anticancer, anti-oxidant, antidiabetic, and anti-inflammatory properties (Lotha et al., 2018).

1.7.1 PAST

Indian and Chinese medicine has used the anticancer effects of different plant and animal derived compounds since ancient times. Many historical civilizations, including ancient Egypt, Greece, and Rome, employed herbal remedies and plants to heal and prevent disease. The oldest written record, which featured various 12 formulas for herbal treatments, was discovered on a Sumerian clay tablet in Nagpur (about 5000 years ago). Dioscorides, the founder of pharmacognosy, published "De Materia Medica." In 77 AD, a book was published that listed 657 plant-derived treatments. Hence human history consist a major portion of herbal products (Andlaur et al., 2002). The rich Indian civilization has offered evidence that food may be utilized as an alternative to prevent and cure human disorders. Ayurveda has indicated the advantages of Ahara for medicinal purposes. It is easily accessible and inexpensive, and it is also available in the form of kitchen treatments. Ayurveda has extensive textual evidence on Ahara and Vihara. Nutritional guidelines have been stated in ancient classical books such as Charak samhita and more recent classics such as Bhavaprakash. Nutraceuticals are not comparable to any of Ayurveda's key ideas. However, it has the concept of nutrition, dietary supplements, food regimen for patients, and health combinations for pediatric to geriatric care in many contexts. Similar references are accessible in seasonal regimens (Ritucharya). We can detect its effect on traditional practice. In Kerala, for example, Oushadha kanji is a popular medicinal meal preparation during the rainy season to avoid loss of appetite. Similarly, gruel formulations with some ash or raw medications are recommended for various sick situations. Acharya Kasyapa, the author of Kasyapa Samhita, mentions Ahara (food) as a maha bheshaja (super medicine) in his literature. Pathya is a comprehensive phrase that encompasses Pathya Ahara and Pathya Vihara (personal hygiene). Pathya Ahara may apply to nutraceuticals. Pathya Kalpana (Ayurvedic dietetics) is indicated for both healthy and ailing people for treating and recouping. Rasayana is yet another Nutraceutical idea. Rasayana is a concept that includes all of the advantages of Nutraceuticals, but in a larger sense. Its inclusion in Ashtangas of Ayurveda demonstrates its significance. Under this heading, Acharyas advocated preventive care, therapy, and patient rehabilitation. Rasayana is not the same as Nutraceutical. Following Rasayana for a certain amount of time, according to Ayurveda, revitalizes a man and extends his life. It should be taken separately before breakfast in the morning, much like a nutritional supplement. In a summary, we may split Ayurvedic Nutraceutical perspectives by illness, age group, and preventive care. Rasayana medications, beverages, and meals in Ritucharya and Pathya Kalpana might be termed Nutraceuticals (Ujaliya et al., 2018).

1.7.2 PRESENT

Nutragenomics is scientific and experimental studies, which studies the correlation of genes and nutrition specialization to cure and prevent disease. The three omics disciplines of gene, protein, and metabolite profiling (transcriptomics, proteomics, and metabolomics) as applied to the subject of nutrition and health are referred to as nutrigenomics. Nutrigenomics is the scientific foundation for creating nutrition that is tailored to the requirements of different consumer groups, whether they are healthy, at risk, or sick. RO Brennan coined the word "nutrigenetics" in his book Nutrigenetics, published in 1975. Nutrigenomics is a brand-new technology that combines numerous genomic and molecular biology methodologies. Nutrigenomics is a technique used in a variety of academic domains, including those listed below, for scientific research of the link between food and food components, health care, and illness prevention. At present major Indian companies which have a greater influence on FMGC and the pharmaceuticals market, such as Himalaya Herbal, GlaxoSmithKline consumer healthcare, Cadila healthcare, and Dabur India, are manufacturing, launching and marketing various nutraceutical products in the Indian market. As India has the upper hand in quality raw materials, world-class Research and Development facilities, and qualified youth with ample of knowledge. Currently researchers are trying various new approaches for delivery of nutraceuticals. As nutraceuticals mainly consists of herbal products or active ingredients from animals, plants, minerals sources they have a specific drawback such as low solubility, fast metabolism, poor permeability, limited tissue distribution, short half-life, and low bioavailability. Researchers are trying to incorporate active constituents of herbal products used in nutraceutical in Novel Drug Delivery System. By addition of various permeation enhancers, surface modifiers, they can be delivered to specific site. Some of formulation system are:

- nanoparticle;
- nanosphere and nanocapsules;
- metal nanoparticles;
- composite nanoparticle;
- A pH-responsive formulations;
- nanohydrogel;
- liposomes;
- solid lipid nanoparticles; and
- nanoemulsion and nanosuspension.

Researchers are majorly focusing on delivering nutraceuticals via nano drug delivery system. These sophisticated delivery technologies are utilized to increase nutraceutical absorption and bioavailability, offer a constant release profile, site specific action and avoid instability of active phytochemicals which are prone to degradation or metabolism (Pandey et al., 2010; Naitr et al., 2010).

In India FSSAI, i.e., food safety and standard authority of India has which is responsible for protecting and promoting public health through regulation and supervision of food safety has enforced rules for obtaining license of nutraceuticals in Indian market. This Act has 21 chapters, and the fourth article, or Article 22, of the Act, deals with nutraceuticals, dietary supplements, and different functional foods, and these items can be produced/manufactured, promoted (sold), or distributed (imported) by any corporation. The percentage of dietary supplement consumed by the United States of America is approximately more than 50%. With a market share of 70%, Japan is Asia's largest nutraceutical market and the world's second largest after the United States. The Japanese ministry of health, labor and welfare has established an agency known as the Consumer Affair agency (CAA) regulates nutraceuticals for safety, efficacy, and labeling. After Japan, China has the second-largest nutraceutical market in Asia Pacific. The Ministry of Health established Healthcare association of China (CHCA) to govern and manage China's nutraceutical business. SFDA, which stands for the state food and drug administration of China is in charge of regulating and registering dietary supplements, similar to the FDA in the United States. CHCA is now renamed to China Food and Drug Administration.

1.7.3 FUTURE

As consumers become more concerned about health and fitness, the Indian nutraceuticals market is predicted to develop around multifarious yearly expansion rate of 21%, approaching $10 billion in 2022 and $18 billion in 2025. The nutraceuticals industry is booming with potential, and manufacturers are helping a lot by introducing multiple nutraceutical products targeted at improving function, building muscles, and healing and repairing damage to the body. End-customers are now loaded for choice, with a wide range of natural products targeted at improving everything from skin and hair health to liver and kidney function, all without the use of harsh chemicals. This sector has grown in recent years, and it has lately gotten a boost from the current epidemic. This industry's growth has been aided by a reliance on preventative healthcare. The Indian public has come to accept in immune-boosting supplements, which has resulted in a significant shift in purchasing habits and market activity. Vitamin capsules, chewable pills, and gummies are indications of healthcare product purchases made with an open mind. During the pandemic, vitamin and zinc supplements were also regularly given by physicians. – According to government figures, 15% of our population is malnourished. Various plan of action, which involve assisting in ensuring that everyone receives adequate nutrition these plans like Integrated Child Development Services (ICDS), the National Health Mission (NHM), and the mid-day meal program. According to the World Bank, malnutrition costs the country roughly US$12 billion in Gross Domestic Product (GDP). Nutraceuticals have the potential to help eradicate malnutrition and provide a link between government initiatives and the general public. The current circumstance suggests that the Indian nutraceutical business may be able to assist the global pharmaceutical industry in growing. FSSAI means Food Safety and Standards Authority of India, is part of the Ministry of Food Processing Industries Nanotechnology-based design and production of nutraceuticals is a significant development direction for the nutraceuticals sector worldwide. Future study should look into how nanodelivery technologies might be used to promote individualized nutrition and novel functionality. Future advances will necessitate regulators and manufacturers judiciously resolving issue related to safety by the sequence of pre-clinical (animal studies) and clinical (human studies) for the investigation which ensure efficacy and safety of nutritional product containing nano drug delivery system. (Gupta et al., 2013; Eric et al., 2015; T'elessy, 2019; Santini et al., 2017).

1.8 CONCLUSION

In recent time patient diagnosed with tumor are getting increased rapidly. Phytomedicines, on the other hand, are becoming increasingly essential as they become more widely utilized. Despite the fact that certain research has shown the beneficial response, the mechanisms of action are yet unknown. Because they are affordable and most of them have no indication of toxicity, nutraceuticals are a viable source of chemicals with chemopreventive properties. More research is needed to identify the most relevant phytochemical targets so that customized clinical studies can produce consistent outcomes for cancer prevention and therapy management. The term "nutraceutical" is inadequately defined around the world, and it is not clearly classed as a food category or as a supplement category from a regulatory standpoint. Medicinal products. Afterward, this is a difficult charge for the governing bodies in various parts of the world. Nutraceuticals, on the other hand, require clear and uniform regulations will be required immediately in the near future to keep up with quickly changing trends, and demands on the global market. By incorporating various herbal crude drugs into various nanosystems can help to achieve reduce the risk of adverse effect of chemotherapy.

KEYWORDS

- **bad quality foods**
- **cancer**
- **daily diet contaminants**
- **nutraceuticals**

REFERENCES

Abnet, C., (2007). Carcinogenic food contaminants. *Cancer Investigation, 25*, 189–196.

Aditya, N. P., Yang, H., Kim, S., & Ko, S., (2015). Fabrication of amorphous curcumin nanosuspensions using β-lactoglobulin to enhance solubility, stability, and bioavailability. *Biointerfaces, 127*, 114–121.

Andic, F., GaripaGaoglu, M., Yurdakonar, E., Tuncel, N., & Kucuk, O., (2009). Lycopene in prevention of gastrointestinal toxicity of radiotherapy. *Nutraceutical Cancer, 61*, 784–788.
Andlaur, W., & Furust, P., (2002). Nutraceuticals: A piece of history, present status and outlook. *Food Research International, 35*, 171–176.
Burns, K., (2010). Therapeutic foods and nutraceuticals in cancer therapy. *Vetlern. Com.*, 1–5.
Campanale, C., Massarilli, C., Savino, I., Vito, L., & Vito, F., (2020). A detailed review study on potential effects of microplastics and additives of concern on human health. *International Journal on Environmental Research and Public Health, 17*(4), 1212.
Cao, J., & Yang, C., (2011). Association between long-term exposure to outdoor air pollution and mortality in China: A cohort study. *Hazard Mater., 186*(2, 3), 1594–1600.
Casey, D., Slawson, C., & Neal, R., (2010). Vitamin D supplementation in infants, children, and adolescents. *American Family Physician, 8*, 745–748.
Cerella, C., Radogna, Dicato, M., & Diederich, M., (2013). Natural compounds as regulators of the cancer cell metabolism. *International Journal of Cell Biology*, 3–11.
Chanda, S., Tiwari, R., Kumar, A., & Singh, K., (2019). Nutraceuticals inspiring the current therapy for lifestyle diseases. *Hindawi Advance in Pharmacological Sciences*, 1–3.
Chu, M., Zheng, C., Cheng, C., Gedi, S., & Xiaoli, H., (2021). *Seminar on Cancer Biology* (pp. 2–5). Elsevier Ltd.
Davenport, D., & Roudebush, F., (2006). The use of nutraceuticals in cancer therapy. *Proceeding of North American Conference, NAVC., 20*, 777, 778.
Dich, J., Zahm, H., Hanberg, A., & Adami, H., (1997). Pesticides and cancer. *Cancer Causes Control, 3*, 420–443. Elsevier Ltd.
Dotto, J., & Abhihudi, S., (2021). Nutraceutical value of *Carica* papaya: A review. *Scientific African, 13*, 3, 4.
Dumitrescu, R., & Shields, G., (2005). The etiology of alcohol-induced breast cancer. *Alcohol. Cancer Investigation, 35*, 213–225.
Eric, B., Daliri, M., & Byoung, L., (2015). *Current Trends and Future Perspectives on Functional Foods and Nutraceuticals*, 230–239. Springer Ltd.
Factual List of Cancer Causing and Cancer Fighting Foods (pp. 1–5). https://www.aetnainternational.com/en/about-us/explore/fit-for-duty-corporate-wellness/cancer-causing-foods-cancer-fighting-foods.html, 2015, Aetna Ltd., 46.05.3431.
FAO and WHO, (2019). *Pesticide Residues in Food 2019 – Report* (Vol. 1–21, pp. 403–623). Food and Agriculture Organization of United States.
Feng, K., Wei, Y., Teng-Gun, H., Linhardt, R., Zong, M., & Hong, W., (2020). *Colon-Targeted Delivery Systems for Nutraceuticals: A Review of Current Vehicles, Evaluation Methods and Future Prospects* (pp. 6, 7). Elsevier Ltd.
George, J., & Shukla, Y., (2011). Pesticides and cancer: Insights into toxicoproteomic-based findings. *Journal of Proteomics, 74*(2011), 2713–2722. Elsevier Ltd.
Gupta, S., Yadav, S., Patil, S., & Mali, S., (2013). Nutraceutical–a bright scope and opportunity of Indian healthcare market. *International Journal of Research and Development in Pharmacy and Life Sciences*, 478–480.
Jarouliya, U., & Keservani, R. K., (2019). Pathways leading to child obesity. In: Debasis, B., (ed.), *Global Perspectives on Childhood Obesity: Current Status, Consequences and Prevention* (2nd edn., pp. 137–146). Academic Press, Elsevier, Chapter 12. ISBN: 9780128128404.
Keservani, R. K., & Sharma, A. K., (2014). Flavonoids: Emerging trends and potential health benefits. *Journal of Chinese Pharmaceutical Sciences, 23*(12), 815.

Keservani, R. K., Kesharwani, R. K., Sharma, A. K., Vyas, N., & Chadoker, A., (2010b). Nutritional supplements: An overview. *International Journal of Current Pharmaceutical Review and Research, 1*(1), 59–75.

Keservani, R. K., Kesharwani, R. K., Vyas, N., Jain, S., Raghuvanshi, R., & Sharma, A. K., (2010a). Nutraceutical and functional food as future food: A review. *Der Pharmacia Lettre, 2*(1), 106–116.

Keservani, R. K., Sharma, A. K., & Jarouliya, U., (2015). Protein and peptide in drug targeting and its therapeutic approach. *Ars Pharmaceutica (Internet), 56*(3), 165–177.

Keservani, R. K., Sharma, A. K., & Kesharwani, R. K., (2016a). Nutraceutical and functional foods for cardiovascular health. In: *Food Process Engineering* (pp. 257–278, 291–312). Apple Academic Press, CRC Press. ISBN: 9781771884020.

Keservani, R. K., Sharma, A. K., & Kesharwani, R. K., (2016b). Medicinal effect of nutraceutical fruits for the cognition and brain health. *Scientifica*, 10. Article ID 3109254. doi: 10.1155/2016/3109254.

Keservani, R. K., Sharma, A. K., & Kesharwani, R. K., (2020). *Nutraceuticals and Dietary Supplements: Applications in Health Improvement and Disease Management*. CRC Press. ISBN: 9781771888738.

Kingsley-Nwosu, O., & Kingsley-Ikechukwu, U., (2020). *Nutraceuticals: History, Classification and Market Demand* (pp. 13–15). Springer Nature Switzerland AG.

Kumar, A., Konar, A., Garg, S., Kaul, S., & Wadhwa, R., (2021). Experimental evidence and mechanism of action of some popular neuro-nutraceutical herbs. *Neurochemistry International, 149*(3–5), 105124.

Kumar, S., Roy, P., & Chakrabarty, S., (2021). Nutraceuticals with pharmaceutics: Its importance and their applications. *International Journal of Drug Development and Research., 1*, 2–7.

Linnewiel-Hermoni, K., Khanin, M., Danilenko, M., Zango, G., Amosi, Y., Levy, J., & Sharoni, Y., (2015). The anticancer effects of carotenoids and other phytonutrients resides in their combined activity. *Arch. Biochem. Biophys., 572*, 28–35.

Lotha, R., & Sivasubramanium, A., (2018). Flavonoids nutraceuticals in prevention and treatment of cancer: A review. *Asian Journal of Pharmaceutical and Clinical Research, 11*(1), 42–46.

Maiuolo, J., Gliozzi, M., Carresi, C., Musolino, V., Oppedisano, F., Scarano, F., Nucera, S., et al., (2021). Nutraceuticals and cancer: Potential for natural polyphenols. *Nutrients, 13*, 4, 5.

Mc Clements, D., & Xiao, H., (2017). *Designing Food Structure and Composition to Enhance Nutraceutical Bioactivity to Support Cancer Inhibition*, 5–18.

Naitr, B., Bokyung, S., Yadav, V., Kannappan, S., Chaturvedi, M., & Aggarwal, B., (2010). Delivery of anti-inflammatory nutraceuticals by nanoparticles for the prevention and treatment of cancer. *Biochemical Pharmacology, 80*, 1833–1844.

Nobili, S., Lippi, D., Witrot, E., Donnini, M., Bausi, L., Mini, E., & Capaciolli, S., (2009). Natural compound for cancer treatment and prevention. *Pharmacological Research*, 365–378.

Pandey, M., & Saraf, S., (2010). Nutraceutical: A new era of medicine and health. *Asian Journal of Pharmaceutical and Clinical Research, 3*(1), 1–5.

Parodi, W., (2007). A role for milk proteins and their peptides in cancer prevention. *Current Pharmaceutical Design, 13*, 813–828.

Poschl, G., & Seitz, K., (2004). Alcohol and cancer. *Alcohol, 39*, 155–165.

Rajamanikam, S., & Agarwal, R., (2008). Natural products and colon cancer: Current status and future prospects. *Drug Development Research, 69*, 460–471.

Rane, B. R., Bharath, M. S., Patil, R. R., Keservani, R. K., & Jain, A. S., (2020b). Novel approaches in nutraceuticals. In: Rajesh, K. K., Raj, K. K., & Anil, K. S., (eds.), *Enhancing the Therapeutic Efficacy of Herbal Formulations Through Novel Drug Delivery Systems* (pp. 241–266). IGI Global International Publisher, Pennsylvania, USA, Chapter 11. ISBN13: 9781799844532.

Rane, B. R., Patil, A. S., Keservani, R. K., & Jain, A. S., (2020a). Novel approaches in herbal formulation. In: Rajesh, K. K., Raj, K. K., & Anil, K. S., (eds.), *Enhancing the Therapeutic Efficacy of Herbal Formulations Through Novel Drug Delivery Systems* (pp. 43–68). IGI Global International Publisher, Pennsylvania, USA, Chapter 2. ISBN13: 9781799844532.

Rane, B., R., Tadavi, S. A., & Keservani, R. K., (2020c). Naturopathy. In: Anil, K. S., Raj, K. K., & Surya, P. G., (eds.), *Herbal Product Development* (pp. 321–347). Apple Academic Press, CRC Press, Taylor & Francis Group, Chapter 12. ISBN: 9781771888776.

Rillig, C., Ingraffia, R., & Machado, A., (2017). Microplastic incorporation into soil in agroecosystems. *Front. Plant Sci., 8*, 1805.

Roudebush, P., Davenport, D., &Novotny, B., (2004). The use of nutraceuticals in cancer therapy. *Vet. Clin. Small Animal., 34*, 249–269. Elsevier Ltd.

Sachdeva, V., Roy, A., & Bharadvaja, N., (2020). Current prospects of nutraceuticals: A review. *Current Pharmaceutical Biotechnology, 21*, 884–896.

Sairin, S., Sharma, M., Sing, R., & Kumar, S., (2012). Nutraceutical: A review. *International Journal of Research and Development in Pharmacy and Life Sciences., 3*(4), 97–99.

Santini, A., Cammarata, S., Capone, G., Ianaro, A., Tenore, G., Pani, L., & Novellino, E., (2018). Nutraceuticals: Opening the debate for a regulatory framework. *British Journal of Clinical Pharmacology*, 3–10.

Sharma, R., (2009). Nutraceuticals and nutraceuticals supplementation criteria in cancer: A literature survey. *The Open Nutraceuticals Journal, 2*, 92–106.

Singh, P., Kesharwani, R. K., & Keservani, R. K., (2017a). Anti-oxidants and vitamins: Roles in cellular function and metabolism. In: *Sustained Energy for Enhanced Human Functions and Activity* (pp. 385–407). Academic Press. ISBN:9780128054130.

Singh, P., Kesharwani, R. K., & Keservani, R. K., (2017b). Protein, carbohydrates, and fats: Energy metabolism. In: *Sustained Energy for Enhanced Human Functions and Activity* (pp. 103–115). Academic Press. ISBN:9780128054130.

Slattery, M., Curtin, K., Edwards, S., & Schaffer, D., (2004). Plant food fiber and rectal cancer. *American Society of Clinical Nutrition, 79*, 274–281.

Souyoul, S., Saussy, K., & Lupo, M., (2017). Nutraceutical: A review. *Dermatol. Ther. (Heidelb)*, 3–15.

T'elessy, G., (2019). *Nutraceutical: Review*, 411–418. Elsevier Ltd.

Turner, M., Andersen, Z., Baccrelli, A., Diver, R., Gapstur, S., Pope, A., Parad, D., et al., (2020). Outdoor air pollution and cancer: An overview of the current evidence and public health recommendations. *CA: Cancer Journal of Clinician*, 3–6.

Ujaliya, N., Dash, S., & Jain, S., (2018). A review on nutraceuticals in ayurveda. *World Journal of Pharmacy and Pharmaceutical Sciences, 7*(5), 277–281.

Wesley, P., Yongling, L., Changmin, L., Monaco, R., Kovavli, G., & Marion, J., (2012). Plastic and carcinogenesis: The example of vinyl chloride. *Journal of Carcinogenesis, 11*(5), 50–57.

CHAPTER 2

NUTRITIONAL STRATEGIES FOR THE PREVENTION OF CANCER

KHEMCHAND SURANA,[1] NISHA SHARMA,[2] EKNATH D. AHIRE,[3] RITESH KHAIRNAR,[4] RITESH PAWAR,[5] SUNIL MAHAJAN,[6] SANJAY KSHIRSAGAR,[3] PRAKASH CHANDRA GUPTA,[2] SWATI G. TALELE,[7] and BHAVANA AHIRE[8]

[1]*Department of Pharmaceutical Chemistry, Shreeshakti Shaikshanik Sanstha, Divine College of Pharmacy, Satana, Nashik, India*

[2]*School of Pharmaceutical Sciences, Chhatrapati Sahu Ji Maharaj University, Kanpur, India*

[3]*Department of Pharmaceutics, MET's Institute of Pharmacy, Adgaon Nashik, India*

[4]*Department of Pharmaceutical Chemistry, St. John Institute of Pharmacy & Research, Palghar, Maharashtra, India*

[5]*Department of Pharmaceutical Chemistry, Poona College of Pharmacy, Pune, Maharashtra, India*

[6]*Department of Pharmaceutical Chemistry, MGV's Pharmacy College, Panchvati, Nashik, India*

[7]*Department of Pharmaceutics, Sandip Institute of Pharmaceutical Sciences, Affiliated to Savitribai Phule Pune University, Nashik, India*

[8]*Department of Quality Assurance Techniques, NDMVP's, College of Pharmacy, Nashik, India*

Nutraceuticals in Cancer Prevention, Management, and Treatment. Raj K. Keservani, Bui Thanh Tung, Sippy Singh, & Rajesh K. Kesharwani, PhD (Eds.)

ABSTRACT

According to accumulating data, nutrition has a role in the etiology of around 1/3 of all fatal occurrences of human cancer in affluent nations. Despite its limitations, the present research lays the groundwork for a successful primary cancer prevention strategy based on dietary changes. Dietary advice suggests lowering the risk of cancer. A cancer-fighting diet should be heavy in vegetables, fruits, legumes, and grains, and low in red meat, salt, and animal-derived saturated fat. Obesity is mostly prevented by increased physical exercise. Regular physical exercise during childhood and adolescence may also help to prevent excessive development, as measured by height, and may have a protective effect against a variety of cancers. In the case of alcoholic beverages, a strategy that would preserve the majority of the health benefits of alcohol consumption while lowering alcohol-related cancer mortality would include: for everyone, reducing heavy alcohol consumption; for smokers, limiting alcoholic beverages to those consumed with meals. Encouragement of moderate drinking (up to two glasses per day) for nonsmoking males; light drinking (one glass per day) for nonsmoking women, unless they are at high risk of breast cancer.

2.1 INTRODUCTION

Cancer is a genome-wide chronic illness that may be influenced by dietary factors at various stages throughout its natural history, affecting not only the prevention but also the progression and treatment of this deadly disease. The phenotype of cancer is the outcome of a combination of hereditary and environmental factors. The evidence for this comes from human population studies as well as animal experiments that mimic the carcinogenesis process. Perhaps the most powerful environmental effect is that it is anticipated that up to 80% of colon, breast, and prostate cancer cases, as well as one-third of all cancer cases, may be influenced by nutrition and related lifestyle variables. We can better specify the particular location at which individual nutrients may impact the development of cancer as our understanding of cancer etiology advances.

Nutrition is crucial for good health and the prevention of diseases like cancer. According to epidermal research, over 35% of cancer cases might be avoided by changing a person's diet. Caloric restriction and the restriction of certain micronutrient groups are examples of these modifications.

The research shows that important foods include micronutrient factors that protect against cancer, including colon, breast, and prostate cancers (Atif et al., 2006).

2.2 EVIDENCE LINKING DIET TO CANCER

According to the predicted prevalence rates for numerous cancers globally in 2002, the maximum common cancers in both women and men had been colon rectum and stomach cancers, in addition to prostate and liver cancers in men and breast and cervical cancers in women. The sample of various cancers distribution is primarily based on prevalence and death rates, wherein is geographical, in general, outstanding cancers in financial early evolved nations, in comparison to the ones in Asia's commercial improvement. In Africa and Latin America, cancers of the higher aerodigestive tract, stomach, and liver are more common, however, cancers of the colon/rectum, breast, and prostate are more common in Europe and North America. The World Cancer Research Fund and the American Institute of Cancer Research (AICR) have extensively reviewed the geographic sample variations in tumor incidences, loose valence, and herbal records as associated with meals eating regimen vitamins, and associated way of life elements in western cancers. In growing countries, such dealers as viral hepatitis and Helicobacter pylori play a key role (Atif et al., 2006; WCRF, 1997).

Epidermal logical research withinside the United States have a unique particular food regimen to issue as having the best effect at the discount of cancers is the maximum regular relation of sheep is an inverse relationship among cancers and an consumption of vegetable and fruit extra nutritional issue with utensils for lowering cancers dangers consist of whole-grain nutritional fiber positive micronutrients (e.g., selenium, vitamin E, vitamin D, and calcium), in addition to positive types of fats (e.g., n-3 fatty acids, in particular n-3/n-6 ratios) and bodily pastime. High intakes of general and diverse types of fats (e.g., saturated fats), alcohol, precise meals coaching techniques including smoking, salting, and pickling ingredients, and excessive-temperature cooking of meats, in addition to obesity (excessive Body Mass Index), are all variables that decorate risk (Atif et al., 2006; Greenwald et al., 2001).

1. To decrease cancers risk, the AICR will bring together specific nutritional guidelines for people. Reduced fats consumption (especially from animal sources), accelerated fiber consumption, and plenty of

veggies and end result withinside the everyday eating regimen are all advocated in those fundamental guidelines. Increasing physical activity and retaining wholesome body weight, proscribing alcoholic beverage consumption, and avoiding salt-cured, salt-pickled, or smoked ingredients are all recommended. The 2005 USDA Dietary Guidelines for Americans are the primary to consist of cancers prevention as final results in reviewing the proof base for growing nutritional guidelines, primarily based totally on a wealth of epidemiological and experimental studies helping the significance of vitamins in cancers prevention (Atif et al., 2006; http://www.healthierus.gov/dietaryguidelines/).

2.3 NUTRITIONAL COMPONENTS

Bioactive dietary components are determined in all traditional nutritional groups, together with carbohydrates, amino acids, fatty acids, structural lipids, minerals, and nutrients. Humans consume over 25,000 extraordinary chemical substances in fruits, vegetables, and exclusive plants. Carotenoids, flavonoids (Keservani et al., 2014), organosulfur compounds, isothiocyanates, indoles, monoterpene, phenolic acids, and chlorophyll are some of the chemical instructions they may be capable of include. For years, researchers have been studying the maximum cancers-preventive homes of macronutrient (carbohydrate, protein, fat, and fiber) and micronutrient (weight loss program and mineral) components of diets, and the National Cancer Institute (NCI) has funded numerous human intervention trials with person vitamins and minerals. However, in modern years, a have a take a observe has centered on non-nutritive phytochemicals. In cellular manner of existence and animal models, the National Cancer Institute located that more than 35 plant-based totally definitely diets and a thousand specific phytochemicals had maximum cancers-preventive potential. Garlic (diallyl sulfide), soybeans (genistein), turmeric (curcumin), tomatoes (lycopene), grapes (resveratrol), inexperienced tea (epigallocatechin-3-gallate [EGCG]), and cruciferous vegetables are all well-studied dietary reasserts and representative phytochemicals (together with broccoli, cabbage, and Brussels sprouts; indole-3-carbinol, sulforaphane). However, the list of chemopreventive phytochemicals is considerable and new foods, dietary supplements, and traditional herbal remedies with previously unknown anti-cancers homes are being located all the time (Keservani et al., 2020; Atif et al., 2006; Rane et al., 2020a; Rane et al., 2020b; Rane et al., 2020c).

2.3 STRATEGIES FOR CANCER PREVENTION

Cancer may be averted through the use of both number one and secondary preventive measures. The intention of number one prevention is to maintain susceptible molecules withinside the human body from being damaged, and it's far achieved in ways:

i. By averting or lowering carcinogenic exposure, including through quitting smoking or switching from excessive to low tar cigarettes; and
ii. By strengthening the body's defenses via immunization, nutritional changes, and chemoprevention. Secondary prevention, which relies upon on presymptomatic illness prognosis and can be achieved via checkups or populace screening, is primarily based totally on secondary prevention. Even while the three strategies are similarly a success in reducing mortality, number one prevention is higher than secondary prevention and medical therapy. This is due to the fact number one prevention isn't always followed through the affliction that includes the analysis and remedy of even presymptomatic cancers and due to the fact number one prevention failure leaves the opposite protective traces intact (Trichopoulos and Willett, 1996; Dimitrios and Pagona, 1996).

2.4 AN OVERVIEW OF CANCER NUTRITIONAL ETIOLOGY

In molecular terms, the influence of nutrition on cancer incidence is poorly understood, but some patterns have emerged. Consumption of fruits and vegetables offers some protection against a variety of cancers in humans. The consumption of red meat is associated with the development of colorectal cancer, and animal-derived saturated fat is linked to the development of prostate cancer and, most likely, colorectal cancer. Excess energy intake in early life, maybe due to a lack of physical exercise, could be to blame for the consistently established positive relationship between height and the risk of breast cancer and probably other cancer types on the one hand, and other cancer types on the other. In adulthood, physical exercise lowers the risk of colon cancer, potentially breast cancer, and maybe other cancers. Obesity in adulthood (Jarouliya and Keservani 2019), caused by either excessive energy intake or decreased expenditure, is a leading cause of endometrial cancer, a proven cause of postmenopausal breast cancer, and a potential cause of kidney and gallbladder cancers. There's also evidence that intrauterine growth is linked to a higher risk of cancer in the children, such as breast and prostate cancer.

Salt appears to be a key factor to stomach cancer in some populations among non-nutrient food additives that have been used. Furthermore, in Southeast Asia, the consumption of salty fish at a young age has been associated with the development of nasopharyngeal cancer. In Central Asia and South America, drinking excessively hot liquids has been linked to an increased risk of esophageal cancer. Large amounts of alcoholic drinks, especially when combined with tobacco smoking, dramatically increase the risk of upper respiratory and digestive tract cancers, whereas alcoholic cirrhosis commonly leads to liver cancer. According to a growing body of evidence, even tiny amounts of alcohol may be associated with the development of breast and colorectal cancer (Trichopoulos and Willett, 1996).

2.5 DIETARY AND PHYSICAL ACTIVITY FACTORS THAT INFLUENCE CANCER RISK

2.5.1 BREAST CANCER

Breast cancer is the maximum common cancers in American women, and it's far second most effective to lung cancer in phrases of cancers mortality. Factors that modify circulating hormone degrees all through life, together with age at the beginning of menstruation, a wide variety of pregnancies, breastfeeding, obesity, and physical activity, all increase breast cancer chance. Many research display that ingesting alcoholic drinks, even in moderation, may also improve the chance of breast cancer. Some studies indicate that consuming an eating regimen wealthy in end result and veggies lowers the chance of breast cancers, albeit the proof is extensively much less than for different cancers. At this time, the pleasant advice for lowering breast cancers chance is to restrict alcohol use, eat an eating regimen wealthy in end result and greens, workout regularly, and keep away from obesity.

2.5.2 PROSTATE CANCER

Prostate cancer is the maximum not unusual place cancer in adult males withinside the United States. Scientists are conscious that male hormones are connected to prostate cancers; however, they may be uncertain of the particular mechanism. The intake of animal fats, purple meats, and dairy merchandise has been related to an elevated risk of prostate cancer, suggesting that saturated fats perform a role. Limit your consumption of animal-primarily based totally foods, especially saturated fat and purple meats, to decrease your chance of prostate cancers.

2.5.3 COLORECTAL CANCER

Colorectal cancer is the second most common reason of cancer mortality withinside the United States. Diets heavy in plant-primarily based totally foods (greens, fruits, complete grains, and legumes) had been related to a decrease threat of colorectal cancer, however diets excessive in fats and pork had been related to an elevated threat. Obesity and inaction have a tendency to elevate the threat as well. Consuming fewer excessive-fats meals, proscribing beef intake, ingesting extra greens, end result, and complete grains, being bodily active, and keeping off weight problems at the moment are the best approaches to lessen the threat of colorectal cancers.

2.5.4 ENDOMETRIUM CANCER

Obesity is continually related to an elevated risk of endometrial cancer in research. The link can be associated with a growth in estrogen degrees in postmenopausal women who're overweight. Maintain a healthful weight through normal physical workout and suitable ingesting selections to decrease the risk of endometrial cancer.

2.5.5 LUNGS CANCER

Lung cancer is the most important purpose of cancer-associated mortality withinside the United States. Tobacco smoking is liable for extra than 80% of lung cancers cases. Many researches have proven that men and women who consume the desired amount of fruits and veggies had a reduced risk of lung cancer, each smokers and non-smokers. Avoid smoking and consume at least five servings of veggies and end result each day to decrease your threat of lung cancer.

2.5.6 ORAL AND ESOPHAGEAL CANCER

Tobacco-including cigarettes, chewing tobacco, and snuff and alcohol, both alone and in combination, raise the risk of oral and esophageal cancers. This risk is reduced by eating the required number of fruits and vegetables. To avoid these malignancies, avoid all forms of tobacco, drink no more than one or two alcoholic beverages per day, and consume at least five servings of fruits and vegetables each day.

2.5.7 STOMACH CANCER

Stomach cancer is becoming less common across the world, particularly in the United States. Fresh food consumption all year, refrigeration, and other advances in food preservation technologies have all contributed to lower danger. Infection with the bacterium Helicobacter pylori can raise the risk of stomach cancer. Eat at least five servings of fruits and vegetables each day to lower your risk of stomach cancer (Atif et al., 2006; Guidelines, 1996).

2.5.8 ANTIOXIDANTS

Certain nutrients included in fruits and vegetables appear to protect the body from oxygen-induced tissue damage, which happens as part of regular metabolism. Antioxidant nutrients are suggested to protect against cancer since such damage is linked to an increased risk of cancer. Vitamin C, vitamin E, selenium, and carotenoids are antioxidant nutrients. According to studies, persons who consume more antioxidant-rich fruits and vegetables had a decreased cancer risk.

2.5.9 BETA-CAROTENE

Because eating fruits and vegetables has been linked to a lower risk of cancer, taking large dosages of beta-carotene supplements appeared to be a viable option. People were given high dosages of synthetic beta carotene in three key studies in the hopes of preventing lung and other malignancies. Two of these trials linked beta-carotene supplements to an increased risk of lung cancer in cigarette smokers, while the third showed no benefit or harm from beta-carotene supplements. As a result, using high-dose beta-carotene supplements has not been shown to replicate the positive effects of fruits and vegetables. Supplements like these may be dangerous to smokers.

2.5.10 CALCIUM

Whether calcium consumption influences cancer risk, consuming calcium-rich foods is critical for preventing osteoporosis. Some study suggests that calcium-rich meals may help lower the incidence of colorectal cancer, although this link has not been proven. Calcium is abundant in low-fat and non-fat dairy products, as well as certain green vegetables and legumes.

2.5.11 CRUCIFEROUS VEGETABLES

Broccoli, cauliflower, and Brussels sprouts are examples of cruciferous vegetables, which belong to the cabbage family. Certain compounds in these veggies are considered to lower the incidence of colorectal cancer. According to the best evidence, eating a wide variety of vegetables, particularly cruciferous and other vegetables, lowers the risk of cancer.

2.5.12 FIBER

Dietary fiber is composed of a variety of non-digestible plant sugars. "Soluble" fiber (like oat bran) and "insoluble" fiber (like psyllium husk) are two types of fiber (like wheat bran). Although the mechanism of action is unknown, insoluble fiber is considered to help lower the incidence of colorectal cancer. Soluble fiber decreases the risk of coronary heart disease by lowering blood cholesterol levels. Beans, vegetables, whole grains, and fruits are all good sources of fiber (Keservani et al., 2020).

2.5.13 SOYBEAN

Soybeans are a high-protein food that may be used in place of meat. Nonfermented soybeans have large quantities of phytoestrogens and other phytochemicals, which have been shown in animal experiments to have positive effects on hormone-dependent malignancies. These effects have yet to be demonstrated in people.

2.5.14 VITAMIN A

Vitamin A (retinol) may be gained from the diet in two ways: through animal food sources of beta carotene in plant foods. Vitamin A is required for the maintenance of healthy tissues. When vitamin A levels are normal, the body does not convert beta carotene to vitamin A, therefore consuming beta carotene-rich fruits and vegetables does not induce vitamin A poisoning. Vitamin A supplementation, on the other hand, has not been proven to reduce cancer risk. Supplements should be taken in suggested amounts, as large quantities of preformed vitamin A can be dangerous, especially to pregnant women.

2.5.15 VITAMIN C

Many fruits and vegetables contain vitamin C. Consumption of vitamin C-rich foods has been associated with a lower risk of cancer in several studies. However, no evidence of a reduced risk of cancer has been shown in the few trials that have used vitamin C as a supplement (Guidelines, 1996).

2.5.16 VITAMIN D

Vitamin D is significant in cancer prevention and may have been recognized for more than 50 years. Even though prolonged sun exposure has been shown to raise the risk of skin cancer, research dating back to 1936 has shown that people with skin cancer had a decreased chance of developing other cancers. Certain forms of cancer, such as prostate, breast, and colon cancers, have been linked to sun exposure. People who live in northern latitudes, such as the United States, have a two to three times higher risk of cancer than those who live in sunnier, equatorial areas. Several epidemiological investigations found an inverse connection between 25-(OH) D3 levels and cancer risk and death, following Apperly fascinating discovery (Atif et al., 2006; Garland et al., 1989; Garland et al., 1990).

2.5.17 GINSENG

Ginseng prepared as an extract or powder was more effective than fresh ginseng in reducing cancers. The risk ratios of gastric (0.33) and lung cancer development were reduced even though these cancers have different mechanisms of carcinogenesis and etiology, again indicating that Ginseng has a non-organ-specific preventative effect against cancer. A prospective cohort study of 4634 people over 40 years of age showed that Koreans had a relative risk of 0.40 (95% confidence interval) compared to non-consumers to develop cancer (Nitenberg and Raynard, 2000; Yun and Choi, 1990; Yun et al., 2001; Yun et al., 1998; Suh et al., 2002).

2.6 PREVENTION OF DIET-RELATED CANCER

Even though we know little about the beneficial or dangerous dietary ingredients, we have a fair concept of what a cancer-prevention diet should consist of. This diet should be heavy in fruits, vegetables, legumes, and grains, low in red meat and salt, and low in saturated fat from animal sources. Added lipids should be of plant origin, and olive oil is one among them, with a long track record of safety. Obesity should be avoided, but the best method to do so is to increase physical activity, which can lower the risk of colorectal cancer and possibly other cancers. Regular physical exercise during childhood and adolescence may also help to prevent excessive development, as measured by height, and may have a protective effect against a variety of cancers. Many civilizations' communal life revolves around alcoholic beverages, and their consumption lowers cardiovascular mortality. Alcohol, on the other hand, interacts with tobacco in the development of cancers of the upper respiratory and gastrointestinal tract; it can induce liver cirrhosis-mediated hepatocellular carcinoma, as well as cancers of the breast and perhaps the large intestine.

An approach that would keep the majority of the health advantages of alcohol use while lowering alcohol-related cancer mortality would include: reducing excessive alcohol consumption for everyone; for smokers who are unable to quit smoking, limitation to alcoholic beverages consumed with meals (primarily wine), which are less likely to damage the mucosa and facilitate the carcinogenic action of tobacco constituents; encouragement of moderate drinking (up to 2 glasses per day) for nonsmoking men; avoidance of drinking for nonsmoking women at high risk for breast cancer, whereas encouragement of light drinking for nonsmoking women at low risk for this disease or at high cardiovascular risk. Encouragement of moderate drinking (one glass per day); for every drinker, encourages high intake of green vegetables that contain folate, since a lack of this vitamin may enhance the possibility for alcohol to raise the risk of colorectal cancer (Dimitrios and Pagona, 1996; DeVita et al., 1997).

2.7 DIETARY GUIDELINES RECOMMENDED FOR REDUCING THE RISK OF CANCER

1. Limit fat consumption to 30% of total calories or less.
2. Increase fiber consumption to 20 to 30 grams per day, with a maximum of 35 grams.
3. Include a variety of fruits and vegetables in your daily diet;
4. Stay away from being overweight;
5. If at all possible, use alcoholic beverages in moderation;
6. Limit your intake of salt-cured, salt-pickled, or smoked foods (Alessandro et al., 1997).
7. Choose food low in fat:

   a) Fruits, vegetables, grains, and beans can be used to replace fat-rich diets.
   b) Reduce the amount of high-fat meals you eat.
   c) Instead of frying, go for baked or broiled dishes.
   d) Non-fat and low-fat milk and dairy products are recommended.
   e) Choose low-fat foods from packaged, snack, convenience, and restaurant items.

8. Limit your meat consumption, especially high-fat meats:

   a) When eating beef, choose lean cuts.
   b) Meats should be consumed in lesser portions.
   c) As an alternative to beef, hog, and lamb, consider beans, shellfish, and poultry.
   d) Instead of frying meats, fish, and poultry, bake or braise them.

High-fat diets have been linked to an increased risk of colon and rectum cancers, prostate cancer, and endometrial cancer. The link between a high-fat diet and breast cancer is much more tenuous. It is yet to be determined if these relationships are caused by the overall quantity of fat, the kind of fat (saturated, monounsaturated, or polyunsaturated), the calories given by fat, or some other element in dietary fats. Because a gram of fat includes more than twice as many calories as a gram of protein or carbohydrate (9 vs. 4 kcal/gram), studies can't simply separate between the effects of fat and the calories it contains. Furthermore, persons who eat high-fat diets tend to be overweight and consume more meat and fewer fruits and vegetables, increasing their risk of cancer for a variety of reasons.

Animal-based foods continue to be key sources of total fat, saturated fat, and cholesterol in the American diet. Meat intake, particularly red meats (beef, hog, and lamb), has been associated with malignancies at various places, most notably colon and prostate cancers, even though meats are rich sources of high-quality protein and provide many vital vitamins and minerals. At this time, it's unclear how much of the link between red meat and cancer is attributable to total fat or saturated fat, and how much is related to other meat or diet components. For example, mutagenic chemicals such as heterocyclic amines, which are formed when protein is cooked, may help explain the link between meat and colon cancer, in addition to fat. Saturated, monounsaturated, and polyunsaturated fats all have the same number of calories, but they may have varied effects on cancer risk. Specific facts, such as those found in vegetable or fish oils, may impact cancer risk differently. The link between different fat forms and cancer risk is still being researched.

According to a growing body of data, saturated fat appears to play a key role in the development of cancer and heart disease. Making intelligent decisions in selecting and preparing animal meals is the greatest approach to limit saturated fat consumption. Choose lean meats and low-fat dairy items, and replace butter or lard with vegetable oils. Food labels can help you choose packaged foods that are lower in saturated fat. Choose lesser servings of meat and serve it as a side dish rather than the main course (Guidelines, 1996).

2.8 NUTRITIONAL ADVICE

According to research, poor dietary characteristics have been linked to worse overall morbidity and quality of life in cancer patients (Ravasco et al., 2004). As a result, even if no nutritional issues are discovered, the need for an appropriate diet should be stressed to prevent nutrient deficiency in cancer patients (Thomas, 2001). Dietary counseling aimed at boosting the food intake of cancer patients through regular meals and drinks is typically the first step in providing nutritional support; this is a crucial function for dieticians and nurses to complete before patients become malnourished (Thomas, 2001; Bloch, 1998). In recent research, individualized dietary counseling has been shown to increase nutrient intake and quality of life (Ravasco et al., 2003; Ravasco et al., 2005).

Found that dietary counseling favorably improved total food intake, especially protein consumption, and overall outcomes such as complications and quality of life in patients with colorectal cancer undergoing radiation, suggesting that dietary interventions should be an integral element of the treatment plan for all patients getting head and neck radiotherapy to prevent nutritional loss (Schueren et al., 2005; Keservani et al., 2010a; Keservani et al., 2010b).

Regular interaction between the healthcare practitioner and the patient, including regular nutritional evaluations and guidance, may help the patient follow dietary instructions (Wickham et al., 1999). Patients (or their families) are sometimes urged to keep a food diary to track what they eat and what influences their appetite. This will encourage early detection of changes in eating patterns and weight loss, as well as highlight another essential role for nurses, who may refer patients to a dietician or clinical nurse specialist for more help and support.

2.9 NUTRITIONAL SUPPORT

2.9.1 ORAL SUPPLEMENTATION

When patients are unable to satisfy their nutritional needs with conventional meals alone, despite dietary guidance, oral nutritional supplements can help. Oral supplementation is the easiest, most natural, and least intrusive way for all patients to increase their nutritional intake (Schueren et al., 2005).

Oral supplementation has been linked to enhanced appetite and weight gain, reduced GI toxicity, and improved performance status. Oral supplementation was also linked to a boost in immunological response as well as an increase in caloric and protein consumption (Schueren et al., 2005; Bounous et al., 1971; Nayel et al., 1992).

To complement the patient's nutritional demands, dietary supplements should supply enough levels of all nutrients, including protein, energy, vitamins, and minerals. Fiber may also be beneficial because it has various good effects on nutritional absorption, gastrointestinal transit time, stool qualities, and perhaps immunological function.

Oral supplementation's efficacy is contingent on sufficient quantities being ingested over a long period. Lean body mass rose in patients who took an EPA-enriched supplement at the recommended amount (1.5–2 cans/day), but not in patients who did not, showing the importance of compliance. Acceptability and palatability of a nutritional supplement are critical variables in its efficacy; flavor, texture, and volume are especially significant. The biggest disadvantage of oral supplements is taste fatigue (Schueren et al., 2005, Fearon et al., 2003; Green et al., 2001).

2.9.2 THE ROLE OF THE DIETICIAN

Managing cancer patients at risk of malnutrition requires regular monitoring by a dietician (Nitenberg and Raynard, 2000). The dietician's job is to assess the patient's nutritional state and predict the nutritional risks associated with cancer and its treatment. The dietician will examine the patient's dietary needs and provide advice in collaboration with other members of the nutritional team. In addition, the dietician can provide supplements, evaluate the efficiency of nutritional guidance, and notify the team of the best feeding strategy.

2.9.3 QUANTITATIVE ESTIMATES

According to the Harvard Center for Cancer Prevention, nutrition in adulthood, particularly obesity, is linked to the etiology of around 30% of cancer deaths in affluent nations. This impending death food additive is primarily salt. On the other hand, sedentary behavior provides an additional 3% of the total. Extremely hot beverages may be able to donate an additional 1% Perinatal impacts, as well as other factors a significant amount of growth that reflects an energy imbalance in early childhood may play a role in a significant number of commonly deadly breast and ovarian cancers, maybe as much as 5% prostate. Finally, the value of alcoholic beverages has been calculated. They account for roughly 3% of overall cancer mortality in the industrialized world.

Diet, physical activity, and obesity are all quantitative factors with no zero exposure categories in practice. Furthermore, absolute measures are difficult to achieve since most measurements depend on the study's design, the databases accessible, and the analytic method used. Individuals are often dispersed in quintiles, or 20%-wide groupings, in the respective frequency distributions. A score is occasionally constructed to incorporate the various diet components. Individuals in all quintiles but the best tend to be driven to improve their diets and increase their physical activity to move to the adjacent "better" quintile, which does not appear to be unreasonable. Both diet-related and sedentary life-related cancer mortality would be lowered by around a quarter if this were to happen. In principle, lowering salt intake might hasten the decline in stomach cancer incidence. Finally, an increase in the popularity of wine and a decrease in the popularity of spirits might result in a 1/3 reduction in alcohol-related cancer mortality. Cancer mortality is attributable to specific factors or groups of factors in developed countries.

TABLE 2.1 Factor or Group of Factors

Sr. No.	Factor or Group of Factor	Percentage
1.	Tobacco	30
2.	Alcohol	3
3.	Diet in Adult life Including Obesity	30
4.	Perinatal Effect and Excessive Growth	5
5.	Food additives and Contamination Salt	1
6.	Sedentary Life	3
7.	Biological Agent, Including Virus	5
8.	Reproductive Factor	3
9.	Medical Product and Procedure	1

2.10 CONCLUSION

The nutritional status of cancer prevention is achievable. In principle, it might prevent around one-third of fatal cancer in industrialized nations, but non-compliance of a wide population segment with dietary standards drastically lowered this theoretical potential. Furthermore, the slow introduction of positive modifications and the confusing impact of other concurrent changes impeded the establishment of a nutritional cancer-preventive approach. At this moment, observation of the best recommendations, which may be described in the suggestion to increase the consumption of vegetables, fruit, legumes, and grain and to minimize the consumption of refined carbohydrates, salt, red meat, and animal fat, to partially substitute animal fat with olive oil and other vegetable oil, to reduce excess calorie in early life to avoid obesity in adulthood, to moderate alcoholic beverage use, and to enhance physical activity levels.

ACKNOWLEDGMENT

We thank the METs, Institute of Pharmacy, BKC, affiliated under Savitribai Phule Pune University, Nashik, Divine College of Pharmacy Satana, and Sandip Institute of Pharmaceutical Science for their constant support and support providing all facilities to complete this work. We are also thankful to the Ministry of Tribal Affairs Govt. of India for providing financial assistance in the form of a fellowship (Award No.: 202021-NFST-MAH-01235).

KEYWORDS

- **cancer etiology**
- **dietary guidelines**
- **nutrition**
- **risk factors**

REFERENCES

Alessandro, L., & Michael, M. M., (1996). Nutritional issues in cancer management. Elsevier Science. *Nutrition, 12*, 358–371.

Atif, B. A., & Peter, G. B., (2006). *Nutrition and Cancer Prevention* (pp. 1–597). CRC Press, Taylor and Francis Group.

Bloch, A. S., (1998). Cancer. In: Matarese, L. E., & Gottschlich, M. M., (eds.), *Contemporary Nutrition Support Practice: A Clinical Guide* (pp. 475–495). W.B. Saunders Company, Philadelphia.

Bounous, G., Gentile, J. M., & Hugon, J., (1971). Elemental diet in the management of the intestinal lesion produced by 5 fluorouracil in man. *Canadian Journal of Surgery, 14*, 312–324.

Vincent T. DeVita, Jr , Samuel Hellman, & Stevan A. Rosenberg (1997). *Cancer: Principles and Practice of Oncology* (5th edn., pp. 231–257). Lippincott-Raven; Philadelphia, PA.

Dimitrios, T., & Pagona, L., (1996). Nutritional strategies for cancer prevention. *Journal of Epidemiology, 6*(4), 111–115.

Fearon, K. C., Von, M. M. F., Moses, A. G., Van, G. R., Roy, A., Gouma, D. J., Giacosa, A., et al., (2003). Effect of a protein and energy dense N-3 fatty acid enriched oral supplement on loss of weight and lean tissue in cancer cachexia: A randomized double-blind trial. *Gut., 52*, 1479–1486.

Garland, C. F., Comstock, G. W., Garland, F. C., Helsing, K. J., Shaw, E. K., & Gorham, E. D., (1989). Serum 25-hydroxyvitamin D and colon cancer: An eight-year prospective study. *Lancet, 2*(8673), 1176–1178.

Garland, F. C., Garland, C. F., Gorham, E. D., & Young, J. F., (1990). Geographic variation in breast cancer mortality in the United States: A hypothesis involving exposure to solar radiation. *Prev. Med., 19*(6), 614–622.

Green, C. J., (2001). The fiber in enteral nutrition. *Clinical Nutrition, 20*(Suppl 1), 23–39.

Greenwald, P., Clifford, C. K., & Milner, J. A., (2001). Diet and cancer prevention. *Eur. J. Cancer 37*(8), 948–965.

Guidelines given by Members of the American Cancer Society 1996 Advisory Committee on Diet, Nutrition, and Cancer Prevention: doi: https://doi.org/10.3322/canjclin.46.6.325.

Jarouliya, U., & Keservani, R. K., (2019). Pathways leading to child obesity. In: Debasis, B., (ed.), *Global Perspectives on Childhood Obesity: Current Status, Consequences and Prevention* (2nd edn., pp. 137–146). Edited by Academic Press, Elsevier, Chapter 12. ISBN: 9780128128404.

Keservani, R. K., & Sharma, A. K., (2014). Flavonoids: Emerging trends and potential health benefits. *Journal of Chinese Pharmaceutical Sciences, 23*(12), 815.

Keservani, R. K., Kesharwani, R. K., Sharma, A. K., Vyas, N., & Chadoker, A., (2010b). Nutritional supplements: An overview. *International Journal of Current Pharmaceutical Review and Research, 1*(1), 59–75.

Keservani, R. K., Kesharwani, R. K., Vyas, N., Jain, S., Raghuvanshi, R., & Sharma, A. K., (2010a). Nutraceutical and functional food as future food: A review. *Der Pharmacia Lettre, 2*(1), 106–116.

Keservani, R. K., Sharma, A. K., & Kesharwani, R. K., (2020). *Nutraceuticals and Dietary Supplements: Applications in Health Improvement and Disease Management*. CRC Press. ISBN: 9781771888738.

Nayel, H., el-Ghoneimy, E., & el-Haddad, S., (1992). Impact of nutritional supplementation on treatment delay and morbidity in patients with head and neck tumors treated with irradiation. *Nutrition, 8*(1), 13–18.

Nitenberg, G., & Raynard, B., (2000). Nutritional support of the cancer patient: Issues and dilemmas. *Critical Revues in Oncology/Hematology, 34*(3), 137–168.

Rane, B. R., Bharath, M. S., Patil, R. R., Keservani, R. K., & Jain, A. S., (2020b). Novel approaches in nutraceuticals. In: Rajesh, K. K., Raj, K. K., & Anil, K. S., (eds.), *Enhancing the Therapeutic Efficacy of Herbal Formulations Through Novel Drug Delivery Systems* (pp. 241–266). IGI Global International Publisher, Pennsylvania, USA, Chapter 11. ISBN13: 9781799844532.

Rane, B. R., Bharath, M. S., Patil, R. R., Keservani, R. K., & Jain, A. S., (2020a). Novel approaches in herbal formulation. In: Rajesh, K. K., Raj, K. K., & Anil, K. S., (eds.), *Enhancing the Therapeutic Efficacy of Herbal Formulations Through Novel Drug Delivery Systems* (pp. 43–68). IGI Global International Publisher, Pennsylvania, USA, Chapter 2. ISBN13: 9781799844532.

Rane, B. R., Tadavi, S. A., & Keservani, R. K., (2020c). Naturopathy. In: Anil, K. S., Raj, K. K., & Surya, P. G., (eds.), *Herbal Product Development* (pp. 321–347). Apple Academic Press, Taylor & Francis Group, Chapter 12. ISBN: 9781771888776.

Ravasco, P. M., Monteiro-Grillo, I., & Camilo, M. E., (2003). Does nutrition influence the quality of life in cancer patients undergoing radiotherapy? *Radiotherapy and Oncology, 67*(2), 213–220.

Ravasco, P., Monteiro-Grillo, I., Vidal, P. M., & Camilo, M. E., (2004). Cancer: Disease and nutrition are key determinants of patients' quality of life. *Supportive Care in Cancer, 12*, 246–252.

Ravasco, P., Monteiro-Grillo, I., Vidal, P. M., & Camilo, M. E., (2005). Dietary counseling improves patient outcomes: A prospective, randomized, controlled trial in colorectal cancer patients undergoing radiotherapy. *Journal of Clinical Oncology, 23*(7), 1431–1438.

van Bokhorst-de van der Schueren, M.A., (2005). Nutritional support strategies for malnourished cancer patients. *European Journal of Oncology Nursing, 9*, S74–S83.

Suh, S. O., Kroh, M., Kim, N. R., Joh, Y. G., & Cho, M. Y., (2002). Effects of red ginseng upon postoperative immunity and survival in patients with stage III gastric cancer. *Am. J. Chin. Med., 30*, 483–494.

Thomas, B., (2001). *Manual of Dietetic Practice* (3rd edn., pp. 637–647). Blackwell Scientific Publications, Oxford.

Trichopoulos, D., & Willett, W. C., (1996). Nutrition and cancer. *Cancer Cause and Control, 7*, 3–180.

U.S. Department of Health and Human Services, U.S. Department of Agriculture, (2005). *Dietary Guidelines Advisory Committee Report–2005.* Departments of Health and Human Services and Agriculture. www.healthierus.gov/dietaryguidelines (accessed on 05 February 2023).

Wickham, R. S., Rehwaldt, M., Kefer, C., Shott, S., Abbas, K., Glynn-Tucker, E., Potter, C., & Blendowski, C., (1999). Taste changes experienced by patients receiving chemotherapy. *Oncology Nursing Forum, 26*, 697–706.

World Cancer Research Fund (WCRF) and American Institute for Cancer Research, (1997). *Food, Nutrition and the Prevention of Cancer: A Global Perspective.* Washington, DC: American Institute for Cancer Research.

Yun, T. K., & Choi, S. Y., (1990). A case-control study of ginseng intake and cancer. *Int. J. Epidemiol., 19*, 871–876.

Yun, T. K., & Choi, S. Y., (1998). Non-organ specific cancer prevention of ginseng: A prospective study in Korea. *Int. J. Epidemiol., 27*, 359–364.

Yun, T. K., Choi, S. Y., & Yun, H. Y., (2001). Epidemiological study on cancer prevention by ginseng: Are all kinds of cancers preventable by ginseng? *J. Korean Med. Sci., 16*, S19–S27.

CHAPTER 3

PHYTOCHEMICALS IN CANCER TREATMENT

K. C. SUMUKHA,[1] RAGHU RAM ACHAR,[1] SHAISTA JABEEN,[2] V. KIRUTHIGA,[3] and A. VINODHINI[3]

[1]*Division of Biochemistry, School of Life Sciences, JSS Academy of Higher Education and Research, Mysuru, Karnataka, India*

[2]*Department of Zoology, Vellore, Tamil Nadu, India*

[3]*Assistant Professor, PG & Research Department of Zoology, D.K.M. College for Women (Autonomous), Vellore–1, Tamil Nadu, India*

ABSTRACT

Cancer was discovered in Egypt in 1500 B.C. Cancer is still dominating, and it is becoming a challenge to the people of the scientific world. Several doctors and scientists are still studying oncology, its anatomy, physiology, chemistry, and the various treatments used to treat this contagious disease. Recently, plant compounds such as flavonoids, polyphenols, isothiocyanate, and triterpenoids have given hope against cancer. The present study highlights phytochemicals proven to have potential in the treatment of various cancers. Natural products, spices, and herbs like ginger (gingerol), garlic (allicin), turmeric (curcumin), black cumin (thymoquinone), *Carum carvi* (limonene), and folic acid, phenolic compounds act as inhibitors in the enzymatic system, metal chelators and scavenging free radicals involved in many chronic conditions like cancer and other inflammatory diseases. They are found in dry fruits like almonds, walnuts, pistachio, hazlenuts, and

Nutraceuticals in Cancer Prevention, Management, and Treatment. Raj K. Keservani, Bui Thanh Tung, Sippy Singh, & Rajesh K. Kesharwani, PhD (Eds.)

vineblastine and vincristine from *Catharanthus roseus*, and are used to treat renal, breast, and testicular cancers.

3.1 INTRODUCTION

Cancer is a major public health problem and the second leading cause of death worldwide. According to the Global Cancer Observatory, there are currently 19 million people around the world suffering from different types of cancer, such as breast cancer, lung cancer, colorectum cancer, prostate cancer, liver cancer, stomach cancer, and other types of cancer (Ferlay et al., 2021). Cancer-related motility rates remain high despite advances in cancer treatments and therapies (Tomeh et al., 2019). An escalatory increase in deaths is due to a person's vulnerability to a wide range of genetic and epigenetic factors that can trigger carcinogenesis. Although there is an increase in the number of therapeutic options, the efficacy of those options is time-limited and non-curative. This creates a demand for therapeutics that are more efficient, with fewer side-effects, and curative.

Natural product compounds have recently attracted significant attention for their potent effects against inflammation-driven diseases, including cancer. Herbal medicines are very safe (Rane et al., 2020a; Rane et al., 2020b), non-toxic, and easily available sources of anticancer treatments. Hence, herbal medicines are a feasible alternative to western medicine (Khan et al., 2019). According to traditional recommendations and experimental studies, numerous medicinal plants have been reported to have anticancer effects. They also have antiproliferative, pro-apoptotic, anti-metastatic, and antiangiogenic effects of several phytochemicals shown in *in vitro* experiments or animal studies (Hosseini & Ghorbani, 2015). Phytochemicals and derivatives are biologically active compounds in herbal medicines with antitumor potential (Choudhari et al., 2020). Phytochemicals exert anticancer effects by killing rapidly dividing cells, inhibiting angiogenesis of cancerous tissue, modulating cell growth factors and inducing apoptosis (Singh et al., 2016).

3.1.1 FACTORS THAT PROMOTE CARCINOGENESIS

3.1.1.1 GENETIC ALTERATIONS

Aging, mutagenic substances, radiation, ultraviolet (UV), oxygen radicals, and other factors all contribute to genetic changes (Takeshima & Ushijima, 2019).

3.1.1.2 MAJOR TYPES OF CANCERS

1. **Breast cancer** refers to cancers originating from breast tissue, most commonly from the inner lining of milk ducts or the lobules that supply the ducts with milk. Family history, alteration in hormonal levels, sedentary lifestyles, intake of high-fat levels in the diet, intake of alcoholic beverages, and exposure to low doses of radiation are some of the common causes of breast cancer (Sharma et al., 2010). High levels of estrogen receptor (ER), progesterone receptor (PR), and human epidermal growth factor receptor 2 (HER2) expression are the most important factors in promoting BC.
2. **Lung cancer** is classified into small cell lung cancer (SCLC) and non-small cell lung cancer (NSCLC). SCLC is a fast-growing cancer and spreads more quickly than NSCLC. Tobacco smoking, inhaling smoke from recreational drugs, and passive smoking are common causes of lung cancer (Dela Cruz et al., 2011). The main signaling pathways that could provide roadmaps for therapy include the following: growth promoting pathways (Epidermal Growth Factor Receptor/Ras/Phosphatidyllnositol 3-Kinase), growth inhibitory pathways (p53/Rb/$P14^{ARF}$, STK11), apoptotic pathways (Bcl-2/Bax/Fas/FasL), DNA repair and immortalization genes.
3. **Colorectal cancer** is the most common malignant cancer in the gastrointestinal tract and is the second most common cause of death related to cancer worldwide. Three molecular pathways have been identified: the chromosomal instability (CIN), the microsatellite instability (MSI), and the CpG Island Methylator Phenotype (CIMP) pathways.

3.1.2 DIFFERENT PHYTOCHEMICALS USED IN CANCER TREATMENTS

3.1.2.1 POLYPHENOLS

They have antitumor effects through a variety of mechanisms, including inducing apoptosis, inhibiting cell cycle events, and modifying cell signaling pathways (Pandey & Rizvi, 2009).

3.1.2.2 FLAVONOIDS

They are responsible for the color and flavor of fruits and vegetables. In addition to their anticancer activities, flavonoids also exert antioxidant, anti-inflammatory, and immunomodulatory properties (Kopustinskiene et al., 2020; Keservani et al., 2010a, 2016).

3.1.2.3 ISOTHIOCYANATES

They are naturally occurring small molecules found in cruciferous vegetables. They are formed from glucosinolate precursors. They affect carcinogenesis by reducing the activation of carcinogens and increasing their detoxification (Anubhuti et al., 2016).

3.1.2.4 TRITERPENOIDS

They are naturally occurring, biologically active phytochemicals found in plants, microorganisms, animals, and marine organisms. They are polymers of isoprene well known for their antitumor, anti-inflammatory, antipyretic, and analgesic effects (Bishayee et al., 2011).

3.2 TARGETING ANTICANCER PATHWAYS BY PHYTOCHEMICALS

3.2.1 ISOTHIOCYANATES TYPES: PHENOL ISOTHIOCYANATES AND BENZYL ISOTHIOCYANATES

PEITC inhibits lung cancer induction by the tobacco-specific carcinogen NNK, mainly by blocking its metabolic activation to intermediates that cause permanent mutations in DNA. Decreased metabolic activation of NNK results in increased urinary excretion of two metabolites: NNAL and NNAL-Gluc. The latter is believed to be a detoxification product of NNK. One good dietary source of PEITC is watercress. In smokers who consumed watercress, levels of NNAL and NNAL-Gluc increased in urine during the watercress consumption period, indicating that inhibition of NNK metabolic activation is occurring in smokers, as observed in rodents. While PEITC may be an effective chemopreventive agent against NNK, it does not inhibit tumorigenesis by BaP, another important tobacco smoke lung carcinogen.

TABLE 3.1 Bioactive Components of Spices and Herbs

Name	Mol wt. (g/mol)	Chemical name	Source	Mechanism	References
10-gingerol	350.5	(5S)-5-hydroxy-1-(4-hydroxy-3-methoxyphenyl)tetradecan-3-one	Ginger	Reduces cell division and induces S phase cell cycle arrest and apoptosis	(Mao et al., 2019)
2' hydroxyflavanone	240.25	2-(2-hydroxyphenyl)-2,3-dihydrochromen-4-one	Diet-derived citrus bioflavonoid	Inhibits the growth of renal cell carcinoma in a VHL-dependent manner	(Awasthi et al., 2018)
Ajoene	234.4	(E)-1-(prop-2-enyldisulfanyl)-3-prop-2-enylsulfinylprop-1-ene	Garlic	Triggers cell apoptosis by activating mitochondria-dependent caspase cascade	(Dirsch et al., 2002)
Allicin	162.3	3-prop-2-enylsulfinylsulfanylprop-1-ene	Garlic	Inhibits the growth of cancer cells, arresting cell cycle at G2/M phase, endoplasmic reticulum (ER) stress, and mitochondria-mediated apoptosis	(Luo et al., 2016)
Allyl isothiocyanate	99.16	3-isothiocyanatoprop-1-ene	Produced by the hydrolysis of sinigrin found in mustard, horseradish and wasabi	Inhibits of cell proliferation, arrests cell cycle, and induces apoptosis	(Zhang, 2010)
Andrographolide	350.4	(3E,4S)-3-[2-[(1R,4aS,5R,6R,8aS)-6-hydroxy-5-(hydroxymethyl)-5,8a-dimethyl-2-methylidene-3,4,4a,6,7,8-hexahydro-1H-naphthalen-1-yl] ethylidene]-4-hydroxyoxolan-2-one	*Andrographis paniculata*	Activates the extrinsic death receptor pathway and induces apoptotic cell death, Induces of Cell-Cycle Arrest	(Varma et al., 2011)
Apigenin	270.24	5,7-dihydroxy-2-(4-hydroxyphenyl) chromen-4-one	Parsley, chamomile, celery, vine-spinach, artichokes, oregano	Regulate p53-Bax-caspase-3 apoptotic pathway, which serves as a treatment for neuroblastoma treatment	(Salehi et al., 2019)

TABLE 3.1 *(Continued)*

Name	Mol wt. (g/mol)	Chemical name	Source	Mechanism	References
Baicalein	270.24	5,6,7-trihydroxy-2-phenylchromen-4-one	Roots of *Scutellariabaicalensis* and *Scutellarialateriflora*	Induces apoptosis, inhibits cancer cell invasion	(Liu et al., 2016)
Benzyl isothiocyanate	149.21	Isothiocyanatomethylbenzene	Garden cress, papaya	Arrests cell cycle as well as disrupts mitochondrial membrane potential to initiate mitochondrial pathway of apoptosis	(Gupta et al., 2014)
Camptothecin	348.4	(19S)-19-ethyl-19-hydroxy-17-oxa-3,13-diazapentacyclo[11.8.0.02,11.04,9.015,20]henicosa-1(21),2,4,6,8,10,15(20)-heptaene-14,18-dione	*Camptotheca acuminata*	Inhibits the action of topoisomerase I and prevents religation of the DNA strand	(*Wishart DS, Knox C, Guo AC, Shrivastava S, Hassanali M, Stothard P, Chang Z, Woolsey J. Drugbank: A Comprehensive Resource for in Silico Drug Discovery and Exploration. Nucleic Acids Res. 2006 Jan 1;34 (Database Issue):D668–72. 16381955.*, n.d.)

TABLE 3.1 *(Continued)*

Name	Mol wt. (g/mol)	Chemical name	Source	Mechanism	References
Chlorogenic acid	354.31	(1S,3R,4R,5R)-3-[(E)-3-(3,4-dihydroxyphenyl)prop-2-enoyl]oxy-1,4,5-trihydroxycyclohexane-1-carboxylic acid	Apples, burdock, carrots, coffee beans, eggplants, grapes, honeysuckle, kiwi fruit	Induces cell differentiation in cancer cells	(Huang et al., 2019)
Chrysin	254.24	5,7-dihydroxy-2-phenylchromen-4-one	Honey, propolis, the passion flowers, *Passiflora caerulea*, and *Passiflora incarnata*	Inhibits proliferation and induces apoptosis in cancer cells and acts via caspase activation and inactivation of the Akt signaling	(Khoo et al., 2010)
Curcumin	368.4	(1E,6E)-1,7-bis(4-hydroxy-3-methoxyphenyl)hepta-1,6-diene-3,5-dione	*Curcuma longa*	Induces apoptosis and inhibits proliferation and invasion of tumors by suppressing a variety of cellular signaling pathways	(Tomeh et al., 2019)
Cyanidin 3-glucoside	484.8	2-[2-(3,4-dihydroxyphenyl)-5,7-dihydroxychromenylium-3-yl]oxy-6-(hydroxymethyl)oxane-3,4,5-triol;chloride	Black soybean, common bean, cowpea, and lentils	Induces apoptosis in breast cancer cells	(Cho et al., 2017)
Daidzein	254.24	7-hydroxy-3-(4-hydroxyphenyl)chromen-4-one	Tofu, soymilk, soy flour, textured soy protein isolates, tempeh, and miso	Inhibits TNF-α induced cellular migration and invasion by downregulating hedgehog–Gli1 signaling	(Ramasamy et al., 2017)
Delphinidin	338.69	2-(3,4,5-trihydroxyphenyl)chromenylium-3,5,7-triol;chloride	Berries, red grapes, purple sweet potatoes, red cabbages, and other pigmented foods, plants and vegetables	Induces apoptosis via activation of caspases, causes G2-M phase cell cycle arrest	(Hafeez et al., 2008)

TABLE 3.1 *(Continued)*

Name	Mol wt. (g/mol)	Chemical name	Source	Mechanism	References
Diallyl trisulfide	178.3	3-(prop-2-enyltrisulfanyl)prop-1-ene	Garlic and onion	Activates metabolizing enzymes that detoxify carcinogens, suppresses the formation of DNA adducts, regulation of cell-cycle arrest, induces of apoptosis and differentiation, histone modification, and inhibits angiogenesis and invasion	(Yi & Su, 2013)
Dicumarol	336.3	4-hydroxy-3-[(4-hydroxy-2-oxochromen-3-yl)methyl]chromen-2-one	Molding sweet-clover hay	Inhibits PDK1, cell viability and induces cell apoptosis	(W. Zhang et al., 2017)
Diindolylmethane	246.31	3-(1H-indol-3-ylmethyl)-1H-indole	Cabbage, Brussels sprouts, cauliflower, and broccoli	Triggers cellular endoplasmic reticulum (ER) stress and apoptosis within cancer cells	(Kim, 2016)
EGCG	458.4 g/mol	[(2R,3R)-5,7-dihydroxy-2-(3,4,5-trihydroxyphenyl)-3,4-dihydro-2H-chromen-3-yl] 3,4,5-trihydroxybenzoate	Green tea, cranberries, strawberries, blackberries, kiwis, cherries, pears, peaches, apples, and avocados	Inhibits carcinogen activity, tumorigenesis, proliferation, and angiogenesis, and induces cell death	(Min & Kwon, 2014)
Ellagic acid	302.19	6,7,13,14-tetrahydroxy-2,9-dioxatetracyclo[6.6.2.04,16.011,15]hexadeca-1(15),4,6,8(16),11,13-hexaene-3,10-dione	Strawberries, raspberries, blackberries, cherries, and walnuts	Inhibits the angiogenesis, migration, and invasion of cancer cells preventing cancer metastasis	(H.-M. Zhang et al., 2014)
Ferulic acid	194.18	(E)-3-(4-hydroxy-3-methoxyphenyl)prop-2-enoic acid	Bamboo, Whole-Grain Rye Bread, Whole-Grain Oat Flakes, Sweet Corn	Inhibits cell proliferation and cell metastasis	(X. Zhang et al., 2016)

TABLE 3.1 *(Continued)*

Name	Mol wt. (g/mol)	Chemical name	Source	Mechanism	References
Fisetin	286.24	2-(3,4-dihydroxyphenyl)-3,7-dihydroxychromen-4-one	Fruits and vegetables such as strawberry, apple, persimmon, grape, onion, and cucumber	Inhibit the proliferation of various cancer cell lines	(Jia et al., 2019)
Galangin	270.24	3,5,7-trihydroxy-2-phenylchromen-4-one	Honey and *Alpinia officinarum*	Anti-proliferation, induction of apoptosis and autophagy, inhibition of metastasis	(Fang et al., 2019)
Gallic acid	170.12	3,4,5-trihydroxybenzoic acid	Blueberry, blackberry, strawberry, plums, grapes, mango, cashew nut, hazelnut, walnut, tea, wine	Induce apoptosis of cancer cells via the mitochondria-mediated pathways	(Nowak et al., 2014)
Genistein	270.24 g/mo	5,7-dihydroxy-3-(4-hydroxyphenyl)chromen-4-one	Soy-based foods, such as soy cheese, soy milk	ER stress through upregulation of glucose-regulated protein 78 (GRP78) expression which finally induces apoptosis	(Tuli et al., 2019)
Hesperidin	610.6	(2S)-5-hydroxy-2-(3-hydroxy-4-methoxyphenyl)-7-[(2S,3R,4S,5S,6R)-3,4,5-trihydroxy-6-[[(2R,3R,4R,5R,6S)-3,4,5-trihydroxy-6-methyloxan-2-yl]oxymethyl]oxan-2-yl]oxy-2,3-dihydrochromen-4-one	Citrus fruits, including lemon, orange, lime, grapefruit	Inhibits cancer cell proliferation by inducing apoptosis and cell cycle arrest	(Aggarwal et al., 2020)
Irinotecan	586.7	[(19S)-10,19-diethyl-19-hydroxy-14,18-dioxo-17-oxa-3,13-diazapentacyclo[11.8.0.02,11.04,9.015,20]henicosa-1(21),2,4(9),5,7,10,15(20)-heptaen-7-yl] 4-piperidin-1-ylpiperidine-1-carboxylate	*Camptotheca acuminata*	Inhibits the action of topoisomerase I	(Wishart et al., 2006)

TABLE 3.1 *(Continued)*

Name	Mol wt. (g/mol)	Chemical name	Source	Mechanism	References
Isorhamnetin	478.4	5,7-dihydroxy-2-(4-hydroxy-3-methoxyphenyl)-3-[(2S,3R,4S,5S,6R)-3,4,5-trihydroxy-6-(hydroxymethyl)oxan-2-yl]oxychromen-4-one	Pears, olive oil, wine, tomato sauce	Inhibits cell proliferation and induces apoptosis via Akt and mitogen-activated protein kinase signaling pathways	(Hu et al., 2015)
Kaempferol	286.24	3,5,7-trihydroxy-2-(4-hydroxyphenyl)chromen-4-one	Green leafy vegetables, dill, chives, and tarragon	Apoptosis, cell cycle arrest at the G2/M phase, downregulation of epithelial-mesenchymal transition (EMT)-related markers, and phosphoinositide 3-kinase/protein kinase B signaling pathways	(Imran et al., 2019)
Limonene	136.23	1-methyl-4-prop-1-en-2-ylcyclohexene	Lemons, limes, and oranges	Induces apoptosis by up-regulating pro-apoptotic factors and down-regulating anti-apoptotic factors	(Mukhtar et al., 2018)
Lovastatin	404.5	[(1S,3R,7S,8S,8aR)-8-[2-[(2R,4R)-4-hydroxy-6-oxooxan-2-yl]ethyl]-3,7-dimethyl-1,2,3,7,8,8a-hexahydronaphthalen-1-yl](2S)-2-methylbutanoate	Oyster mushrooms, red yeast rice, and Pu-erh	Regulate the proliferation, apoptosis, and drug resistance in different types of cancer cells	(Xie et al., 2021)
Luteolin	286.24	2-(3,4-dihydroxyphenyl)-5,7-dihydroxychromen-4-one	Celery, parsley, broccoli, onion leaves, carrots, peppers, cabbages, apple skins, and chrysanthemum flowers	Acts as a novel HGF/c-Met inhibitor by suppressing phosphorylation of c-Met tyrosine kinase	(Tuorkey, 2016)

TABLE 3.1 *(Continued)*

Name	Mol wt. (g/mol)	Chemical name	Source	Mechanism	References
Lycopene	536.9	(6E,8E,10E,12E,14E,16E,18E,20E,22E,24E,26E)-2,6,10,14,19,23,27,31-octamethyldotriaconta-2,6,8,10,12,14,16,18,20,22,24,26,30-tridecaene	Watermelon, pink grapefruit, pink guava, papaya, tomatoes, and tomato products	Interferes with growth factor receptor signaling and cell cycle progression specifically in prostate cancer cells	(Heber & Lu, 2002)
Malvidin	528.9	(2S,3R,4S,5R,6R)-2-[5,7-dihydroxy-2-(4-hydroxy-3,5-dimethoxyphenyl)chromenylium-3-yl]oxy-6-(hydroxymethyl)oxane-3,4,5-triol;chloride	American cranberry, bilberry, blueberry	Suppresses the growth and metastasis potential of hepatocellular carcinoma cell	(Lin et al., 2020)
Myricetin	318.23	3,5,7-trihydroxy-2-(3,4,5-trihydroxyphenyl)chromen-4-one	Cranberry Sweet potato leaves, Chard, Swiss, Broadbeans, immature seeds, Rutabagas	Suppresses cancer cell invasion and metastasis, induces cell cycle arrest and apoptosis, and inhibit cell proliferation	(Jiang et al., 2019)
Nimbolide	466.5	methyl 2-[(1R,2S,4R,6R,9R,10S,11R,15R,18R)-6-(furan-3-yl)-7,9,11,15-tetramethyl-12,16-dioxo-3,17-dioxapentac yclo[9.6.1.02,9.04,8.015,18]octadeca-7,13-dien-10-yl]acetate	Leaves of the neem tree	Disturbs the cell cycle of cancer cells	(Wang et al., 2016)
Paclitaxel	853.9	[(1S,2S,3R,4S,7R,9S,10S,12R,15S)-4,12-diacetyloxy-15-[(2R,3S)-3-benzamido-2-hydroxy-3-phenylpropanoyl]oxy-1,9-dihydroxy-10,14,17,17-tetramethyl-11-oxo-6-oxatetracyclo[11.3.1.03,10.04,7]heptadec-13-en-2-yl] benzoate	Bark of the Pacific yew tree (*Taxus brevifolia*)	In vitro, it enhances the polymerization of tubulin to stable microtubules and also interacts directly with microtubules	(Horwitz, 1994)

TABLE 3.1 *(Continued)*

Name	Mol wt. (g/mol)	Chemical name	Source	Mechanism	References
Pelargonidin	271.24	2-(4-hydroxyphenyl) chromenylium-3,5,7-triol	Blueberries, blackberries, cranberries, ripe raspberries, and strawberries	Inhibits the expression of MMP-2 and MMP-9 by inhibiting the PI3K/Akt pathway in cancer cells	(Lin et al., 2017)
Peonidin	301.27	2-(4-hydroxy-3-methoxyphenyl) chromenylium-3,5,7-triol	SWEET potato, *Eugenia jambolana*	Induces cell-cycle arrest, antiproliferative, pro-apoptotic	(Lin et al., 2017)
Perillyl alcohol	152.23	(4-prop-1-en-2-ylcyclohexen-1-yl) methanol	Lavender, peppermint, cherries, sage, and lemongrass	Induces cell differentiation and cell apoptosis in cancer cells	(Belanger, 1998)
Petunidin	317.27	2-(3,4-dihydroxy-5-methoxyphenyl) chromenylium-3,5,7-triol	Jamun, Blackberry, Blueberry, Black soybean	Antiproliferative, controls metastasis	(Lin et al., 2017)
Phenyl isothiocyanate	135.19	Isothiocyanatobenzene	Bok choy, broccoli, cabbage, cauliflower, kale, and others, are rich sources of glucosinolate precursors of isothiocyanates	Depression of activation of carcinogens, Acceleration of carcinogen disposal	(Wu et al., 2009)
Piceatannol	244.24	4-[(E)-2-(3,5-dihydroxyphenyl)ethenyl] benzene-1,2-diol	Red wine, grapes, passion fruit, white tea, and Japanese knotweed	Induce apoptosis and suppress cell cycle progression	(Hu et al., 2020)

TABLE 3.1 *(Continued)*

Name	Mol wt. (g/mol)	Chemical name	Source	Mechanism	References
Procyanidins	594.5	2-(3,4-dihydroxyphenyl)-2-[[2-(3,4-dihydroxyphenyl)-5,7-dihydroxy-3,4-dihydro-2H-chromen-3-yl]oxy]-3,4-dihydrochromene-3,4,5,7-tetrol	Cranberry, blackcurrant, elderberry, and aronia	Inhibit the proliferation of various cancer cells	(Lee, 2017)
Pterostilbene	256.3	4-[(E)-2-(3,5-dimethoxyphenyl)ethenyl]phenol	Almonds, grape leaves, and vines, *Pterocarpus marsupium* heartwood	Inhibit cancer cell viability, induce cell cycle arrest, alter apoptosis expression gene, promote autophagy-related proteins, and inhibit cancer cells from metastasizing	(Tsai et al., 2017)
Quercetin	302.23	2-(3,4-dihydroxyphenyl)-3,5,7-trihydroxychromen-4-one	Apples, honey, raspberries, onions, red grapes, cherries, citrus fruits, green leafy vegetables	Inhibits tyrosine kinases leading to inhibition of the growth of tumor cells	(Shafabakhsh & Asemi, 2019)
Resveratrol	228.24	5-[(E)-2-(4-hydroxyphenyl)ethenyl]benzene-1,3-diol	Peanuts, pistachios, grapes, red and white wine, blueberries, cranberries, and even cocoa and dark chocolate	Affects diverse signal-transduction pathways that control cell growth and division, inflammation, apoptosis, metastasis, and angiogenesis	(Ko et al., 2017)
Rosmarinic acid	360.3	(2R)-3-(3,4-dihydroxyphenyl)-2-[(E)-3-(3,4-dihydroxyphenyl)prop-2-enoyl]oxypropanoic acid	Rosemary, sage, Spanish sage, basil, oregano, marjoram	Inhibits several important steps of angiogenesis, including proliferation, migration, adhesion	(Huang & Zheng, 2006)

TABLE 3.1 *(Continued)*

Name	Mol wt. (g/mol)	Chemical name	Source	Mechanism	References
S-allylcysteine	161.22	(2R)-2-amino-3-prop-2-enylsulfanylpropanoic acid	Garlic	Suppresses cell proliferation, alters cell cycle in cancer cells	(Ho et al., 2018)
S-allylmercaptocystein	193.3	(2R)-2-amino-3-(prop-2-enyldisulfanyl)propanoic acid	Soft-necked garlic	Promotes cell apoptosis	(Zhang et al., 2014)
Secoisolariciresinoldiglucoside	686.7	(2R,3R,4S,5S,6R)-2-[(2R,3R)-2,3-bis[(4-hydroxy-3-methoxyphenyl)methyl]-4-[(2R,3R,4S,5S,6R)-3,4,5-trihydroxy-6-(hydroxymethyl)oxan-2-yl]oxybutoxy]-6-(hydroxymethyl)oxane-3,4,5-triol	Flax, sunflower, sesame, and pumpkin seeds	Prevents malignancies, has antiproliferative and antiangiogenic properties	(Kezimana et al., 2018)
Sesamin	354.4	5-[(3S,3aR,6S,6aR)-3-(1,3-benzodioxol-5-yl)-1,3,3a,4,6,6a-hexahydrofuro[3,4-c]furan-6-yl]-1,3-benzodioxole	Bark of Fagara plants, sesame oil	It has antiproliferative, pro-apoptotic, anti-inflammatory, anti-metastatic, anti- and pro-angiogenic, and pro-autophagocytic activities	(Majdalawieh et al., 2017)
Sulforaphane	177.3	1-isothiocyanato-4-methylsulfinylbutane	Broccoli, kale, cabbage, and watercress	Blocks of phase I metabolic enzymes, and arrests cell cycle in the G2/M and G1 phase to inhibit cell proliferation	(Kamal et al., 2020)
Thymol	150.22	5-methyl-2-propan-2-ylphenol	Extracted from *Thymus vulgaris, ajwain*	Induces apoptosis, anti-proliferation, inhibits angiogenesis and migration	(Nagoor Meeran et al., 2017)
Thymoquinone	164.2	2-methyl-5-propan-2-ylcyclohexa-2,5-diene-1,4-dione	Seeds of *Nigella sativa L.*	Induces apoptosis in cancer cells via generating reactive oxygen species (ROS), DNA damage, telomeric attrition and inhibits cancer metastasis	(Asaduzzaman Khan et al., 2017)

TABLE 3.1 *(Continued)*

Name	Mol wt. (g/mol)	Chemical name	Source	Mechanism	References
Topotecan	421.4	(19S)-8-[(dimethylamino)methyl]-19-ethyl-7,19-dihydroxy-17-oxa-3,13-diazapentacyclo[11.8.0.02,11.04,9.015,20]henicosa-1(21),2,4(9),5,7,10,15(20)-heptaene-14,18-dione	*Camptotheca acuminata*	Exert its cytotoxic effects during the S-phase of DNA synthesis	(Wishart et al., 2006)
Triterpenoids	552.8	(4aS,6aR,6aS,6bR,8aR,9R,10S,12aR,14bS)-10-hydroxy-2,2,6a,6b,9,12a-hexamethyl-9-(sulfooxymethyl)-1,3,4,5,6,6a,7,8,8a,10,11,12,13,14b-tetradecahydropicene-4a-carboxylic acid	Beans, soybeans, spinach, lentils, and oats	Activate or deactivate nuclear receptors and G-protein coupled receptors which contribute to their antitumorigenic activity	(Safe et al., 2012)
Ursolic acid	456.7	(1S,2R,4aS,6aR,6aS,6bR,8aR,10S,12aR,14bS)-10-hydroxy-1,2,6a,6b,9,9,12a-heptamethyl-2,3,4,5,6,6a,7,8,8a,10,11,12,13,14b-tetradecahydro-1H-picene-4a-carboxylic acid	Leaves of rosemary, marjoram, lavender, thyme, organum	Induces apoptosis, inhibits cell proliferation, prevents tumor angiogenesis and metastatic	(Zou et al., 2019)
Withaferin-A	470.6	(1S,2R,6S,7R,9R,11S,12S,15R,16S)-6-hydroxy-15-[(1S)-1-[(2R)-5-(hydroxymethyl)-4-methyl-6-oxo-2,3-dihydropyran-2-yl]ethyl]-2,16-dimethyl-8-oxapentacyclo[9.7.0.02,7.07,9.012,16]octadec-4-en-3-one	Ashwagandha	Induces apoptosis through activation of p53 family members	(Lee & Choi, 2016)

TABLE 3.1 *(Continued)*

Name	Mol wt. (g/mol)	Chemical name	Source	Mechanism	References
Wogonin	284.26	5,7-dihydroxy-8-methoxy-2-phenylchromen-4-one	*Scutellaria radix, Scutellariabaicalensis*	Modulates various cell signaling pathways, including serine-threonine kinase Akt (also known as protein kinase B) and AMP-activated protein kinase (AMPK) pathways, p53-dependent/independent apoptosis, and inhibition of telomerase activity	(Huynh et al., 2017)

BITC inhibits lung tumorigenesis induced by BaP in mice. It is likely that combinations of agents, including blocking agents such as PEITC and BITC, as well as suppressing agents, will be necessary for the chemoprevention of lung cancer in smokers.

3.2.1.1 POLYPHENOLS

Polyphenols show anticancer effects through different signaling pathways, including the tumor suppressor gene tumor protein 53 (p53). Various types of cancers are caused by the silencing of endogenous p53. Polyphenols from dietary sources (Rane and Keservani, 2020; Keservani et al., 2020; Keservani et al., 2015) could upregulate expression of p53 through various mechanisms. Polyphenols stabilize p53 protein through p53 phosphorylation, p53 acetylation, and reduction of oxidative stress (Khan et al., 2020). Tyrosine kinase and other protein kinases are enzymes involved in cell proliferation. Plant phenolics could be useful dietary inhibitors of these kinases by reducing hyperproliferation of epithelial cells, thus lowering cancer risk. For example, quercetin is an inhibitor of protein kinase C, tyrosine-protein kinase, and a specific protein kinase in rat colonic epithelium (Keservani et al., 2010b).

3.2.1.2 ANTHOCYANIDINES

Anthocyanidins inhibit cell proliferation by blocking various stages of cell cycles through cell regulator proteins (e.g., p53, p27, cyclin D1). Anthocyanidins have the ability to induce phase II antioxidants and detoxifying enzymes. Anthocyanidins have pro-apoptotic properties that include increasing mitochondrial membrane potential, cytochrome c release and modulating caspase dependent pro-apoptoic proteins, which they perform intrinsically, wherein extrinsically, anthocyanidins modulate expression of FAS and FASL, resulting in apoptosis (Wang & Stoner, 2008).

3.3 ACTIVE COMPOUNDS: ROLES IN INHIBITION AND SUPPRESSION OF TUMOR CELLS

Culinary herbs and spices and nuts are packed with therapeutic phytochemicals that are being used in traditional medicines such as Ayurveda (Indian Traditional Medicine System), Chinese traditional medicines, and Unani

(Persian Traditional Medicine System). These three systems are considered to be the most primitive based on their evidence-documented and scriptures. Some of the most common spices used in cuisines are black cumin seeds (Nigella sativa), cumin seeds (cuminum cyminum), carum carvi seeds, saffron, ginger, etc. Some of the spices and their major chemical compounds, molecular structures, and therapeutic potentials are given in Table 3.2.

TABLE 3.2 Spices and Herbs Major Chemical Compounds and Therapeutics

S. No.	Medicinal plants/ Common Names	Bioactive Compounds	Molecular Structure	Therapeutic properties
1.	*Nigella Sativa* / Black cumin seeds	Thymoquinone	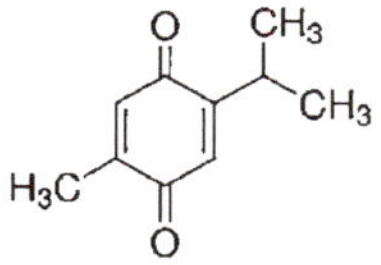	Antitumor, anticancer, cytotoxic, anti-inflammatory, antidiabetic, hypoglycemic etc.
2	*Ciminum cyminum*/Cumin seeds	Cuminaldehyde	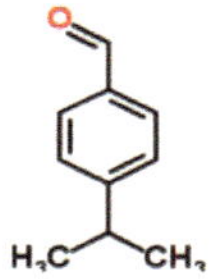	Antitumor activity, antidiabetic, inhibitor of squamous carcoma and hepatomas
3.	*Moringa peregrine*/Parsley	Apigenin	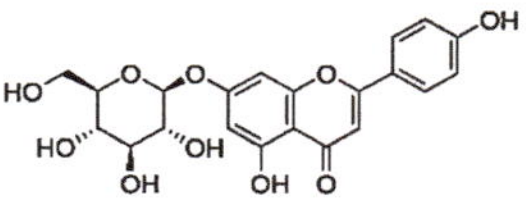	Cytotoxic activity, breast & colon cancer cell line
4	Carum carvi/ Caraway seeds	Carvone	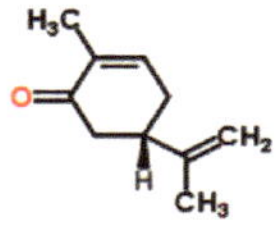	Antitumor/anti-mutagenic, anticolitis, hepatoprotective, inhibition and suppression of colon & rectal tumor cells
5.	*Curcuma longa* L/ Turmeric	Curcumin	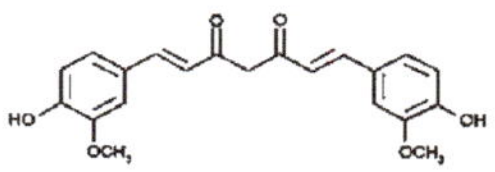	Antitumor activities colon, breast, lung and brain tumors induce apoptosis in tumor cells
6	*Saffron crocus*/ *Saffron*	Crocetin	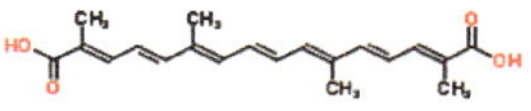	Pancreatic, skin carcinoma, colorectal breast and lung carcinoma (Bathaie and Mousavi, 2007)
7	*Zingiber Officinale*/Ginger	Gingerol	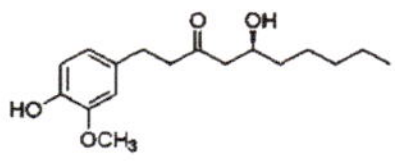	Anti-emetic, antitumor activity (skin carcinoma)

TABLE 3.2 *(Continued)*

S. No.	Medicinal plants/ Common Names	Bioactive Compounds	Molecular Structure	Therapeutic properties
8	Broccoli, tea, W-itch-hazel	Kaempferol	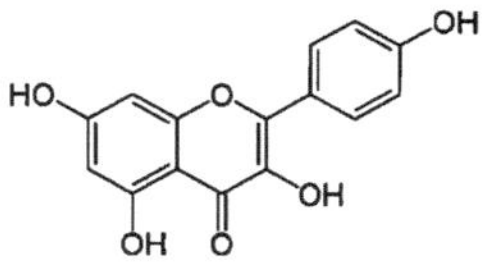	Chemoprevent agent, antioxidant prevent arteriosclerosis (Jan Kowalski et al., 2005)
9	Various berries, grapes	Cyanidins	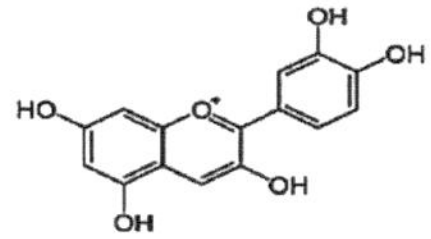	Antioxidant, inhibit breast metastasis
10	Bioflavonoid-Flavonols/tea, apple, fruits, vegetables, beverages	Quercetin	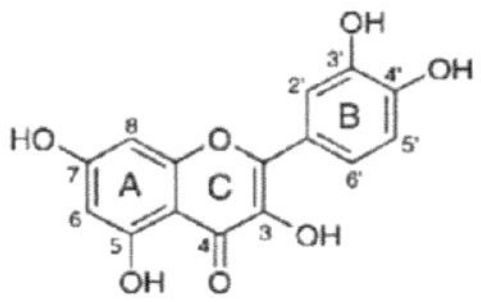	Antioxidant, anti-inflammatory activity
11	*Carum carvi* L seeds	Carvone, limonene	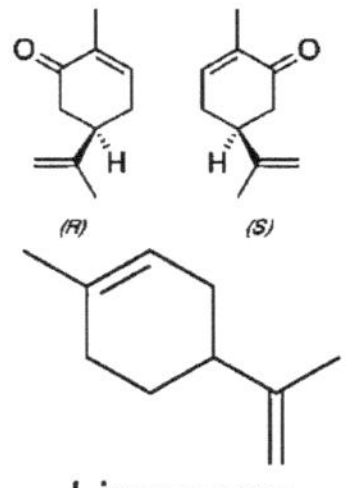 Limonene	Antidiabetic, antifertility, antioxidant, antispasmodic antihemolytic, bowel motility, gastric action, hypoglycemic, hypolipidemic, hypothyroidism, bepgro-protective
12	Strawberries, Apples *Acacia greggii*, *Acacia berlandieri*	Fisetin	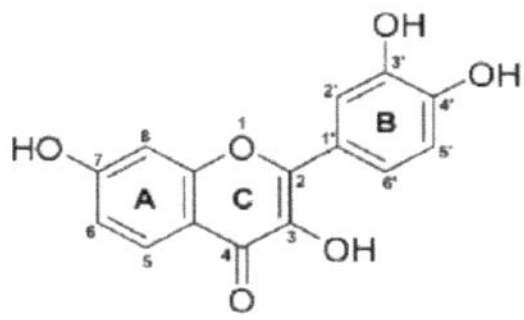	Antihyperalgesic, nephrotoxicity, antioxidant, anti-inflammatory, anticancer activity, hypolipidemic
13	*Flemingiavestita, Soybean, Kudzu, Psoralea*	Genistein	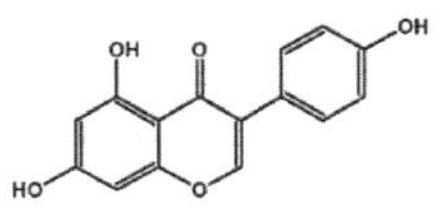	Anticancer activity, antihelminthic, antiangiogenic
14	Tomatoes, red-carrots, watermelons	Lycopene	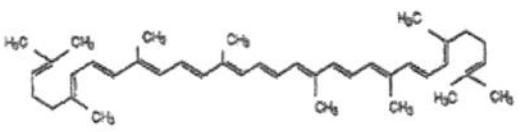	Anticancer activity (prostate cancer)
15	Red grapes skin, Peanuts (Jang et al.)	Resveratrol	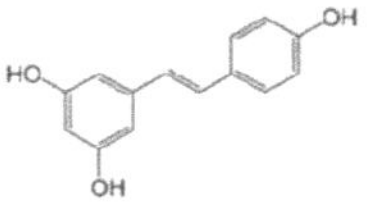	Cancer chemopreventive activity, anti-initiation activity

3.4 MEDICINAL PLANTS AND THEIR ACTIVE COMPOUNDS ACT AS ANTITUMOR ACTIVITY

3.4.1 *NIGELLA SATIVA* SEEDS (BLACK CUMIN)

Nigella sativa seeds, commonly called Hebbatul Baraka in the Middle East, Black cumin in English and Kalonji in India and Pakistan originated from Turkey, the Mediterranean, the Middle East, Pakistan, and India. This plant has been a great focus for research for many centuries. "Hold on to the use of the black seeds for it is healing for all diseases except death," as narrated in the following hadith (Sahih Bukhari vol. 7 book 71 # 592).

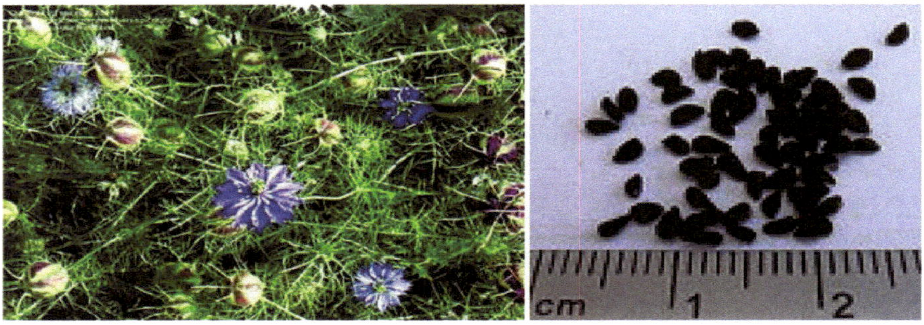

FIGURE 3.1 *Nigella sativa* (black cumin plant and seeds).

3.4.1.1 ANTICANCER ACTIVITY OF NIGELLA.SATIVA SEEDS

The major constituent of Nigella sativa seeds and oil contains many chemical compounds, but the seeds and oil exhibited antitumor activity due to their major active constituent, thymoquinone. Thymoqinone exerts anti-prolifertive, antiangiogenic, anti-metastatic and antioxidant effects on various tumor cells. The compound thymoquinone seems to mediate its anticancer effects by targeting a number of cellular pathways involving p53, NF-kB, PPARg, STAT3, MAPK, and PI3K/AKT transducing signals. Moreover, thymol, thymohydroquinone, dithymoquinone, nigellimine-N-oxide, nigellicine, nigellidine, and carvacrol are phytoconstituents of N. sativa that have been demonstrated to have anticancer and cytotoxic functions. Despite the antitumor activity of Nigella sativa seeds and its oil, which are attributed to many other antioxidant and hepatoprotective Nephroprotective, immunomodulator, bronchodilatory, antibacterial, antifungal, neuroprotective, cardioprotective, etc. Thus, thymoquinone is also compared with many antibiotics like paclitaxol, ampicillin, ciproflaxcin, taxol, etc. Hence, intense study is required by isolating the compound thymoquinone. In the future, it may lead to novel drug discovery and certainly it will become an elixir for those who are affected by this deadly disease.

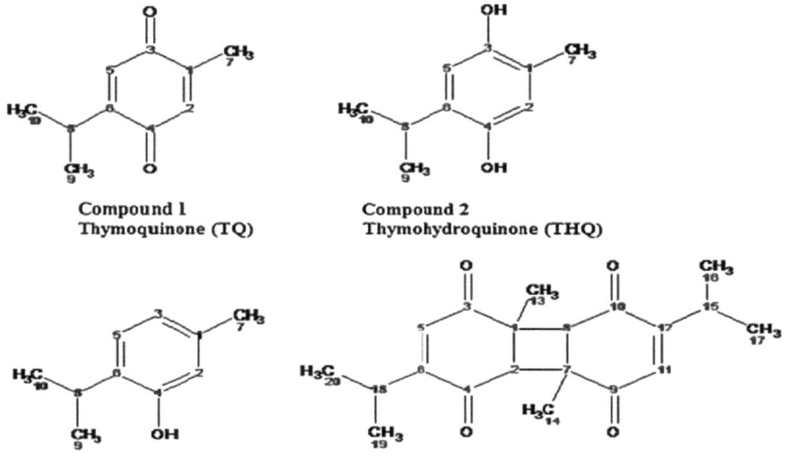

Compound 1
Thymoquinone (TQ)

Compound 2
Thymohydroquinone (THQ)

Compound 3
Thymol (THY)

Compound 4
Dithymoquinone (DTQ)

FIGURE 3.2 Chemical compounds molecular structure of *Nigella sativa.*

3.4.2 CUMINUM CYMINUM SEEDS (ZEERA)

Cumin seeds (family Apiaceae) are a popular culinary spice, and there is no kitchen without these seeds almost all over the world. Besides, cumin seeds are used in folklore medicines because of the presence of therapeutic compounds. Cumin seed is used in many ethano-medicinal systems such as gynecological, gastrointestinal, respiratory disorders, etc. The other pharmacological activities of cumin have been used as anti-inflammatory, diuretic, carminative, and antispasmodic treatments for toothaches and epilepsy, and also as an aid for treating dyspepsia, jaundice, diarrhea, flatulence, and indigestion.

3.4.2.1 ANTITUMOR ACTIVITY OF CUMINUM CYMINUM

Cumin seeds dietary supplements prevent colorectal carcenoma. It decreases the β-glucoronidase and mucinase enzyme activity. The major constituent of cumin seeds the cuminaldehyde attributes to the cytotoxic activity. Such natural aldehyde possess the therapeutic properties. The aroma of cumin is due to the presence of cuminaldehyde. Cumin seeds inhibit 79% HeLa cells it is proved to be chemopreventive potentials.

3.4.2.2 CUMINALDEHYDE: A POTENTIAL DRUG ELEMENT

As per the report of Rihawy et al. (2014) cuminaldehyde is a major component of the EO of cuminum cyminum, an oxidized aldehyde monoterpene found in green cumin seeds (Cuminum cyminum Linn, Family Apiaceae) cultivated in Egypt and the most commonly used spice. According to Nostro et al. (2005) the pharmacological activity of cuminaldehyde (cuminum cyminum) is used to treat diarrhea, jaundice, dyspepsia, and abdominal colic. It also possesses antibacterial, antifungal, and anti-convulsant effects.

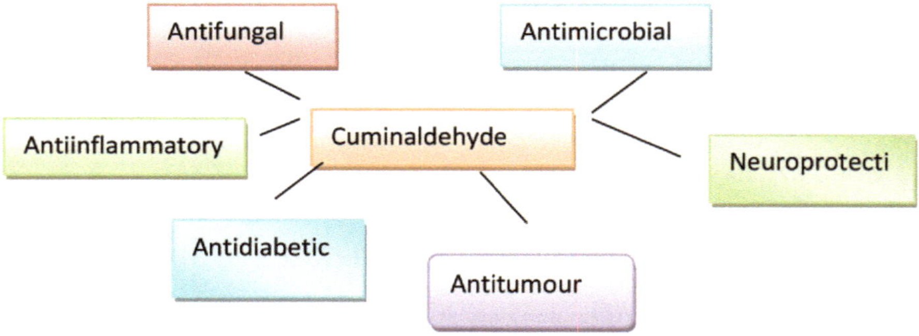

FIGURE 3.3 Anticancer activity of cuminaldehyde.

3.4.2.3 ANTICANCER EFFECTS OF CUMINALDEHYDE

Recent studies shed light on the cytotoxic activity of cuminaldehyde. As per the reports of Nitoda *et al.* (2008), antineoplastic activity of cumin aldehyde was detected by the inhibitory effect on melanin synthesis by a mouse melanoma cell line at a low concentration. Previously, Tsai et al. (2016) reported that cumin aldehyde triggered pro-apoptotic proteins such as caspase 3 and 9, altered the integrity of mitochondria, and inhibited malignancy. Human colorectal adenocarcinoma cells showed increased activity of DNA integrity-conserving enzymes, including topoisomerase I and II, thereby enhancing apoptosis and growth inhibition. Such anticancer effects of cumin aldehyde were validated in a mouse model of colorectal cancer, demonstrating reduced tumor size elicited by cumin aldehyde-enhanced apoptosis.

3.4.3 APIGENIN FROM PARSLEY

Apigenin is a family of flavonoids and is available in leafy vegetables such as parsley, celery, and many plants. It acts as a chemopreventive agent in the process of cancerous treatment, and it is also used to treat hypopigmentation disorders. It has cytotoxic activities and has the potential to inhibit breast cell carcinoma and colon carcinoma cells.

3.4.4 CARVONE FROM CARUM CARVI SEEDS

The culinary spice *Carum carvi* seeds was evaluated for anticancer activity. Carvone and D-limonene were also found to have high fumigant toxicity. The Carum carvi seeds' histopathological studies of colon tissues showed a tremendous inhibition (70–90%) inhibition. Apoptotic activities were observed in *Carum carvi* seeds. Caraway oil contains (50–60%) of carvone specific to Tunisian *Carum carvi* seeds, which exhibit chemopreventive effects. Carvone is responsible for its aroma and flavor and shows antimicrobial activity.

3.4.5 CURCUMIN FROM TURMERIC

Curcumin is a major chemical constituent of *Curcuma longa L. (turmeric)* and other Indian spices. No dish is complete without the use of turmeric. Turmeric possesses a wide range of medicinal properties and it has great apoptotic activity. Curcumin modulates the growth of cancer cells by regulating multiple cell signaling pathways. It does not inhibit the tumor cells but suppresses the target cells without damaging the normal cells. Curcumin is non-toxic to humans and has numerous antioxidant, anti-inflammatory, and cytotoxic activities in addition to antitumor activity.

3.4.5.1 ANTICANCER ACTIVITY OF CURCUMIN

According to Nagahama K et al. (2016), curcumin, the most important chemical compound of the rhizome of *Curcuma longa* L. (turmeric) in the Zingiberaceae family, has piqued the interest of most researchers due to its immense pharmacological effects on multiple cancers as well as antitumor, anti-inflammatory, and antioxidant activities. Curcumin is a drug candidate and naturally derived compound, constituted of two phenyl rings substituted with hydroxyl and methoxyl groups connected through a 7-carbon and keto-enol linker. A reaction between aryl-aldehyde and acetyl-acetone produces its derivatives. As per the reports of Shi et al. (2009), dimethylcurcumin enhances androgen receptor degradation and has been used for the treatment of prostate cancer. Moreover, it also has a significant antiproliferation effect on estrogen-dependent breast cancer cells.

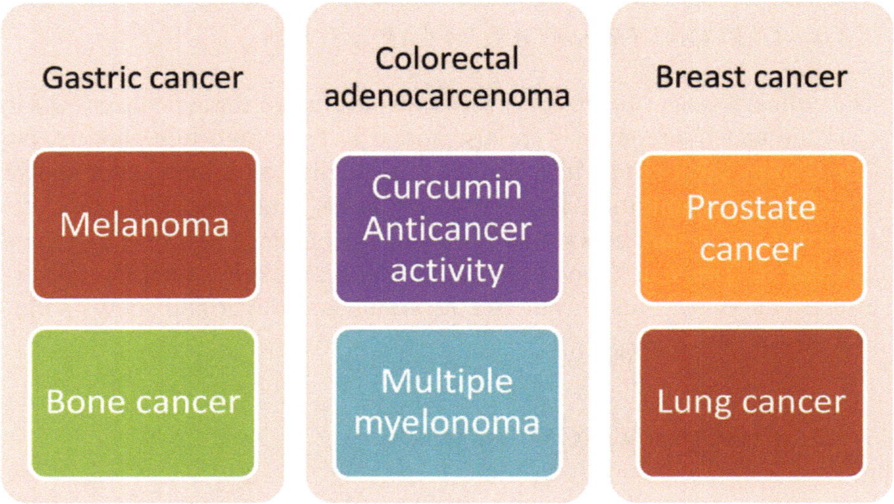

FIGURE 3.4 Anticancer activity of curcumin.

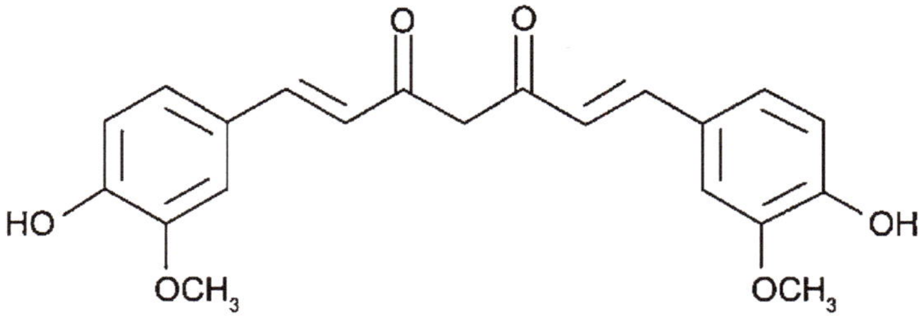

FIGURE 3.5 Molecular structure of curcumin.

Sandur et al. (2007) stated that based on the evidence, turmeric contains three major compounds, namely curcumin, demethoxycurcumin and bisdemethoxycurcumin. Among which, curcumin is the most potent and abundant element, showing anti-inflammatory and antiproliferative activities. Curcumin's antitumor activity is mediated by its antiproliferative effects on a variety of cancers, as well as its inhibitory effects on transcription factors and cell adhesion molecules involved in angiogenesis and metastasis.

3.5 CONCLUSION

Natural products have proven to be effective, inexpensive, and easily accessible for the treatment of cancer, even for the average person. Natural products, in particular, play an important role in chemotherapy medicines, exhibiting their actions on target proliferative tumor cells. Bioactive components such as thymoquinone (black cumin), curcumin (turmeric), gingerol (ginger), cuminaldehyde (*Cuminum cyminum*), and allicine (garlic) among others, have shown a promising role in the treatment of various types of cancers.

KEYWORDS

- **cancers**
- **herbs**
- **phytochemicals**
- **spices and treatment of cancer**

REFERENCES

Aggarwal, V., Tuli, H. S., Thakral, F., Singhal, P., Aggarwal, D., Srivastava, S., Pandey, A., et al., (2020). Molecular mechanisms of action of hesperidin in cancer: Recent trends and advancements. *Experimental Biology and Medicine, 245*(5), 486–497. https://doi.org/10.1177/1535370220903671.

Anubhuti, S., Ashok, S., Prashant, Y., & Dhiraj, S., (2016). Isothiocyanates in brassica: Potential anticancer agents. *Asian Pacific Journal of Cancer Prevention: APJCP, 17*(9), 4507–4510.

Asaduzzaman, K. M., Tania, M., Fu, S., & Fu, J., (2017). Thymoquinone, as an anticancer molecule: From basic research to clinical investigation. *Oncotarget, 8*(31), 51907–51919. PubMed. https://doi.org/10.18632/oncotarget.17206.

Awasthi, S., Singhal, S. S., Singhal, J., Nagaprashantha, L., Li, H., Yuan, Y. C., Liu, Z., et al., (2018). Anticancer activity of 2'-hydroxyflavanone towards lung cancer. *Oncotarget, 9*(90), 36202–36219. PubMed. https://doi.org/10.18632/oncotarget.26329.

Belanger, J. T., (1998). Perillyl alcohol: Applications in oncology. *Alternative Medicine Review: A Journal of Clinical Therapeutic, 3*(6), 448–457.

Bishayee, A., Ahmed, S., Brankov, N., & Perloff, M., (2011). Triterpenoids as potential agents for the chemoprevention and therapy of breast cancer. *Frontiers in Bioscience (Landmark Edition), 16*, 980–996. PubMed. https://doi.org/10.2741/3730.

Cho, E., Chung, E. Y., Jang, H. Y., Hong, O. Y., Chae, H. S., Jeong, Y. J., Kim, S. Y., etal., (2017). Anticancer effect of cyanidin-3-glucoside from mulberry via caspase-3 cleavage and DNA fragmentation *in vitro* and *in vivo*. *Anticancer Agents in Medicinal Chemistry, 17*(11), 1519–1525. https://doi.org/10.2174/1871520617666170327152026.

Choudhari, A. S., Mandave, P. C., Deshpande, M., Ranjekar, P., & Prakash, O., (2020). Phytochemicals in cancer treatment: From preclinical studies to clinical practice. *Frontiers in Pharmacology, 10*, 1614. https://doi.org/10.3389/fphar.2019.01614.

Dela, C. C. S., Tanoue, L. T., & Matthay, R. A., (2011). Lung cancer: Epidemiology, etiology, and prevention. *Clinics in Chest Medicine, 32*(4), 605–644. PubMed. https://doi.org/10.1016/j.ccm.2011.09.001.

Dirsch, V., Antlsperger, D., Hentze, H., & Vollmar, A., (2002). Ajoene, an experimental anti-leukemic drug: Mechanism of cell death. *Leukemia, 16*(1), 74–83. https://doi.org/10.1038/sj.leu.2402337.

Fang, D., Xiong, Z., Xu, J., Yin, J., & Luo, R., (2019). Chemopreventive mechanisms of galangin against hepatocellular carcinoma: A review. *Biomedicine & Pharmacotherapy, 109*, 2054–2061. https://doi.org/10.1016/j.biopha.2018.09.154.

Ferlay, J., Colombet, M., Soerjomataram, I., Parkin, D. M., Piñeros, M., Znaor, A., & Bray, F., (2021). Cancer statistics for the year 2020: An overview. *International Journal of Cancer*. https://doi.org/10.1002/ijc.33588.

Gupta, P., Kim, B., Kim, S. H., & Srivastava, S. K., (2014). Molecular targets of isothiocyanates in cancer: Recent advances. *Molecular Nutrition & Food Research, 58*(8), 1685–1707. PubMed. https://doi.org/10.1002/mnfr.201300684.

Hafeez, B. B., Siddiqui, I. A., Asim, M., Malik, A., Afaq, F., Adhami, V. M., Saleem, M., et al., (2008). A dietary anthocyanidin delphinidin induces apoptosis of human prostate cancer PC3 cells *in vitro* and *in vivo*: Involvement of nuclear factor-kappaB signaling. *Cancer Research, 68*(20), 8564–8572. PubMed. https://doi.org/10.1158/0008-5472.CAN-08-2232.

Heber, D., & Lu, Q. Y., (2002). Overview of mechanisms of action of lycopene. *Experimental Biology and Medicine (Maywood, N.J.), 227*(10), 920–923. https://doi.org/10.1177/153537020222701013.

Ho, J. N., Kang, M., Lee, S., Oh, J. J., Hong, S. K., Lee, S. E., & Byun, S. S., (2018). Anticancer effect of S-allyl-L-cysteine via induction of apoptosis in human bladder cancer cells. *Oncology Letters, 15*(1), 623–629. PubMed. https://doi.org/10.3892/ol.2017.7280.

Horwitz, S. B., (1994). Taxol (paclitaxel): Mechanisms of action. *Annals of Oncology: Official Journal of the European Society for Medical Oncology, 5*(6), S3–6.

Hosseini, A., & Ghorbani, A., (2015). Cancer therapy with phytochemicals: Evidence from clinical studies. *Avicenna Journal of Phytomedicine, 5*(2), 84–97.

Hu, S., Huang, L., Meng, L., Sun, H., Zhang, W., & Xu, Y., (2015). Isorhamnetin inhibits cell proliferation and induces apoptosis in breast cancer via Akt and mitogen-activated protein kinase signaling pathways. *Molecular Medicine Reports, 12*(5), 6745–6751. PubMed. https://doi.org/10.3892/mmr.2015.4269.

Hu, W. H., Dai, D. K., Zheng, B. Z. Y., Duan, R., Dong, T. T. X., Qin, Q. W., & Tsim, K. W. K., (2020). Piceatannol, a natural analog of resveratrol, exerts antiangiogenic efficiencies by blockage of vascular endothelial growth factor binding to its receptor. *Molecules (Basel, Switzerland), 25*(17), 3769. PubMed. https://doi.org/10.3390/molecules25173769.

Huang, S., & Zheng, R., (2006). Rosmarinic acid inhibits angiogenesis and its mechanism of action *in vitro*. *Cancer Letters, 239*(2), 271–280. https://doi.org/10.1016/j.canlet.2005.08.025.

Huang, S., Wang, L. L., Xue, N. N., Li, C., Guo, H. H., Ren, T. K., Zhan, Y., et al., (2019). Chlorogenic acid effectively treats cancers through induction of cancer cell differentiation. *Theranostics, 9*(23), 6745–6763. PubMed. https://doi.org/10.7150/thno.34674.

Huynh, D. L., Sharma, N., Kumar, S. A., Singh, S. S., Zhang, J. J., Mongre, R. K., Ghosh, M., et al., (2017). Antitumor activity of wogonin, an extract from *Scutellaria baicalensis*, through regulating different signaling pathways. *Chinese Journal of Natural Medicines, 15*(1), 15–40. https://doi.org/10.1016/S1875-5364(17)30005-5.

Imran, M., Salehi, B., Sharifi-Rad, J., Aslam, G. T., Saeed, F., Imran, A., Shahbaz, M., et al., (2019). Kaempferol: A key emphasis to its anticancer potential. *Molecules (Basel, Switzerland), 24*(12), 2277. PubMed. https://doi.org/10.3390/molecules24122277.

Jia, S., Xu, X., Zhou, S., Chen, Y., Ding, G., & Cao, L., (2019). Fisetin induces autophagy in pancreatic cancer cells via endoplasmic reticulum stress – and mitochondrial stress-dependent pathways. *Cell Death & Disease, 10*(2), 142. https://doi.org/10.1038/s41419-019-1366-y.

Jiang, M., Zhu, M., Wang, L., & Yu, S., (2019). Antitumor effects and associated molecular mechanisms of myricetin. *Biomedicine & Pharmacotherapy, 120*, 109506. https://doi.org/10.1016/j.biopha.2019.109506.

Kamal, M. M., Akter, S., Lin, C. N., & Nazzal, S., (2020). Sulforaphane as an anticancer molecule: Mechanisms of action, synergistic effects, enhancement of drug safety, and delivery systems. *Archives of Pharmacal Research, 43*(4), 371–384. https://doi.org/10.1007/s12272-020-01225-2.

Keservani, R. K., Kesharwani, R. K., Sharma, A. K., & Jarouliya, U., (2015). Dietary supplements, nutraceutical and functional foods in immune response (Immunomodulators). In: Debasis, B., Harry, G. P., & Anand, S., (eds.), *Nutraceutical and Functional Foods in Human Life and Disease Prevention* (pp. 343–358). Boca Raton, Fl. Taylor and Francis, Chapter 20. ISBN: 9781482237214.

Keservani, R. K., Kesharwani, R. K., Sharma, A. K., Vyas, N., & Chadoker, A., (2010b). Nutritional supplements: An overview. *International Journal of Current Pharmaceutical Review and Research, 1*(1), 59–75.

Keservani, R. K., Kesharwani, R. K., Vyas, N., Jain, S., Raghuvanshi, R., & Sharma, A. K., (2010a). Nutraceutical and functional food as future food: A review. *Der Pharmacia Lettre, 2*(1), 106–116.

Keservani, R. K., Sharma, A. K., & Kesharwani, R. K., (2016). Medicinal effect of nutraceutical fruits for the cognition and brain health. *Scientifica, 2016*, 10. Article ID 3109254. doi: 10.1155/2016/3109254.

Keservani, R. K., Sharma, A. K., & Kesharwani, R. K., (2020). *Nutraceuticals and Dietary Supplements: Applications in Health Improvement and Disease Management*. CRC Press. ISBN: 9781771888738.

Kezimana, P., Dmitriev, A. A., Kudryavtseva, A. V., Romanova, E. V., & Melnikova, N. V., (2018). Secoisolariciresinol diglucoside of flaxseed and its metabolites: Biosynthesis and potential for nutraceuticals. *Frontiers in Genetics, 9*, 641. PubMed. doi: 10.3389/fgene.2018.00641.

Khan, H., Reale, M., Ullah, H., Sureda, A., Tejada, S., Wang, Y., Zhang, Z. J., & Xiao, J., (2020). Anticancer effects of polyphenols via targeting p53 signaling pathway: Updates and future directions. *Biotechnology Advances, 38*, 107385. https://doi.org/10.1016/j.biotechadv.2019.04.007.

Khan, T., Ali, M., Khan, A., Nisar, P., Jan, S. A., Afridi, S., & Shinwari, Z. K., (2019). Anticancer plants: A review of the active phytochemicals, applications in animal models, and regulatory aspects. *Biomolecules, 10*(1), 47. PubMed. https://doi.org/10.3390/biom10010047.

Khoo, B. Y., Chua, S. L., & Balaram, P., (2010). Apoptotic effects of chrysin in human cancer cell lines. *International Journal of Molecular Sciences, 11*(5), 2188–2199. PubMed. https://doi.org/10.3390/ijms11052188.

Kim, S. M., (2016). Cellular and molecular mechanisms of 3,3'-diindolylmethane in gastrointestinal cancer. *International Journal of Molecular Sciences, 17*(7), 1155. PubMed. https://doi.org/10.3390/ijms17071155.

Ko, J. H., Sethi, G., Um, J. Y., Shanmugam, M. K., Arfuso, F., Kumar, A. P., Bishayee, A., & Ahn, K. S., (2017). The role of resveratrol in cancer therapy. *International Journal of Molecular Sciences, 18*(12), 2589. PubMed. https://doi.org/10.3390/ijms18122589.

Kopustinskiene, D. M., Jakstas, V., Savickas, A., & Bernatoniene, J., (2020). Flavonoids as anticancer agents. *Nutrients, 12*(2), 457. PubMed. https://doi.org/10.3390/nu12020457.

Lee, I. C., & Choi, B. Y., (2016). Withaferin-A--A natural anticancer agent with pleitropic mechanisms of action. *International Journal of Molecular Sciences, 17*(3), 290. PubMed. https://doi.org/10.3390/ijms17030290.

Lee, Y., (2017). Cancer chemopreventive potential of procyanidin. *Toxicological Research, 33*(4), 273–282. PubMed. https://doi.org/10.5487/TR.2017.33.4.273.

Lin, B. W., Gong, C. C., Song, H. F., & Cui, Y. Y., (2017). Effects of anthocyanins on the prevention and treatment of cancer. *British Journal of Pharmacology, 174*(11), 1226–1243. https://doi.org/10.1111/bph.13627.

Lin, J., Tian, J., Shu, C., Cheng, Z., Liu, Y., Wang, W., Liu, R., et al., (2020). Malvidin-3-galactoside from blueberry suppresses the growth and metastasis potential of hepatocellular carcinoma cell Huh-7 by regulating apoptosis and metastases pathways. *Food Science and Human Wellness, 9*(2), 136–145. https://doi.org/10.1016/j.fshw.2020.02.004.

Liu, H., Dong, Y., Gao, Y., Du, Z., Wang, Y., Cheng, P., Chen, A., & Huang, H., (2016). The fascinating effects of baicalein on cancer: A review. *International Journal of Molecular Sciences, 17*(10), 1681. PubMed. https://doi.org/10.3390/ijms17101681.

Luo, R., Fang, D., Hang, H., & Tang, Z., (2016). The mechanism in gastric cancer chemoprevention by allicin. *Anticancer Agents in Medicinal Chemistry, 16*(7), 802–809. https://doi.org/10.2174/1871520616666151111115443.

Majdalawieh, A. F., Massri, M., & Nasrallah, G. K., (2017). A comprehensive review on the anticancer properties and mechanisms of action of sesamin, a lignan in sesame seeds (*Sesamum indicum*). *European Journal of Pharmacology, 815*, 512–521. https://doi.org/10.1016/j.ejphar.2017.10.020.

Mao, Q. Q., Xu, X. Y., Cao, S. Y., Gan, R. Y., Corke, H., Beta, T., & Li, H. B., (2019). Bioactive compounds and bioactivities of ginger (*Zingiber officinale* Roscoe). *Foods (Basel, Switzerland), 8*(6), 185. PubMed. https://doi.org/10.3390/foods8060185.

Min, K. J., & Kwon, T. K., (2014). Anticancer effects and molecular mechanisms of epigallocatechin-3-gallate. *Integrative Medicine Research, 3*(1), 16–24. PubMed. https://doi.org/10.1016/j.imr.2013.12.001.

Mukhtar, Y. M., Adu-Frimpong, M., Xu, X., & Yu, J., (2018). Biochemical significance of limonene and its metabolites: Future prospects for designing and developing highly potent anticancer drugs. *Bioscience Reports, 38*(6), BSR20181253. PubMed. https://doi.org/10.1042/BSR20181253.

Nagoor, M. M. F., Javed, H., Al Taee, H., Azimullah, S., & Ojha, S. K., (2017). Pharmacological properties and molecular mechanisms of thymol: Prospects for its therapeutic potential and pharmaceutical development. *Frontiers in Pharmacology, 8*, 380. PubMed. https://doi.org/10.3389/fphar.2017.00380.

Nowak, R., Olech, M., & Nowacka, N., (2014). Chapter 97—Plant polyphenols as chemopreventive agents. In: Watson, R. R., Preedy, V. R., & Zibadi, S., (eds.), *Polyphenols in Human Health and Disease* (pp. 1289–1307). Academic Press. https://doi.org/10.1016/B978-0-12-398456-2.00086-4.

Pandey, K. B., & Rizvi, S. I., (2009). Plant polyphenols as dietary antioxidants in human health and disease. *Oxidative Medicine and Cellular Longevity, 2*(5), 270–278. PubMed. https://doi.org/10.4161/oxim.2.5.9498.

Ramasamy, K., Samayoa, C., Krishnegowda, N., & Tekmal, R. R., (2017). Chapter six—Therapeutic use of estrogen receptor β agonists in prevention and treatment of endocrine therapy resistant breast cancers: Observations from preclinical models. In: Lakshmanaswamy, R., (ed.), *Progress in Molecular Biology and Translational Science* (Vol. 151, pp. 177–194). Academic Press. https://doi.org/10.1016/bs.pmbts.2017.08.002.

Rane, B. R., & Keservani, R., (2020). Introduction to nutraceuticals and dietary supplements. In: *Nutraceuticals and Dietary Supplements* (pp. 35–56). Apple Academic Press. ISBN: 9781771888738.

Rane, B. R., Bharath, M. S., Patil, R. R., Keservani, R. K., & Jain, A. S., (2020b). Novel approaches in nutraceuticals. In: Rajesh, K. K., Raj, K. K., & Anil, K. S., (eds.), *Enhancing the Therapeutic Efficacy of Herbal Formulations Through Novel Drug Delivery Systems* (pp. 241–266). IGI Global International Publisher, Pennsylvania, USA, Chapter 11. ISBN13: 9781799844532.

Rane, B. R., Patil, A. S., Keservani, R. K., & Jain, A. S., (2020a). Novel approaches in herbal formulation. In: Rajesh, K. K., Raj, K. K., & Anil, K. S., (eds.), *Enhancing the Therapeutic Efficacy of Herbal Formulations through Novel Drug Delivery Systems* (pp. 43–68). IGI Global International Publisher, Pennsylvania, USA, Chapter 2. ISBN13: 9781799844532.

Safe, S. H., Prather, P. L., Brents, L. K., Chadalapaka, G., & Jutooru, I., (2012). Unifying mechanisms of action of the anticancer activities of triterpenoids and synthetic analogs. *Anticancer Agents in Medicinal Chemistry, 12*(10), 1211–1220. PubMed. https://doi.org/10.2174/187152012803833099.

Salehi, B., Venditti, A., Sharifi-Rad, M., Kręgiel, D., Sharifi-Rad, J., Durazzo, A., Lucarini, M., et al., (2019). The therapeutic potential of apigenin. *International Journal of Molecular Sciences, 20*(6), 1305. PubMed. https://doi.org/10.3390/ijms20061305.

Shafabakhsh, R., & Asemi, Z., (2019). Quercetin: A natural compound for ovarian cancer treatment. *Journal of Ovarian Research, 12*(1), 55. https://doi.org/10.1186/s13048-019-0530-4.

Sharma, G. N., Dave, R., Sanadya, J., Sharma, P., & Sharma, K. K., (2010). Various types and management of breast cancer: An overview. *Journal of Advanced Pharmaceutical Technology & Research, 1*(2), 109–126. PubMed.

Singh, S., Sharma, B., Kanwar, S. S., & Kumar, A., (2016). Lead phytochemicals for anticancer drug development. *Frontiers in Plant Science, 7*, 1667. PubMed. https://doi.org/10.3389/fpls.2016.01667.

Takeshima, H., & Ushijima, T., (2019). Accumulation of genetic and epigenetic alterations in normal cells and cancer risk. *NPJ Precision Oncology, 3*(1), 7. https://doi.org/10.1038/s41698-019-0079-0.

Tomeh, M. A., Hadianamrei, R., & Zhao, X., (2019). A review of curcumin and its derivatives as anticancer agents. *International Journal of Molecular Sciences, 20*(5), 1033. PubMed. https://doi.org/10.3390/ijms20051033.

Tsai, H. Y., Ho, C. T., & Chen, Y. K., (2017). Biological actions and molecular effects of resveratrol, pterostilbene, and 3′-hydroxypterostilbene. *Dietary Natural Compounds, 25*(1), 134–147. https://doi.org/10.1016/j.jfda.2016.07.004.

Tuli, H. S., Tuorkey, M. J., Thakral, F., Sak, K., Kumar, M., Sharma, A. K., Sharma, U., et al., (2019). Molecular mechanisms of action of genistein in cancer: Recent advances. *Frontiers in Pharmacology, 10*, 1336–1336. PubMed. https://doi.org/10.3389/fphar.2019.01336.

Tuorkey, M. J., (2016). Molecular targets of luteolin in cancer. *European Journal of Cancer Prevention: The Official Journal of the European Cancer Prevention Organization (ECP), 25*(1), 65–76. PubMed. https://doi.org/10.1097/CEJ.0000000000000128.

Varma, A., Padh, H., & Shrivastava, N., (2011). Andrographolide: A new plant-derived antineoplastic entity on horizon. *Evidence-Based Complementary and Alternative Medicine: ECAM, 2011*, 815390, 1–9. PubMed. https://doi.org/10.1093/ecam/nep135.

Wang, L. S., & Stoner, G. D., (2008). Anthocyanins and their role in cancer prevention. *Cancer Letters, 269*(2), 281–290. PubMed. https://doi.org/10.1016/j.canlet.2008.05.020.

Wang, L., Phan, D. D. K., Zhang, J., Ong, P. S., Thuya, W. L., Soo, R., Wong, A. L. A., et al., (2016). Anticancer properties of nimbolide and pharmacokinetic considerations to accelerate its development. *Oncotarget, 7*(28), 44790–44802. PubMed. https://doi.org/10.18632/oncotarget.8316.

Wishart, D. S., Knox, C., Guo, A. C., Shrivastava, S., Hassanali, M., Stothard, P., Chang, Z., & Woolsey, J., (n.d.). DrugBank: A comprehensive resource for in silico drug discovery and exploration. *Nucleic Acids Res.,34* (Database issue), D668–672. 16381955.

Wu, X., Zhou, Q., & Xu, K., (2009). Are isothiocyanates potential anticancer drugs? *Acta Pharmacologica Sinica, 30*(5), 501–512. PubMed. https://doi.org/10.1038/aps.2009.50.

Xie, L., Zhu, G., Shang, J., Chen, X., Zhang, C., Ji, X., Zhang, Q., & Wei, Y., (2021). An overview on the biological activity and anticancer mechanism of lovastatin. *Cellular Signaling, 87*, 110122. https://doi.org/10.1016/j.cellsig.2021.110122.

Yi, L., & Su, Q., (2013). Molecular mechanisms for the anticancer effects of diallyl disulfide. *Food and Chemical Toxicology: An International Journal Published for the British Industrial Biological Research Association, 57*, 362–370. https://doi.org/10.1016/j.fct.2013.04.001.

Zhang, H. M., Zhao, L., Li, H., Xu, H., Chen, W. W., & Tao, L., (2014). Research progress on the anticarcinogenic actions and mechanisms of ellagic acid. *Cancer Biology & Medicine, 11*(2), 92–100. PubMed. https://doi.org/10.7497/j.issn.2095–3941.2014.02.004.

Zhang, H., Wang, K., Lin, G., & Zhao, Z., (2014). Antitumor mechanisms of S-allyl mercaptocysteine for breast cancer therapy. *BMC Complementary and Alternative Medicine, 14*, 270–270. PubMed. https://doi.org/10.1186/1472-6882-14-270.

Zhang, W., Su, J., Xu, H., Yu, S., Liu, Y., Zhang, Y., Sun, L., et al., (2017). Dicumarol inhibits PDK1 and targets multiple malignant behaviors of ovarian cancer cells. *PloS One, 12*(6), e0179672–e0179672. PubMed. https://doi.org/10.1371/journal.pone.0179672.

Zhang, X., Lin, D., Jiang, R., Li, H., Wan, J., & Li, H., (2016). Ferulic acid exerts antitumor activity and inhibits metastasis in breast cancer cells by regulating epithelial to mesenchymal transition. *Oncology Reports, 36*(1), 271–278. https://doi.org/10.3892/or.2016.4804.

Zhang, Y., (2010). Allyl isothiocyanate as a cancer chemopreventive phytochemical. *Molecular Nutrition & Food Research, 54*(1), 127–135. PubMed. https://doi.org/10.1002/mnfr.200900323.

Zou, J., Lin, J., Li, C., Zhao, R., Fan, L., Yu, J., & Shao, J., (2019). Ursolic acid in cancer treatment and metastatic chemoprevention: From synthesized derivatives to nanoformulations in preclinical studies. *Current Cancer Drug Targets, 19*(4), 245–256. https://doi.org/10.2174/1568009618666181016145940.

CHAPTER 4

NANOTECHNOLOGY IN NUTRACEUTICALS DELIVERY FOR THE PREVENTION AND TREATMENT OF CANCER

OZAN E. EYUPOGLU[1] and KALSOOM SALEEM[2]

[1]*Department of Biochemistry, School of Pharmacy, Istanbul Medipol University, Istanbul, Turkey*

[2]*Department of Pharmaceuticals Sciences, Riphah Institute of Pharmaceutical Sciences, Islamabad, Pakistan*

ABSTRACT

Nanotechnology has received significant progress in the field of oncology in recent years. Nanomedicine is at the forefront to limit the shortcomings associated with traditional or conventional chemotherapeutic agents and chemotherapies. Nutraceutical delivery through nanotechnology has made great advancement in the field of oncology. Nutraceuticals are any food containing substances that have some medicinal benefits. They prevent the cancer progression by different mechanisms and are delivered to their target cancer cells without causing harm to healthy/normal cells. There have been multiple implications and advancement to the use of nanotechnology in delivering nutraceuticals to prevent and treat cancer. Nanotechnology-based formulations that include different kinds of polymeric, lipid and inorganic formulations have been explored to enhance nutraceuticals' bioavailability and anticancer potential. To exploit their full potential, further preclinical and clinical studies are required to be carried out.

Nutraceuticals in Cancer Prevention, Management, and Treatment. Raj K. Keservani, Bui Thanh Tung, Sippy Singh, & Rajesh K. Kesharwani, PhD (Eds.)

4.1 INTRODUCTION

Over the past two decades, nanoscale sciences, nanotechnology, and nanomedicine, have evolved tremendously, incorporating various sectors such as chemistry, physics, biotechnology, engineering, material sciences, cosmetics, bioremediation, pharmaceutical production and food industry (Logothetidis, 2012; Salama et al., 2020). Nanomedicine is at the forefront in limiting the shortcomings of traditional medicines. With the emerging role of nanomedicine, scientists discovered the intrinsic of nanotechnology and nanomedicine to circumvent most shortcomings associated with traditional medicines, such as unavoidable off-target drug side effects, non-specific drug targeting, both causing severe toxicities, drug instability, etc. Besides that, a major breakthrough has been achieved in multi-drug resistance (MDR) associated with chemotherapy and chemotherapeutic agents (Choudhury et al., 2019).

Nutraceuticals are defined as substances with physiological benefits and provide protection against chronic diseases (Kalra, 2003). They can also be defined as mixture of "nutrition" and "pharmaceuticals" based on natural substances with food and herbal (Rane et al., 2020a; Rane et al., 2020b, 2020c) products that deliver therapeutic and health benefits and are used as pharmaceutical formulations (Shahidi, 2012; Keservani et al., 2010a, 2010b, 2020). Nutraceuticals have gained considerable interest due to applications in prophylaxis and cure of diseases like cancer (Shirzad et al., 2011), cardiovascular diseases (Khosravi-Boroujeni et al., 2012; Keservani et al., 2016a), obesity, diabetes (Nasri, 2013), infectious diseases, neurological disorders (Akhlaghi et al., 2011) and osteoporosis and have gained attention in delivery of diverse bioactive compounds such as vitamin D, vitamin B-complex, zinc, calcium, magnesium, flavones, polyphenols, coenzyme Q-10, dietary fibers, probiotics, carotenoids, etc. (Wang et al., 2016). However, they have certain limitations, i.e., poor stability, solubility, absorption, bioavailability and higher first pass metabolism, which can be overcome by formulating nano-nutraceuticals.

Recently, they have been widely used to overcome major challenges associated with chemotherapy and chemotherapeutic agents (Surve et al., 2019) as well as for prevention and treatment. Nano-nutraceuticals prevent cancer by multiple mechanisms such as inhibition of cell proliferation and differentiation, inhibiting efflux transporters involved in MDR (P-glycoproteins (P-gp)), breast cancer resistance proteins (BCRP), multi-drug resistance proteins (MDR), or reducing toxicities of chemotherapeutic agents (Trottier et al., 2010).

In the field of oncology, nanotechnology has been used drastically to deliver nutraceuticals for prevention and treatment of different types of cancer. Emphasis has been made to present nano-nutraceuticals effective on cancer. This chapter presents the latest concepts about nano-nutraceuticals based on their disease-modifying applications.

4.2 NANOTECHNOLOGY-BASED DELIVERY OF NUTRACEUTICALS FOR CANCER PREVENTION AND TREATMENT

Growing evidences demonstrate that nutraceuticals have potential anticancer properties that exhibit promising results. They have been shown to modulate miRNAs, cellular signaling, epigenome, and pleiotropic (ability to downregulate multiple signaling pathways) (Huang et al., 2015), hence, can be treated as ideal candidates for inhibiting carcinogenesis and to achieve better treatment outcomes in patients (Piermartiri et al., 2015). Several nutraceuticals, such as fatty acids, carotenoids, vitamins, minerals, probiotics, and phenolics, including dietary fibers and different phytochemicals, have been developed in nano-nutraceutical formulations for use as an alternative for pharmaceuticals in cancer chemotherapy.

Nanotechnology used for the delivery of nutraceuticals range from polymer-based nanoformulations such as polymeric nanoparticles, polymeric micelles, dendrimers, polymeric hydrogels, polymeric conjugates, lipid-based nanoformulations such as liposomes, solid lipid nanoparticles (SLNs), nanoemulsions, self-emulsifying drug delivery system (SEDDs) to inorganic nanoformulations, such as quantum dots, carbon nanotubes, magnetic nanoparticles, silica nanoparticles, and gold nanoparticles (Surve et al., 2019). The subsequent sections briefly illustrate nanotechnology used for nutraceuticals along with their potential applications in different types of cancer. A summary of nano technology-based delivery of nutraceuticals in presented in Table 4.1 along with their application in oncology.

4.2.1 POLYMER-BASED NANOFORMULATIONS

Among the polymers, biodegradable polymers such as poly lactic-co-glycolic acid (PLGA) and polylactic acid (PLA) have gained much attention apart from poly ε-caprolactone (PCL), poly ethylene-glycol (PEG) (Coelho et al., 2010). Polysaccharides-based polymers such as chitosan, alginate, pectin, etc., have also been used in the delivery of nutraceuticals. These polymers

TABLE 4.1 Nanotechnology Used For Nutraceuticals Delivery in Cancer

S. No.	Nanotechnology	Nutraceutical(s)	Target(s)/Application	References
I	**Polymer-based Nano formulations**			
1	Polymeric nanoparticles	Epigallocetachin-3-gallate (EGCG)	Colon cancer	(Teong et al., 2015)
		Ferulic acid (FA)	Colon cancer	(Zheng et al., 2019)
		Honokiol (HK) + EGCG	Liver cancer	(Tang et al., 2018)
2	Polymeric micelles	β-lapachone	NQO1-overexpressing, H596 lung cancer	(Blanco et al., 2007)
		Curcumin	HeLa cells, HepG2 cells	(Cao et al., 2015; Gallien et al., 2021; Wang et al., 2015)
3	Dendrimers	Curcumin	Glioblastoma cell line, A549 cell lines (Lung carcinoma), SKBr3 and BT549 (Breast cancer cells)	(Gallien et al., 2021; Surve et al., 2019)
		Resveratrol (Chen et al., 2015)	HeLa cell lines	(Chen et al., 2015)
4	Polymeric hydrogels	Ellagic acid	MCF-7 breast cancer cells	(Trombino et al., 2013)
		Curcumin	A549 cells (lung adenocarcinoma cells)	(Wang et al., 2017)
5	Polymer-drug conjugates	Curcumin	L929 fibroblast cells	(Gallien et al., 2021)
		Resveratrol (Yee, 2018)	Melanoma cells	(Yee, 2018)
		EGCG	Not studied against any cancer model	(Dutta et al., 2018)
II	**Lipid-based nanotechnology**			
1	Liposomes	EGCG	Caco-2 cell lines, MDA-MB-231 (Breast cancer cells)	(Luo et al., 2014; Ramadass et al., 2015; Song et al., 2014)
		Curcumin	Pancreatic cancer	(Dutta et al., 2018)
		Beta-cryptoxanthin	Leukemia K562 cell lines	(Gharib et al., 2015)
		Triptolide	MCF-7 and 4TI (Breast cancer cell lines)	(Zheng et al., 2019)
		β-glucan	A549 (Epithelial cell line)	(Halwani et al., 2015)
		Ursolic acid	MDA-MB-231, LNCaP (Prostate cancer cell lines), EC-304 cells (Gastric cancer cells)	(Caldeira de Araújo Lopes et al., 2013; Zhao et al., 2015)
		Berberine	Breast cancer stem cells	(Wang et al., 2017)

TABLE 4.1 *(Continued)*

S. No.	Nanotechnology		Nutraceutical(s)	Target(s)/Application	References
2	SLNs		Beta-carotene	MCF-7 (Breast cancer cell lines)	(Jain et al., 2019)
			Aloe-emodin	HepG2 (Human hepatoma cells), MCF-7 (Breast cancer cells)	(Chen et al., 2015)
			Resveratrol	MDA-MB-231 (Breast cancer cells)	(Wang et al., 2017)
			EGCG	DU-145 (Prostate cancer cells), MDA-MB-231 (Breast cancer cells)	(Radhakrishnan et al., 2016)
3	SEDDS	SNEDDS	Curcumin	Caco-2 cells, colon cancer cells	(Kanwal et al., 2021)
			Berberine	Anticancer activity to be studied for developed formulation	(Ke et al., 2015)
			Quercetin	S180 (sarcomaros sarcoma cell)	(Sun et al., 2018)
			Apigenin	Anticancer activity to be studied for developed formulation	(Ahmed et al., 2021)
		SMEDDS	Lecithin	Lung cancer cell line	(Ishak & Osman, 2015)
			Quercetin + Resveratrol	AGS, Caco-2 and HT-29 cancer cells	(De Matos et al., 2018)
			Curcumin	Metastatic 4TI breast cancer	(Liu et al., 2019)
4	Nanoemulsions		Curcumin	Cervical carcinoma cell lines, MDA-MB-231 (Breast cancer cells)	(Bharmoria et al., 2021; De Matos et al., 2018)
			Quercetin	MDA-MB-231(Breast cancer cells)	(Ceramella et al., 2021)
			Ursolic acid + Oleanic acid	Melanoma cells	(Alvarado et al., 2018)
III	**Inorganic Nanoformulations**				
3	AuNPs		Resveratrol	Breast, prostate, and pancreatic cancer	(Thipe et al., 2019)
			Berberin	Breast cancer	(Chiu et al., 2021)
			Curcumin	HCT-116 (Colon cancer cell lines), MCF-7 (Breast cancer cell lines)	(Elbialy et al., 2019)

TABLE 4.1 *(Continued)*

S. No.	Nanotechnology	Nutraceutical(s)	Target(s)/Application	References
4	CNTs	Curcumin	Less work done on anticancer activities of developed formulations	(Li et al., 2019)
		Berberin		(Geto et al., 2013)
		Quercetin		(Dolatabadi et al., 2011)
5	Magnetic nanoparticles	Curcumin	Ovarian cancer, MCF-7 (Breast cancer cell lines)	(Mancarella et al., 2015; Nosrati et al., 2018)
		Resveratrol	A549 (Human lung cancer), LLC (Lewis lung carcinoma)	(Dai et al., 2017)
6	QDs	Resveratrol	L929 Fibroblasts cells	(Wu et al., 2017)
		Curcumin	HCT-116 (Colon cancer cells), MCF-7 (Breast cancer cells)	(Khan et al., 2020)

have been demonstrated to be non-immunogenic, non-toxic *in vivo,* protect nutraceuticals from enzymatic degradation, and provide better stability and sustained release. Many promising nutraceuticals with anticancer properties have been delivered using polymer, for instance, curcumin-loaded PLGA nanoparticles showed a tenfold increase in solubility and three folds increase anticancer activity (Khan et al., 2018).

4.2.1.1 POLYMERIC NANOPARTICLES

Various preclinical and epidemiological reports show that epigallocetachin-3-gallate (EGCG) (a polyphenol) can decrease the risk of cancer owing to its inhibitory effects on enzyme activities, signal transduction and antioxidants properties but is unstable *in vivo* leading to its low bioavailability. Polymeric nanoparticles made up of gallic acid (GA) grafted with chitosan (CS) and caseinophosphopeptides (CPP) developed for delivery of EGCG showed intense activity against colon cancer improving its bioavailability and anti-cancer property and preventing degradation (Teong et al., 2015).

Ferulic acid (FA) (a hydroxycinnamic acid) possess strong antioxidant and anticancer activities but has low bioavailability due to low permeability and solubility. FA when incorporated in polymeric nanoparticles, not only showed improved bioavailability but also possessed sustained release properties, high tumor accumulation and ability to deliver chemotherapeutic drug, paclitaxel in colon cancer (Zheng et al., 2019). Honokiol (HK) (a biphenol) has been reported to show several pharmacological properties such as anti-thrombosis, antioxidant, anti-bacterial and most importantly, anti-cancerous activities but with limited solubility and bioavailability. EGCG functionalized chitin (CH) nanoparticles loaded with HK exhibited effective inhibition of cell proliferation, tumor selectivity, growth reduction both *in vitro* and *in vivo* in liver cancer, as compared to free HK (Tang et al., 2018).

4.2.1.2 POLYMERIC MICELLES

Polymeric micelles are formed by self-aggregation of co-polymeric amphiphiles above critical micelle concentration (CMC). Micelles have been widely used for nutraceuticals delivery in cancer. Recently, β-lapachone encapsulated in PEG-PLGA polymeric micelles were developed in order to enhance its circulation time, reduce systemic toxicity and exhibited substantial increase half-life and cytotoxicity (Surve et al., 2019) against NQO1-overexpressing H596 lung cancer (Blanco et al., 2007). In addition, curcumin loaded redox sensitive micelles demonstrated higher cellular uptake in HeLa cells as compared to control micelles (Cao et al., 2015) and HepG2 cells (Wang et al., 2015).

4.2.1.3 DENDRIMERS

Dendrimers are highly branched nanoscale macromolecules with functional terminal end groups (Gallien et al., 2021). Their nanoscale size and potential to manipulate and control separate components, make them suitable for delivery of nutraceuticals in the field of oncology. They have also been utilized for increasing the bioavailability of nutraceuticals, besides that, protecting them from harsh environmental conditions such as enzymatic degradation, pH variations and controlling their release. Recently, curcumin (a phenolic) with potential antioxidant and anti-inflammatory activity has been used for the treatment of glioblastoma, a deadly and aggressive cancer of the central nervous system (CNS). To facilitate efficient delivery of therapeutic doses of curcumin into cancer cells, surface-modified polyamidoamine (PAMAM) dendrimers were used to encapsulate it and were studied against three species of glioblastoma cell line viz mouse-GL261, rat-F98, and human-U87 (rodent and non-rodent cell lines). The study demonstrated that delivering curcumin-loaded dendrimers were lethal to only cancer cells and, therefore, could be a new alternative to treatment of devastating glioblastoma. Results with curcumin suggest that antioxidant are good candidates for treating glioblastoma (Gallien et al., 2021).

Similarly, another study with curcumin-loaded dendrimer revealed enhanced *in vitro* cytotoxicity against A549 cell lines (human lung carcinoma), SKBr3 and BT549 breast cancer cells, generation of ROS (reactive oxygen species) and loss in mitochondrial membrane potential (Surve et al., 2019). Resveratrol, another phenolic with antioxidant and anticancer potential with low bioavailability, poor metabolic stability, and instability at high pH. Dendrimer nanotechnology used for delivery of resveratrol had tremendous improvements in its solubility, stability and pharmacokinetics intended to enhance bioavailability (Chauhan, 2015). Yousefi et al. (2020) summarized dendritic applications in the delivery of various nutraceuticals.

4.2.1.4 POLYMERIC HYDROGELS

Hydrogels are cross-linked hydrophilic polymeric structures having great affinity towards water or biological fluids due to which they are thermodynamically compatible with water. They provide sustained and local delivery of nutraceuticals. For instance, ellagic acid has been presented with anticancer, anti-viral, antioxidant and anti-bacterial properties. Ellagic acid-based hydrogel functionalized with folic acid used as a subcutaneous implant for the treatment of breast cancer. Cytotoxicity against MCF-7 breast cancer cells was evaluated and results showed a slow kinetic release with reduction in cell viability (Trombino et al., 2013). Another nutraceutical, curcumin was delivered using folate-functionalized PEG cross-linked acrylic polymer (FA-CLAP) hydrogel. Results suggested that synthesized curcumin-loaded FA-CLAP hydrogel exhibited higher anticancer proliferation activities in A549 cells (lung adenocarcinoma cells). In addition, synthesized formulation provided ease of uptake of curcumin by cells and enhanced apoptotic effect. Studies showed that hydrogels can be used as an efficient delivery vehicle of curcumin into cells (Teong et al., 2015).

4.2.1.5 POLYMER-DRUG CONJUGATES

In polymer-drug conjugate, the drug or nutraceutical is not encapsulated within the polymer rather attached to polymeric macromolecular carrier which is stable in systemic circulation and releases drug at target under specific stimuli. For example, recently hyaluronic acid conjugation with curcumin showed enhanced solubility and stability of curcumin. Furthermore, *in vitro* cytotoxicity in L929 fibroblast cells showed higher cytotoxicity as compared to curcumin alone. Another nutraceutical, resveratrol was also conjugated with mPEG-PCL that demonstrated an increase in half-life from 7.8 minutes to 10 minutes. A similar study was also performed on resveratrol that undergoes rapid metabolism under physiological conditions resulting in low bioavailability. Studies performed on resveratrol conjugated with polymeric methoxy-poly (ethylene glycol)-block-poly (ε-caprolactone) (mPEG-PCL) was found to have improved stability and solubility as compared to resveratrol alone (Ng et al., 2015). Yuting et al., synthesized β-Lactoglobulin–chlorogenic acid conjugate-based nanoparticles for delivery of (−)-epigallocatechin-3-gallate (EGCG) (Fan et al., 2017). Besides that, Jun et al., combined several phenolic-protein conjugates with their potential applications (Liu et al., 2019).

4.2.2 LIPID-BASED NANOTECHNOLOGY

4.2.2.1 LIPOSOMES

Conventional liposomes are spherical amphiphilic phospholipid vesicles, containing a bilayer lipid membrane surrounding an aqueous interior compartment. This feature is advantageous in the delivery of both hydrophilic and lipophilic nutraceuticals in chemotherapy (Salama et al., 2020). Such delivery is suitable through liposomes as they delay the clearance and increase circulation time, thereby, enhancing bioavailability (Dutta et al., 2018). Various nutraceuticals formulated in liposomes have been shown to efficiently target cancerous cells. For example, EGCG has been delivered via liposomal formulation showing enhanced anti-MRSA activity *in vitro* and *in vivo* and enhanced inhibitory effect on tumor cell viability (Luo et al., 2014). Another liposomal formulations for EGCG presented high stability in neutral pH and enhanced cellular permeability in caco-2 cell lines (Song et al., 2014) and enhancing synergistic effects between EGCG and paclitaxel in inducing apoptosis in MDA-MB-231 breast cancer cells (Ramadass et al., 2015).

Curcumin, the widely studied nutraceuticals for cancer potential, was studied against human pancreatic cells *in vitro* and *in vivo*. Liposomal curcumin downregulated nuclear factor κB (NF-κB) machinery, suppressed growth and induced apoptosis from which Lan et al., concluded that anticancer and anti-angiogenesis effect of developed formulation provided a biological rational for treatment of patients suffering with pancreatic cancer (Dutta et al., 2018). Beta-cryptoxanthin, a carotenoid, plays important in preventing free radical damage to biomolecules and treatment of several other cancers. Beta-cryptoxanthin-loaded nanoliposomes were evaluated for anti-proliferative activity against leukemia K562 cell lines. The results of the study showed that the greater anti-proliferative activity as compared to free beta-cryptoxanthin. Furthermore, in presence of developed formulation, the proportion of apoptotic cells was higher. Amir et al., concluded that beta-cryptoxanthin-loaded nanoliposomes may provide a basis for development of leukemia therapies (Gharib et al., 2015).

Recently, triptolide-loaded cationic liposomes developed to investigate their effect in MCF-7, 4TI, HepG2, 293T cell lines. Developed liposomes showed inhibitory activity against MCF-7 and 4TI breast cancer cell lines and indicated no signs of toxicity in liver and kidney tumor bearing mouse models (Zheng et al., 2019). Besides that, several other nutraceuticals have also been developed in nanoliposomal formulations such as liposomal β-glucan effective against human lung carcinoma epithelial cell line A549(Halwani et al., 2015), long-circulating and pH-sensitive liposomes containing ursolic acid effective against breast (MDA-MB-231) and prostate (LNCaP) cancer cell lines (Caldeira de Araújo Lopes et al., 2013), PEG-modified ursolic acid liposomes effective against EC-304 cells (gastric cancer cells) (Zhao et al., 2015), berberine liposomes effective against breast cancer stem cells (Wang et al., 2017), etc. A summary about different formulations of liposome encapsulation of nutraceuticals is presented by Dutta et al. (2018).

4.2.2.2 SOLID-LIPID NANOPARTICLES (SLNS)

Solid-lipid nanoparticles (SLNs) are colloidal carriers consisting of lipids dispersed in aqueous surfactant solution (Arora & Jaglan, 2016). Many nutraceuticals delivered through SLNs have been shown to provide effective prevention and treatment potential against several types of cancers. Several research works have been done regarding the loading of nutraceuticals in SLNs. For example, beta-carotene (a carotenoid) is widely investigated carotenoid for its anticancer, antioxidant, and provitamin-A activity. Beta-carotene-loaded solid lipid nanoparticles (BC-SLNs) formulated, were studied for cytotoxicity in human breast cancer cell lines (MCF-7). Studies confirmed that encapsulation of beta-carotene in SLNs did not affect its anticancer activity rather it improved its activity against MCF-7 cell lines. Similarly, encapsulation of aloe-emodin into SLNs enhanced its *in vitro* cytotoxicity against human hepatoma cells (HepG2) and human breast cancer cells (MCF-7) as compared to aloe-emodin alone (Chen et al., 2015). Hence, Jain et al. (2019) concluded that SLNs could be an effective and promising strategy to improve the anticancer effects of carotenoids.

More recently, to improve the bioavailability, stability and solubility of resveratrol, Palmitic acid (PA)-decorated resveratrol-loaded SLNs were prepared. The *in vitro* release studies demonstrated negligible release of resveratrol in simulated gastric and sustained release in simulated intestinal conditions. Hence, the bioavailability of resveratrol was found to be 3.8-fold higher in SLNs than that from resveratrol suspension (Ramalingam & Ko, 2016). SLNs developed for delivery of EGCG were successful in increasing its stability, provided sustained release, a sharp decrease in cell viability and apoptosis in breast cancer cells MDA-MB-231 and prostate cancer cells DU-145 as compared to free EGCG (Radhakrishnan et al., 2016).

4.2.2.3 SELF-EMULSIFYING DRUG DELIVERY SYSTEMS (SEDDS)

Among SEDDS, self-nanoemulsifying drug delivery system (SENDDS) have drawn substantial attention due to thermodynamic stability, industrial scalability, solubilizing amphiphilic compounds (super-solvents). SNEDDS are anhydrous isotropic mixtures of oil, surfactant and co-surfactants at nanoscale that spontaneously emulsify to give oil-in-water nanoemulsion when in contact with gastrointestinal tract (GIT) fluids. Curcumin when formulated into SNEDDS, was found to have increased oral bioavailability and anticancer activity in colon cancer cells and cellular uptake in Caco-2 cells. The formulation was highly stable and results indicated the applicability of novel SNEDDS in improving curcumin anticancer activity and bioavailability (Kanwal et al., 2021). Berberine's oral bioavailability was improved after encapsulating in SNEDDS (Ke et al., 2015) but its anticancer effect on various cancer types (Sun et al., 2009) is yet to be investigated. Using quercetin loaded SEDDS, the study was carried out to investigate the anti-tumor effect on mice sarcomaros sarcoma cell S180. Quercetin-SNEDDS could inhibit the growth of tumor cells and the rate of inhibition was higher than quercetin alone (Sun et al., 2018). More recently, Ahmed et al., developed quercetine in novel α-tocopherol PEG-100 succinate based SNEDDS formulation (Ahmed et al., 2021). Kazi et al., synthesized SNEDDS of apigenin (a phenolic nutraceutical) to enhance its oral bioavailability and provide it *in vitro* and *in vivo* stability (Kazi et al., 2020). Testing of anticancer activity of developed formulation against multiple cancers (Imran et al., 2020) remains a future perspective.

Self-microemulsifying systems drug delivery systems (SMEDDS), another class of SEDDS, are widely used for nutraceuticals (Maji et al., 2021). SMEDDS are isotropic mixtures of oil, surfactant and/or co-solvent at nanoscale that spontaneously emulsify to give oil-in-water microemulsion when in contact with GIT fluids. Lecithin (a fatty acid) was delivered in SMEDDS formulation and studied against lung cancer cell line. Rania et al., concluded that Lecithin based SMEDDS showed the highest cytotoxicity against lung cancer cell line as compared to free drug solution and other SMEDDS formulations developed in the study (Ishak & Osman, 2015). Recently, SMEDDS in combination of quercetin and resveratrol were prepared that showed nine folds increase in area under the curve (AUC), slightly increased antioxidant and anticancer activity on AGS, Caco-2 and HT-29 cells and successfully enhanced oral bioavailability of both the nutraceuticals (Jaisamut et al., 2021). Ying et al., developed hybrid curcumin-phospholipid SMEDDS to test their potential against breast cancer metastasis. In metastatic 4TI breast cancer, developed formulation induced significant cytotoxicity and inhibited invasion and migration of 4TI cells. Besides that, in orthotropic 4TI tumor bearing nude mice, a combination of orally administered SMEDDS with near infrared (NIR) laser irradiation inhibited tumor progression and suppressed lung metastasis of breast cancer (Liu et al., 2019).

4.2.2.4 NANOEMULSIONS

Nanoemulsions have considerable potential in encapsulating, protecting, and delivering of nutraceuticals. They are heterogeneous mixtures of two or more immiscible liquids in which one phase is dispersed in the second immiscible/partially miscible phase (Arora & Jaglan, 2016). De Matos et al. (2018) synthesized a novel nanoemulsion of curcumin and studied its effect with photodynamic therapy in cervical carcinoma cell lines. Nanoemulsion was shown to be internalized inside cells and a high phototoxic effect was observed after photodynamic therapy suggesting cell death by apoptosis. Another studied carried out, developed protein-olive oil-in-water nanoemulsion of curcumin which proved as successful application of curcumin as anticancer agent against MDA-MB-231 breast cancer cells (Bharmoria et al., 2021).

Recently, nanoemulsion was formulated in combination with cisplatin and quercetin as a strategy to reduce oxidative stress responsible for cisplatin induced cytotoxicity. The study demonstrated that the developed nanoemulsion improved the anticancer properties of both the molecules and provided a synergistic effect against MDA-MB-231 breast cancer cells. Antioxidant properties of quercetin improved while cytotoxic effects of cisplatin against human renal HEK-293 cells diminished (Ceramella et al., 2021). Similarly, nanoemulsions of ursolic and oleanic acid improved antioxidant and cytotoxic activities in melanoma cells. Alvarado et al. concluded that ursolic and oleanic acid-based nanoemulsion could be considered as a new potential tool for further investigation as anticancer agents (Alvarado et al., 2018).

4.2.3 INORGANIC NANOFORMULATIONS

Inorganic nanocarriers, such as gold nanoparticles, magnetic nanomaterials, carbon nanotubes, nanosilica, and quantum dots, have been extensively used due to their unique physicochemical properties (Arora & Jaglan, 2016).

4.2.3.1 GOLD NANOPARTICLES (AUNPS)

Gold nanoparticles, like other nano-delivery systems, are also widely studied for their potential in carrying nutraceuticals for treatment and prevention of cancer. Recently, resveratrol conjugated gold nanoparticles were developed. These AuNPs were effective against breast, pancreatic and prostate cancer (Thipe et al., 2019). The apoptotic effects of berberin were enhanced against breast cancer when delivered through AuNP (Chiu et al., 2021). Similarly, the anti-tumor activity of curcumin was greatly enhanced when formulated as AuNPs (Elbialy et al., 2019).

4.2.3.2 CARBON NANOTUBES (CNTS)

Carbon nanotube are tubular network of carbon atoms having diameter approximately 1–4 nm and length approximately 1–100 nm (Arora & Jaglan, 2016). A theoretical study was done for delivery of quercetin as an anticancer agent in carbon nanotubes (Daneshmehr, 2015). Carbon nanotubes for curcumin (Li et al., 2019), berberin (Geto et al., 2013), quercetin (Dolatabadi et al., 2011), etc., but less work has been done with regards to explore the anticancer potential of nutraceuticals when delivered as carbon nanotubes.

4.2.3.3 MAGNETIC NANOPARTICLES

Magnetic nanoparticles have also been demonstrated as interesting nanodelivery systems along with other systems. Magnetic nanoparticles bear magnetic properties and are at nanoscale range. Nostari et al. developed Bovine Serum Albumin (BSA) coated iron oxide magnetic nanoparticles as biocompatible carriers for curcumin-anticancer drug and studied their cytotoxic activity against MCF-7 cancer cells. Results showed significant cytotoxicity against MCF-7 cancer cells (Nosrati et al., 2018). A similar formulation was developed for ovarian cancer (Mancarella et al., 2015). Magnetic nanoparticles developed for resveratrol (Almagro et al., 2020) studied for A549 (Human lung cancer), and LLC (Lewis lung carcinoma) showed enhanced anticancer activity, enhanced *in vitro* release and stability, better tumor reduction and decreased side effects as compared to resveratrol alone (Dai et al., 2017).

4.2.3.4 QUANTUM DOTS (QDS)

Quantum dots are semi-conducting nanocrystals at nanometer scale (2–10 nm in size) with an inorganic core and organic coated shell. They emit fluorescence when stimulated by light (Salama et al., 2020). This unique property of QDs make them useful in the delivery of nutraceuticals. The protective effect of resveratrol-QDs was studied. Results showed resveratrol-QDs were capable of attenuating cell apoptosis and intracellular ROS production in fibroblasts (L929) cells (Wu et al., 2017). Recently, curcumin-QDs have been synthesized to study their potential against several cancers. Curcumin-QDs profoundly inhibited the growth of colon cancer cells (HCT-116) and breast cancer cells (MCF-7) (Khan et al., 2020). QDs have limited studied established for detecting the anticancer potential of nutraceuticals delivered through QDs.

4.3 CONCLUSION

With the growing population worldwide, there is an increase in the prevalence of various diseases among which cancer is the most rapidly growing disease condition. Nowadays, nutraceuticals have received considerable interest due to their safety, nutritional and therapeutic effects. Nutraceuticals seek their application in prophylaxis, cure, and treatment of cancers. However, they have certain limitations, such as poor stability, solubility, bioavailability, absorption, and higher first-pass metabolism, which can be overcome by nanodelivery of nutraceuticals. Various nanotechnological formulations have been used to deliver nutraceuticals to overcome such limitations as well as achieve their potential in cancer. Thorough research has been carried out for use of nanotechnology to deliver nutraceuticals for prevention and treatment of different types of cancers, such as polymer-based nanoformulations, lipid-based nanoformulations, inorganic nanoformulations, etc. These nanoformulations can further be surface functionalized with targeting ligands to achieve site specific targeting. Recently, co-delivery of nutraceuticals and pharmaceuticals (or chemotherapeutic agents) has gained much interest. Although *in vitro* and *in vivo* studies conducted for several nutraceuticals have proved their anticancer potential and other health benefits, their clinical use is yet limited.

KEYWORDS

- **anticancer**
- **breast cancer resistance proteins**
- **chemotherapeutic agents**
- **multi-drug resistance proteins**
- **nanotechnology**

REFERENCES

Ahmed, O. A., El-Bassossy, H. M., El-Sayed, H. M., & El-Hay, S. S. A., (2021). Rp-HPLC determination of quercetin in a novel D-α-tocopherol polyethylene glycol 1000 succinate based SNEDDS formulation: Pharmacokinetics in rat plasma. *Molecules, 26*(5), 1435.

Akhlaghi, M., Shabanian, G., Rafieian-Kopaei, M., Parvin, N., Saadat, M., & Akhlaghi, M., (2011). Citrus aurantium blossom and preoperative anxiety. *Rev. Bras. Anestesiol., 61*, 707–712.

Almagro, L., Gea-Abellán, A. D., Rodríguez-López, M. I., Núñez-Delicado, E., Gabaldón, J. A., & Pedreño, M. A., (2020). A Smart strategy to improve t-resveratrol production in grapevine cells treated with cyclodextrin polymers coated with magnetic nanoparticles. *Polymers, 12*(4), 991.

Alvarado, H. L., Calpena, A. C., Garduno-Ramirez, M. L., Ortiz, R., Melguizo, C., Prados, J. C., & Clares, B., (2018). Nanoemulsion strategy for ursolic and oleanic acids isolates from *Plumeria obtusa* improves antioxidant and cytotoxic activity in melanoma cells. *Anticancer Agents Med Chem (Formerly Current Med Chemistry-Anti-Cancer Agents), 18*(6), 847–853.

Arora, D., & Jaglan, S., (2016). Nanocarriers based delivery of nutraceuticals for cancer prevention and treatment: A review of recent research developments. *Trends Food Sci. & Technol., 54*, 114–126.

Bharmoria, P., Bisht, M., Gomes, M. C., Martins, M., Neves, M. C., Mano, J. F., Bdikin, I., et al., (2021). Protein-olive oil-in-water nanoemulsions as encapsulation materials for curcumin acting as anticancer agent towards MDA-MB-231 cells. *Sci. Rep., 11*(1), 1–12.

Blanco, E., Bey, E. A., Dong, Y., Weinberg, B. D., Sutton, D. M., Boothman, D. A., & Gao, J., (2007). β-lapachone-containing PEG–PLA polymer micelles as novel nanotherapeutics against NQO1-overexpressing tumor cells. *J. Control. Release, 122*(3), 365–374.

Caldeira De, A. L. S., Vinícius, M. N. M., Salviano, T. C., Honorato-Sampaio, K., Tadeu, P. M., Ferreira, L. A. M., Braga, F. C., & Cristina, O. M., (2013). Preparation, physicochemical characterization, and cell viability evaluation of long-circulating and pH-sensitive liposomes containing ursolic acid. *Biomed Res. Int., 2013.*

Cao, Y., Gao, M., Chen, C., Fan, A., Zhang, J., Kong, D., Wang, Z., Peer, D., & Zhao, Y., (2015). Triggered-release polymeric conjugate micelles for on-demand intracellular drug delivery. *Nanotechnology, 26*(11), 115101.

Ceramella, J., Groo, A. C., Iacopetta, D., Séguy, L., Mariconda, A., Puoci, F., Saturnino, C., et al., (2021). A winning strategy to improve the anticancer properties of cisplatin and quercetin based on the nanoemulsions formulation. *J. Drug Deliv. Sci. Technol.*, 102907.

Chauhan, A. S., (2015). Dendrimer nanotechnology for enhanced formulation and controlled delivery of resveratrol. *Ann. N. Y. Acad. Sci., 1348*(1), 134–140.

Chen, R., Wang, S., Zhang, J., Chen, M., & Wang, Y., (2015). Aloe-emodin loaded solid lipid nanoparticles: Formulation design and *in vitro* anticancer study. *Drug Deliv, 22*(5), 666–674.

Chiu, C. F., Fu, R. H., Hsu, S. H., Yu, Y. H., Yang, S. F., Tsao, T. C. Y., Chang, K. B., et al., (2021). Delivery capacity and anticancer ability of the berberine-loaded gold nanoparticles to promote the apoptosis effect in breast cancer. *Cancers (Basel), 13*(21), 5317.

Choudhury, H., Pandey, M., Yin, T. H., Kaur, T., Jia, G. W., Tan, S. Q. L., Weijie, H., et al., (2019). Rising horizon in circumventing multidrug resistance in chemotherapy with nanotechnology. *Mater. Sci. Eng. C, 101*, 596–613.

Coelho, J. F., Ferreira, P. C., Alves, P., Cordeiro, R., Fonseca, A. C., Góis, J. R., & Gil, M. H., (2010). Drug delivery systems: Advanced technologies potentially applicable in personalized treatments. *EPMA Journal, 1*(1), 164–209.

Dai, L., Liu, R., Hu, L. Q., Zou, Z. F., & Si, C. L., (2017). Lignin nanoparticle as a novel green carrier for the efficient delivery of resveratrol. *ACS Sustain. Chem. Eng., 5*, 8241–8249.

Daneshmehr, S., (2015). Carbon nanotubes for delivery of quercetin as anticancer drug: Theoretical study. *Procedia Manuf. Sci., 11*, 131–136.

De Matos, R. P. A., Calmon, M. F., Amantino, C. F., Villa, L. L., Primo, F. L., Tedesco, A. C., & Rahal, P., (2018). Effect of curcumin-nanoemulsion associated with photodynamic therapy in cervical carcinoma cell lines. *Biomed Res. Int., 2018*.

Dolatabadi, J. E. N., Jamali, A. A., Hasanzadeh, M., & Omidi, Y., (2011). Quercetin delivery into cancer cells with single walled carbon nanotubes. *Int. J. Biosci. Biochem. Bioinforma, 1*(1), 21.

Dutta, S., Moses, J. A., & Anandharamakrishnan, C., (2018). Encapsulation of nutraceutical ingredients in liposomes and their potential for cancer treatment. *Nutr. Cancer, 70*(8), 1184–1198.

Elbialy, N. S., Abdelfatah, E. A., & Khalil, W. A., (2019). Antitumor activity of curcumin-green synthesized gold nanoparticles: *In vitro* study. *BioNano Science, 9*(4), 813–820.

Fan, Y., Zhang, Y., Yokoyama, W., & Yi, J., (2017). β-Lactoglobulin–chlorogenic acid conjugate-based nanoparticles for delivery of (−)-epigallocatechin-3-gallate. *RSC Advances, 7*(35), 21366–21374.

Gallien, J., Srinageshwar, B., Gallo, K., Holtgrefe, G., Koneru, S., Otero, P. S., Bueno, C. A., et al., (2021). Curcumin loaded dendrimers specifically reduce viability of glioblastoma cell lines. *Molecules, 26*(19), 6050.

Geto, A., Pita, M., De Lacey, A. L., Tessema, M., & Admassie, S., (2013). Electrochemical determination of berberine at a multi-walled carbon nanotubes-modified glassy carbon electrode. *Sens. Actuators B Chem., 183*, 96–101.

Gharib, A., Faezizadeh, Z., & Godarzee, M., (2015). Preparation and characterization of nanoliposomal beta-cryptoxanthin and its effect on proliferation and apoptosis in human leukemia cell line K562. *Trop. J. Pharm. Res., 14*(2), 187–194.

Halwani, M., Hossain, Z., Khiyami, M. A., & Omri, A., (2015). Liposomal β-glucan: Preparation, characterization and anticancer activities. *J. Nanomed. Nanotechnol., 6*(319), 2.

Huang, D., Lan, H., Liu, F., Wang, S., Chen, X., Jin, K., & Mou, X., (2015). Anti-angiogenesis or pro-angiogenesis for cancer treatment: Focus on drug distribution. *International Journal of Clinical and Experimental Medicine, 8*(6), 8369.

Imran, M., Aslam, G. T., Atif, M., Shahbaz, M., Batool, Q. T., Hanif, M. M., Salehi, B., et al., (2020). Apigenin as an anticancer agent. *Phytother. Res., 34*(8), 1812–1828.

Ishak, R. A., & Osman, R., (2015). Lecithin/TPGS-based spray-dried self-microemulsifying drug delivery systems: *In vitro* pulmonary deposition and cytotoxicity. *Int. J. Pharm., 485*(1, 2), 249–260.

Jain, A., Sharma, G., Thakur, K., Raza, K., Shivhare, U., Ghoshal, G., & Katare, O. P., (2019). Beta-carotene-encapsulated solid lipid nanoparticles (BC-SLNs) as promising vehicle for cancer: An investigative assessment. *AAPS PharmSciTech, 20*(3), 1–7.

Jaisamut, P., Wanna, S., Limsuwan, S., Chusri, S., Wiwattanawongsa, K., & Wiwattanapatapee, R., (2021). Enhanced oral bioavailability and improved biological activities of a quercetin/resveratrol combination using a liquid self-microemulsifying drug delivery system. *Planta Med., 87*(04), 336–346.

Kalra, E. K., (2003). Nutraceutical-definition and introduction. *AAPS Pharmsci., 5*(3), 27–28.

Kanwal, T., Saifullah, S., Ur Rehman, J., Kawish, M., Razzak, A., Maharjan, R., Imran, M., et al., (2021). Design of absorption enhancer containing self-nanoemulsifying drug delivery system (SNEDDS) for curcumin improved anticancer activity and oral bioavailability. *J. Mol. Liq., 324*, 114774.

Kazi, M., Alhajri, A., Alshehri, S. M., Elzayat, E. M., Al Meanazel, O. T., Shakeel, F., Noman, O., et al., (2020). Enhancing oral bioavailability of apigenin using a bioactive self-nanoemulsifying drug delivery system (Bio-SNEDDS): *In vitro, in vivo* and stability evaluations. *Pharmaceutics, 12*(8), 749.

Ke, Z., Zhu, Z., Xu, Z., Fang, C., & Hu, S., (2015). Formulation design and *in vitro* evaluation of berberine-loaded self-nanoemulsifying drug delivery system. *Trop. J. Pharm. Res., 14*(5), 747–752.

Keservani, R. K., Kesharwani, R. K., Sharma, A. K., Vyas, N., & Chadoker, A., (2010b). Nutritional supplements: An overview. *International Journal of Current Pharmaceutical Review and Research, 1*(1), 59–75.

Keservani, R. K., Kesharwani, R. K., Vyas, N., Jain, S., Raghuvanshi, R., & Sharma, A. K., (2010a). Nutraceutical and functional food as future food: A review. *Der Pharmacia Lettre, 2*(1), 106–116.

Keservani, R. K., Sharma, A. K., & Kesharwani, R. K., (2016a). Nutraceutical and functional foods for cardiovascular health. In: *Food Process Engineering* (pp. 257–278, 291–312,). Apple Academic Press. ISBN: 9781771884020.

Keservani, R. K., Sharma, A. K., & Kesharwani, R. K., (2020). *Nutraceuticals and Dietary Supplements: Applications in Health Improvement and Disease Management*. CRC Press. ISBN: 9781771888738.

Khan, F. A., Lammari, N., Muhammad, S. A. S., Alkhater, K. M., Asiri, S., Akhtar, S., Almansour, I., et al., (2020). Quantum dots encapsulated with curcumin inhibit the growth of colon cancer, breast cancer and bacterial cells. *Nanomedicine, 15*(10), 969–980.

Khan, M. N., Haggag, Y. A., Lane, M. E., McCarron, P. A., & Tambuwala, M. M., (2018). Polymeric nano-encapsulation of curcumin enhances its anticancer activity in breast (MDA-MB231) and lung (A549) cancer cells through reduction in expression of HIF-1α and nuclear p65 (REL A). *Curr. Drug. Deliv., 15*(2), 286–295.

Khosravi-Boroujeni, H., Mohammadifard, N., Sarrafzadegan, N., Sajjadi, F., Maghroun, M., Khosravi, A., Alikhasi, H., et al., (2012). Potato consumption and cardiovascular disease risk factors among Iranian population. *Int. J. Food Sci. Nutr., 63*(8), 913–920.

Li, H., Zhang, N., Hao, Y., Wang, Y., Jia, S., & Zhang, H., (2019). Enhancement of curcumin antitumor efficacy and further photothermal ablation of tumor growth by single-walled carbon nanotubes delivery system *in vivo*. *Drug Deliv., 26*(1), 1017–1026.

Liu, J., Yong, H., Yao, X., Hu, H., Yun, D., & Xiao, L., (2019). Recent advances in phenolic–protein conjugates: Synthesis, characterization, biological activities and potential applications. *RSC Advances, 9*(61), 35825–35840.

Liu, Y., Huang, P., Hou, X., Yan, F., Jiang, Z., Shi, J., Xie, X., et al., (2019). Hybrid curcumin–phospholipid complex-near-infrared dye oral drug delivery system to inhibit lung metastasis of breast cancer. *Int. J. Nanomedicine, 14*, 3311.

Logothetidis, S., (2012). *Nanostructured Materials and Their Applications*. Springer Science & Business Media.

Luo, X., Guan, R., Chen, X., Tao, M., Ma, J., & Zhao, J., (2014). Optimization on condition of epigallocatechin-3-gallate (EGCG) nanoliposomes by response surface methodology and cellular uptake studies in Caco-2 cells. *Nanoscale Res. Lett., 9*(1), 1–9.

Maji, I., Mahajan, S., Sriram, A., Medtiya, P., Vasave, R., Khatri, D. K., Kumar, R., et al., (2021). Solid self-emulsifying drug delivery system: Superior mode for oral delivery of hydrophobic cargos. *J. Control. Release*.

Mancarella, S., Greco, V., Baldassarre, F., Vergara, D., Maffia, M., & Leporatti, S., (2015). Polymer-coated magnetic nanoparticles for curcumin delivery to cancer cells. *Macromol. Biosci., 15*(10), 1365–1374.

Nasri, H., (2013). Impact of diabetes mellitus on parathyroid hormone in hemodialysis patients. *J. Parathyr. Dis., 1*(1), 9–11.

Ng, Y. J., Benson, H. A. E., Brown, D. H., & Chen, Y., (2015). Synthesis and characterization of novel copolymeric resveratrol conjugates. *J. Chem., 2015*, 245625.

Nosrati, H., Sefidi, N., Sharafi, A., Danafar, H., & Manjili, H. K., (2018). Bovine serum albumin (BSA) coated iron oxide magnetic nanoparticles as biocompatible carriers for curcumin-anticancer drug. *Bioorg. Chem., 76*, 501–509.

Piermartiri, T., Pan, H., Figueiredo, T. H., & Marini, A. M., (2015). α-Linolenic acid, a nutraceutical with pleiotropic properties that targets endogenous neuroprotective pathways to protect against organophosphate nerve agent-induced neuropathology. *Molecules, 20*(11), 20355–20380.

Radhakrishnan, R., Kulhari, H., Pooja, D., Gudem, S., Bhargava, S., Shukla, R., & Sistla, R., (2016). Encapsulation of biophenolic phytochemical EGCG within lipid nanoparticles enhances its stability and cytotoxicity against cancer. *Chem. Phys. Lipids, 198*, 51–60.

Ramadass, S. K., Anantharaman, N. V., Subramanian, S., Sivasubramanian, S., & Madhan, B., (2015). Paclitaxel/epigallocatechin gallate coloaded liposome: A synergistic delivery to control the invasiveness of MDA-MB-231 breast cancer cells. *Colloids Surf B, 125*, 65–72.

Ramalingam, P., & Ko, Y. T., (2016). Improved oral delivery of resveratrol from N-trimethyl chitosan-g-palmitic acid surface-modified solid lipid nanoparticles. *Colloids Surf B, 139*, 52–61.

Rane, B. R., Bharath, M. S., Patil, R. R., Keservani, R. K., & Jain, A. S., (2020b). Novel approaches in nutraceuticals. In: Rajesh, K. K., Raj, K. K., & Anil, K. S., (eds.), *Enhancing the Therapeutic Efficacy of Herbal Formulations Through Novel Drug Delivery Systems* (pp. 241–266). IGI Global International Publisher, Pennsylvania, USA, Chapter 11. ISBN13: 978179984453.

Rane, B. R., Patil, A. S., Keservani, R. K., & Jain, A. S., (2020a). Novel approaches in herbal formulation. In: Rajesh, K. K., Raj, K. K., & Anil, K. S., (eds.), *Enhancing the Therapeutic Efficacy of Herbal Formulations Through Novel Drug Delivery Systems* (pp. 43–68). IGI Global International Publisher, Pennsylvania, USA, Chapter 2. ISBN13: 9781799844532.

Rane, B. R., Tadavi, S. A., & Keservani, R. K., (2020c). Naturopathy In: Anil, K. S., Raj, K. K., & Surya, P. G., (eds.), *Herbal Product Development* (pp. 321–347). Apple Academic Press, Taylor & Francis Group, Chapter 12. ISBN: 9781771888776.

Salama, L., Pastor, E. R., Stone, T., & Mousa, S. A., (2020). Emerging nanopharmaceuticals and nanonutraceuticals in cancer management. *Biomedicines, 8*(9), 347.

Shahidi, F., (2012). Nutraceuticals, functional foods and dietary supplements in health and disease. *J Food Drug Anal., 20*(1), 226–230.

Shirzad, H., Burton, R., Smart, Y., Rafieian-Kopaei, M., & Shirzad, M., (2011). Natural cytotoxicity of NC-2+ cells against the growth and metastasis of WEHI-164 fibrosarcoma. *Scand. J. Immunol., 73*(2), 85–90.

Song, Q., Li, D., Zhou, Y., Yang, J., Yang, W., Zhou, G., & Wen, J., (2014). Enhanced uptake and transport of (+)-catechin and (−)-epigallocatechin gallate in niosomal formulation by human intestinal Caco-2 cells. *Int. J. Nanomedicine, 9*, 2157.

Sun, Y., Xun, K., Wang, Y., & Chen, X., (2009). A systematic review of the anticancer properties of berberine, a natural product from Chinese herbs. *Anticancer Drugs, 20*(9), 757–769.

Sun, Y., Yu, S. L., Wu, B. Y., Che, Y. X., & Wang, X., (2018). Anti-tumor effect and mechanisms of quercetin self-nanoemulsifying drug delivery system. *Chinese Journal of Experimental Traditional Medical Formulae*.

Surve, D. H., Paul, A. T., & Jindal, A. B., (2019). Nanotechnology based delivery of nutraceuticals. In: Dasgupta, N., Ranjan, S., & Lichtfouse, E., (eds.), *Environmental Nanotechnology* (Vol. 2, pp. 63–107). Cham: Springer International Publishing.

Tang, P., Sun, Q., Yang, H., Tang, B., Pu, H., & Li, H., (2018). Honokiol nanoparticles based on epigallocatechin gallate functionalized chitin to enhance therapeutic effects against liver cancer. *Int. J. Pharm., 545*(1, 2), 74–83.

Teong, B., Lin, C. Y., Chang, S. J., Niu, G. C. C., Yao, C. H., Chen, I. F., & Kuo, S. M., (2015). Enhanced anticancer activity by curcumin-loaded hydrogel nanoparticle derived aggregates on A549 lung adenocarcinoma cells. *J. Mater. Sci. Mater. Med., 26*(1), 49.

Thipe, V. C., Panjtan, A. K., Bloebaum, P., Raphael, K. A., Khoobchandani, M., Katti, K. K., Jurisson, S. S., & Katti, K. V., (2019). Development of resveratrol-conjugated gold nanoparticles: Interrelationship of increased resveratrol corona on anti-tumor efficacy against breast, pancreatic and prostate cancers. *Int. J. Pharm., 14*, 4413–4428.

Trombino, S., Ferrarelli, T., Pellegrino, M., Ricchio, E., Mauro, L., Ando, S., Picci, N., & Cassano, R., (2013). Anticancer activity of a hydrogel containing folic acid towards MCF-7 and MDA-MB-231 cells. *Anticancer Res., 33*(11), 4847–4854.

Trottier, G., Boström, P. J., Lawrentschuk, N., & Fleshner, N. E., (2010). Nutraceuticals and prostate cancer prevention: A current review. *Nat. Rev. Urol., 7*(1), 21–30.

Wang, L., Wang, W., Rui, Z., & Zhou, D., (2016). The effective combination therapy against human osteosarcoma: Doxorubicin plus curcumin co-encapsulated lipid-coated polymeric nanoparticulate drug delivery system. *Drug Deliv., 23*(9), 3200–3208.

Wang, W., Zhang, L., Chen, T., Guo, W., Bao, X., Wang, D., Ren, B., et al., (2017). Anticancer effects of resveratrol-loaded solid lipid nanoparticles on human breast cancer cells. *Molecules, 22*(11), 1814.

Wang, X., Wang, Q., Liu, Z., & Zheng, X., (2017). Preparation, pharmacokinetics and tumor-suppressive activity of berberine liposomes. *J. Pharm. Pharmacol., 69*(6), 625–632.

Wang, Z., Chen, C., Zhang, Q., Gao, M., Zhang, J., Kong, D., & Zhao, Y., (2015). Tuning the architecture of polymeric conjugate to mediate intracellular delivery of pleiotropic curcumin. *Eur. J. Pharm. Biopharm., 90*, 53–62.

Wu, T., Zhan, Q., Zhang, T., Ang, S., Ying, J., He, K., Zhang, S., et al., (2017). The protective effects of resveratrol, H2S and thermotherapy on the cell apoptosis induced by CdTe quantum dots. *Toxicol. in Vitro, 41*, 106–113.

Yee, Y. J., (2018). *Evaluation of Novel Resveratrol Conjugate and Nanoparticle Formulations for Enhanced Anticancer Activity*. Curtin University.

Yousefi, M., Narmani, A., & Jafari, S. M., (2020). Dendrimers as efficient nanocarriers for the protection and delivery of bioactive phytochemicals. *Adv. Colloid Interface Sci., 278*, 102125.

Zhao, T., Liu, Y., Gao, Z., Gao, D., Li, N., Bian, Y., Dai, K., & Liu, Z., (2015). Self-assembly and cytotoxicity study of PEG-modified ursolic acid liposomes. *Mater. Sci. Eng. C., 53*, 196–203.

Zheng, W., Wang, C., Ding, R., Huang, Y., Li, Y., & Lu, Y., (2019). Triptolide-loaded nanoparticles targeting breast cancer *in vivo* with reduced toxicity. *Int. J. Pharm., 572*, 118721.

Zheng, Y., You, X., Guan, S., Huang, J., Wang, L., Zhang, J., & Wu, J., (2019). Poly (ferulic acid) with an anticancer effect as a drug nanocarrier for enhanced colon cancer therapy. *Adv. Funct. Mater., 29*(15), 1808646.

CHAPTER 5

OXIDATIVE STRESS IN CANCER

MUHAMMAD BILAL HUSSAIN,[1] RABIA SHABIR AHMAD,[1]
SADIA HASSAN,[2,3] MARWA WAHEED,[1] and AMNA JAVED[1]

[1]*Department of Food Science, Government College University Faisalabad, Faisalabad, Pakistan*

[2]*Department of Nutritional Sciences, Faculty of Science and Technology, Government College Women University Faisalabad, Faisalabad, Pakistan*

[3]*Department of Dietetics and Nutritional Sciences, The University of Faisalabad, Faisalabad, Pakistan*

ABSTRACT

Free radicals have secured immense importance in biological studies owing to their role in different physiological conditions and their implications in numerous life-threatening maladies. Free radicals including ROS (reactive oxygen species) and RNS (reactive nitrogen species) are derived both from internal sources (endoplasmic reticulum, mitochondria, peroxisomes, etc.) and from external ones (tobacco smoke, alcohol, pollution, heavy metals, etc.). They can severely affect various biological molecules, which are of key importance, such as lipids, proteins, and nucleic acids, resultantly alter the normal redox status of the body causing increased oxidative stress. This condition is believed to be responsible for a disease like neurodegenerative disorder, cardiovascular diseases, diabetes mellitus, and various types of cancers.

Nutraceuticals in Cancer Prevention, Management, and Treatment. Raj K. Keservani, Bui Thanh Tung, Sippy Singh, & Rajesh K. Kesharwani, PhD (Eds.)

5.1 INTRODUCTION

In this era of mechanization, sedentary lifestyle and constant stress have led humanity on the verge of the prevalence of numerous life-threatening ailments, including cardiovascular diseases, diabetes, hypertension, and most significant of all is cancer. Cancer is referred to as an illness triggered by the malignant growth of abnormal cells in any part of the human body. It ranks among the 2nd most significant source of death in developed states and the leading one both in developing and under-developed countries (Ferlay et al., 2012; Mosby et al., 2012). According to the statistics presented by IARC (International Agency for Research on Cancer), every year 10 million fatal cases of this drastic disease have been reported, along with more than a million new cases of the onset of cancer, globally (Torre et al., 2015). Numerous factors which play a crucial role in the onset of cancer include an inactive lifestyle, unhealthy dietary habits, alcohol use, smoking, and oxidative stress (Troselj et al., 2016; Keservani et al., 2020; Rane et al., 2020).

Epidemiological studies have revealed that extra production of ROS (Reactive Oxygen Species) may cause changes in intracellular homeostasis. This could lead to damage to the vital cell components, as the excess of oxidants cannot be neutralized by the antioxidant defense system and/or DNA repair mechanisms (Kruk and Aboul-Enein, 2017). Oxidative stress is mainly instigated by the discrepancy in the redox status of the human body, which is not detoxified by the natural defense system, thus originating huge damage to the cells and tissues. The ROS comprises singlet oxygen ($1O_2$), superoxide anion radical (O_2), hydroxyl radical (OH^-), and hydrogen peroxide (H_2O_2). The main factors contributing towards the production of these ROS include extreme environmental conditions and an unhealthy lifestyle (Pan and Ho, 2008). Prolonged oxidative stress could be responsible for carcinogenesis, by changing the expressions of genes resulting in mutations (Kruk and Aboul-Enein, 2017). ROS can have manifold effects at the initial phase of carcinogenesis, facilitating the activation of carcinogen, damaging the DNA, and also hinder the DNA damage response (DDR) (Waris and Ahsan, 2006). It can disrupt many pathways working in the human body like mitosis, the process of proliferation of cells, which then can cause their wild growth, thus causing carcinogenesis. Elevated levels of oxidative stress can weaken the defense system of the body, operated by antioxidants against catastrophic processes of angiogenesis and metastasis, playing a key role in cancer progression in the human body (Nourazarian et al., 2014).

5.1.1 FREE RADICALS IN OXIDATIVE STRESS

Free radicals play a crucial role in the process of oxidative stress, and they have gathered the great attention of biologists, not only due to their key role in the normal working of numerous physiological functions but also because of their contribution to the onset of many ailments. Free radicals are the products of metabolic processes, which are normally taking place in the human body at the cellular level. They can be defined as the molecules or atoms having one or more electrons in the unpaired condition in the outermost orbit and are having the ability to exist independently. The main reason for the instability of free radicals is the presence of an odd number of electrons, which makes them highly reactive and short-lived. Owing to their reactive nature, they tend to abstract electrons from neighboring compounds, to make themselves stable. This makes the attacked atom lose an electron, having less stability, and thus convert into a free radical. This creates a chain reaction, which results in the disruption of a living cell (Lobo et al., 2010).

Both ROS and RNS can generate free radicals and non-radical components. Both of them play a dual role in the human body, having beneficial and harmful effects, depending upon their concentration. At low or moderate levels, they used to contribute to several bodily functions such as in mitogenic response, in the immune system, in several cellular signaling pathways, and redox regulation (Valko et al., 2007). Contrary to it, the elevated levels of ROS and RNS impart drastic effects on the biomolecules by generating oxidative and nitrosative stress, respectively. This condition arises owing to the lack of balance between higher production of ROS/ RNS, which is not being counteracted by the enzymatic and non-enzymatic antioxidants, generating at a lower rate. Higher levels of ROS can impart detrimental effects on the biomolecules like proteins, lipids, and DNA, which could lead to ailments including rheumatoid arthritis, cardiovascular diseases, neurodegenerative diseases, cataracts, aging, and in diabetes mellitus (Phaniendra et al., 2015).

5.1.1.1 MECHANISM OF FREE RADICALS

Free radicals can start reversible changes due to the decomposition and dissipation reactions as well as their formation with low intensity. Oxygen activation is the factor that determines the increase in the formation of free radicals. The reaction between free radicals and oxygen is predictable because of its presence in the atmosphere and also in the body. The free radicals attack the existing pro-oxidants for which they have an affinity and this action is neutralized by the antioxidants (Molyneux, 2004). The assumption of the aging theory is linked with the reaction of free radicals, which are involved in the modifications triggered by aging. The intrinsic aging process, the disease, and the environment are the factors that are associated with the proposed modifications. Hydroxyl is the most reactive of all oxygen-free radicals which respond to the deoxyribose and the bases of DNA. Through the hypothesis of aging theory, two main concluding points have been achieved on the connection between the maximum life span and DNA deterioration. The oxidative modifications of proteins because of the ROS action could result in the inactivation of proteins as well as membrane enzymes and could also be able to change the structure and destabilize the morphology of cells (Casado et al., 2007; Galloway et al., 2008).

5.1.1.1.1 Physiological Activities of Free Radicals

Free radicals have numerous beneficial functions for human health at low or moderate levels. They are used to manufacture cellular structures and to fight against pathogens through the defense system. Phagocytic cells can synthesize and store free radicals, and in case of invading pathogenic microbes' phagocytic cells are also able to release free radicals to destroy those microbes (Droge, 2002). In patients suffering from granulomatous disease, oxygen reactive species demonstrated their fundamental function for the immune system. Due to the imperfect NADPH oxidase system, these individuals cannot produce O_2. Therefore they are susceptible to various persistent infections (Valko et al., 2007; Droge, 2002).

In the intracellular signaling system, free radicals have a key regulatory function in various cells like cardiac myocytes, endothelial cells, fibroblasts, thyroid tissue, and vascular smooth muscle cells. Free radicals also have their role in the signaling pathway of cellular systems and can be produced through nonphagocytic NADPH oxidase isoforms (Pacher et al., 2007; Halliwell, 2007). Nitric oxide (NO) plays a role as an important free radical in the signaling system including normal neural activity, modulation of proper blood flow, and also in thrombosis. Nitric oxide (NO) is also important for the host defense system, required to eradicate tumor cells and intracellular pathogens and to initiate a mitogenic response (Genestra, 2007).

5.2 METHODS FOR EVALUATION OF OXIDATIVE STRESS

Oxidative stress can be evaluated by different methods like (i) quantification of antioxidants, (ii) measurement of active oxygen species themselves, and

(iii) detection of oxidized DNA and lipids. But detection and measurement of these agents show different issues due to the involvement of a range of substances in the oxidation-reduction reactions (Halliwell, 1998). Additionally, these agents are also entangled through cross-linkage in a complex way. Thus, explanation of the results necessitates the understanding of sample type, sampling location, substances to be evaluated, and method of evaluation. It's not easy and simple to attain exact measurement because the target substances mostly have unstable nature. In 1986, oxidized DNA was detected by using an 8-hydroxydeoxyguanosine assay. This assay is now extensively used due to its simplicity, which originates from high-performance liquid chromatography (Floyd et al., 1986). Different substances have been recommended as markers for oxidative stress like DNA oxides and lipid peroxides. Range of antioxidants including β-carotene, catalase, uric acid, glutathione, superoxide dismutase, vitamins E and C are used as in measurements as markers of redox status. To examine the oxidative stress related to carcinogenesis, for future clinical practice, evaluation of consistent markers of oxidative stress is very essential. Based on the concentration level, antioxidants and free radicals can cause different effects on cells, thus emphasizing the importance of new developments in studies to introduce simple, easy, accurate methods of quantification. It's also important to know that during interpretation of results which substance of the redox system has to be evaluated (Noda and Wakasugi, 2001).

5.2.1 MOLECULAR DAMAGE THROUGH OXIDATIVE STRESS

Set up of oxidative stress originates from an imbalance between antioxidants and oxidants, favoring the production of free radicals. So, the production of free radicals causes oxidation of biomolecules resulting in loss of their biological activities and homeostatic imbalances, which is the probable oxidative damage to cells and tissues. The range of harmful effects (DNA damage, lipid peroxidation, and protein oxidation) can be developed through the accumulation of ROS and RNS (Lushchak, 2014).

5.3 NUCLEIC ACIDS DAMAGE

Nucleic acids like DNA and RNA are not chemically stable and show susceptibility for hydrolysis, oxidation, and nonenzymatic methylation because of being vulnerable to endogenous and exogenous agents. Endogenous factors are mostly produced through lipid peroxidation (aldehydes and estrogen metabolites) and cellular metabolism (reactive oxygen species and reactive nitrogen species) (Ranchoux et al., 2016; Marengo et al., 2016). Hydroxyl radicals and peroxynitrite are the main endogenous oxidants that are responsible for damaging nucleic acids. Mitochondrial respiration is the main cause of reactive oxygen species, through respiration almost five percent of oxygen produces superoxide anion radical by undergoing single electron transfer. The superoxide anion radical is converted into hydrogen peroxide through a superoxide dismutase. Produced hydrogen peroxide further undergoes reduced reaction by catalase or glutathione peroxidase, while it is reduced to hydroxyl radicals in the presence of transition metals. Hydroxyl radicals are very reactive therefore to oxidize DNA or RNA these radicals must be produced close to them. Nitric oxide and superoxide are generated instantaneously in macrophages and both react together to produce peroxynitrite. Oxidation of nucleic acids is also facilitated through a synergic mechanism of RNS to enhance oxidative imbalance. RNS causes inhibition of enzyme FAPY glycosylase involved in DNA repair mechanism to oxidation (De Bont and Van Larebeke, 2004).

DNA structure endures various lesions by oxidative stress such as alteration of nucleotide bases, training sites, breaking single-strand and double strands. Guanine is more vulnerable to oxidative stress among all nucleotide bases; this is due to its lesser potential for reduction (Smith et al., 2013). Mostly considered DNA oxidation marker is 8-hydroxydeoxyguanosine produced by oxidation of guanosine oxidation through hydroxyl radicals. 8-hydroxydeoxyguanosine can pair with adenine and upon replication generate a GC/ TA mutation (De Bont and Van Larebeke, 2004). Likewise, to detect RNA oxidation the homolog 8-hydroxyguanosine is the most appropriate marker. RNA is more susceptible to oxidation than DNA, due to having a cellular location closer to ROS and RNS. Strand breakage, ribosomal dysfunction, and incorrect protein production are the main results of RNA oxidation (Pisoschi and Pop, 2015).

5.3.1 PROTEIN DAMAGE

Protein oxidation can negatively influence backbone fragmentation, side-chain oxidation, and protein folding. All of these reactions can affect the biochemical reactions and thus losing cellular functions. Most easily oxidizable amino acids include cysteines and methionines, but through disulfite reductases activity this oxidation reaction can be reversed. Yet, cysteine can undergo irretrievable oxidation reactions which lead to the formation of S-(2-Succinyl) cysteine and S-carboxymethyl cysteine, resulting in the development of dicarbonyl and fumarate groups which are covalently bound with cysteine residues. Oxidation of arginine, lysine, proline, and threonine produce the carbonyl derivatives used as markers for the measurement of oxidative stress. Aromatic amino acids (tyrosine) on oxidation form various products through interaction with RNS – 3-nitrotyrosine or ROS – dityrosine (Pisoschi and Pop, 2015). These modified oxidized proteins can undergo degradation in the cells or can be accumulated leading to cellular malfunctioning. For example, iron-catalyzed oxidation of lipids and proteins can produce lipofuscin (brown-yellow pigment), this pigment shows resistance for proteolysis reaction, it becomes accumulated in cells and is used as a marker for aging (Aslani and Ghobadi, 2016).

5.3.2 LIPID DAMAGE

Two mediums are involved in lipid peroxidation one is through an enzymatic medium while the other is a non-enzymatic medium. The enzymatically induced method has the involvement of cyclooxygenase and lipoxygenase in the oxidation of fatty acids while the non-enzymatically induced method has the contribution of reactive species oxygen, nitrogen, and transition metals (Ayala et al., 2014). Peroxidation reactions in excess can be very harmful to the cells thus effects of free radicals on lipids cause the formation of lipid hydroperoxides and aldehydes (isoprostanes, 4-hydroxynonenal, and malondialdehyde) contributing to increased cellular toxicity. These produced lipid hydroperoxides and aldehydes can be used in biological samples to detect oxidative stress. Lipid bilayers surround both the cell itself and the membranes of organelles, so lipid peroxidation disturbs the normal functioning and structure of these lipid bilayers. Lipid peroxidation can cause alterations in fluidity, permeability, and transportation of membrane (Morita et al., 2016). The chronic state of this process can influence many chronic diseases such as atherosclerosis, cancer, diabetes, neurodegenerative disorders, and obesity (Lobo et al., 2010; Jarouliya and Keservani 2019).

5.4 CANCER INDUCTION

The process of cancer induction is triggered by a series of different reactions which further involves several molecular and cellular functions that alter the normal cells into malignant neoplastic cells. All these pieces of evidence came through in recent years showed multiple stages and steps in the process of chemical carcinogenesis. In this process, two of the very early steps are initiation that results when a normal cell sustains a DNA mutation followed by a round of DNA synthesis to produce an initiated cell and promotion.

5.4.1 INVOLVEMENT OF DIFFERENT FACTORS

The responsible factors for the production of the initiated mutated cell are physical carcinogens including UV light and radiation, and chemical carcinogens. The genotoxic agent is defined as that includes both physical carcinogens and chemical carcinogens damaging DNA to make mutagenic properties. Faulty repair of damaged DNA can also cause spontaneous mutation of cells. The chemicals as well as endogenous physiological events are directly associated with subsequent selective clonal growth of initiated cells through the progression of tumor promotion. The promotion process does not engross DNA reactivity and damage. However, this phase involves modulation of gene expression resulting in amplified cell numbers processed through cell division and might be due to a decrease in the apoptotic process (Klaunig and Kamendulis, 2007).

5.5 INFLUENCE OF ENVIRONMENTAL AGENTS

The non-DNA reactive carcinogens can produce ROSs by cell metabolism. This process might occur by activating endogenous sources of ROSs. Chlorinated compounds, radiation, barbiturates, and phorbol esters are some classes of compounds involved in oxidative stress and damage. Through research, it has been shown that oxidative stress from chronic inflammation is allied with carcinogenesis (Hwang and Bowen, 2007). In this way, a high incidence of colorectal cancer is associated with ulcerative colitis and gastric cancer with chronic gastritis (Seril et al., 2003; Konturek et al., 2006). In living organisms, DNA damage through oxidative stress is a chief cause of the mutation. The probable frequency of oxidative DNA damage in human cells is 104 lesions per cell per day.

5.6 ANTIOXIDANT DEFENSE SYSTEM

A wide antioxidant variety in the human body is serving to balance the counter-effect of oxidants. For the practical purposes to understand the application, working, and collaboration, antioxidants are divided into two categories which are enzymatic and non-enzymatic division.

5.7 ENZYMATIC DIVISION

The enzymatic antioxidants include superoxide dismutases, catalase, and GSH-Px which fall in major class while heme oxygenase-1 and redox proteins, such as thioredoxins, peroxiredoxins, and glutaredoxins also found to play vital roles in pulmonary antioxidant defenses. The enzymes involved in the redox process played important role in H_2O_2 and lipid hydroperoxides reduction include GSH-Pxs. The tetrameric enzymes family contains GSH-Pxs which have unique amino acid selenocysteine in the active sites. They use low-molecular-weight thiols to reduce H_2O_2 and lipid peroxides for corresponding alcohols. The GSH-Pxsare encoded by various genes including GSHPx- 1 that is cellular GSH-Px (ubiquitous) which reduces H_2O_2 and fatty acid peroxides. The only member of the GSH-Px family, the GSH-Px-3 that is extracellular GSH-Px, known as the most essential extracellular antioxidant enzyme present in mammals and diversely studied in human lungs (Arthur, 2005).

5.8 NON-ENZYMATIC DIVISION

The non-enzymatic antioxidants class includes compounds with low molecular weight for instance vitamin C, vitamin E, and b-carotene. However, uric acid and GSH (glutathione) are also included in this group. Ascorbic acid provides very effective antioxidant capacity by catching antioxidant capacity on a primary basis. It can shift vitamin E free radicals into vitamin E as its level of plasma decreased over age (Mezzetti et al., 1996).

Vitamin E or a-tocopherol, a lipid-soluble vitamin, is concerted in the cell membrane hydrophobic interior site. This system provides principal defense against oxidant-induced membrane injury by donating an electron to peroxyl-radical (generated during lipid peroxidation). The most energetic form of vitamin E is a-tocopherol, which is the membrane-bounded antioxidant in cells and triggers cancer cells towards apoptosis. This process also resists free radical production.

The major soluble antioxidant is glutathione which is highly copious in all cell compartments and played an important role in the determination of oxidative stress in different ways. It has the ability to detoxification of hydrogen peroxide and lipid peroxides through specific action. It can convert vitamin C and E into their active forms (Masella et al. 2005).

5.9 TRANSCRIPTION FACTORS

Different transcription factors are activated and regulated including AP-1, NF-kB, and Sp-1. Carotenoids such as b-carotene, also known as pigments present in plants, also showed vital functionality. They showed antioxidant effects in low oxygen partial pressure (OPP) but might have pro-oxidant effects at higher OPP. Retinoic acids also showed the capacity to regulate transcription factors. Mammary carcinoma cells, retinoic acid receptors showed triggering effects in growth inhibition by bringing cell cycle arrest and apoptosis (Donato and Noy, 2005; Niizuma et al., 2006).

5.10 CONCLUSION

Oxidative stress causes severe injury to cells and induces gene mutation resulting in carcinogenesis involving intracellular signal transduction and transcription factors related to antioxidants. There is an indispensable need to adapt easy and accurate methods to measure oxidative stress in the human body. This approach is indispensable for investigating the association between the human body and disease and the application of the outcome to implement research as clinical practice. However, technology needs to improve for better methods of measurements and construal of more accurate results. A series of complex reactions and interactions involve various substances, carcinogenesis, and tumor-bearing conditions during oxidative stress. Furthermore, novel investigating techniques are anticipated to make the prevention and treatment of cancer in the clinical setting. The molecular alterations, accumulation in the crucial signaling pathways of several organs are linked with postprandial oxidative stress. The oxidative stress and nutrition pathophysiological roles are still indefinable for targeted therapeutic modalities.

KEYWORDS

- **cancer**
- **free radicals**
- **oxidative stress**
- **reactive nitrogen species**
- **reactive oxygen species**

REFERENCES

Arthur, J. R., (2000). The glutathione peroxidases. *Cell Mol. Life Sci., 57*, 1825–1835.

Aslani, B. A., & Ghobadi, S., (2016). Studies on oxidants and antioxidants with a brief glance at their relevance to the immune system. *Life Sci., 146*, 163–173.

Ayala, A., Muñoz, M. F., & Argüelles, S., (2014). Lipid peroxidation: Production, metabolism, and signaling mechanisms of malondialdehyde and 4-hydroxy-2-nonenal. *Oxid. Med. Cell. Longev.*, 1–31.

Casado, M. F., Cecchini, A. L., Simão, A. N., Oliveira, R. D., & Cecchini, R., (2007). Free radical-mediated pre-hemolytic injury in human red blood cells subjected to lead acetate as evaluated by chemiluminescence. *Food Chem. Toxicol., 45*, 945–952.

De Bont, R., & Van, L. N., (2004). Endogenous DNA damage in humans: A review of quantitative data. *Mutagenesis, 19*, 169–185.

Donato, L. J., & Noy, N., (2005). Suppression of mammary carcinoma growth by retinoic acid: Proapoptotic genes are targets for retinoic acid receptor and cellular retinoic acid-binding protein II signaling. *Cancer Res., 65*, 8193–8199.

Droge, W., (2002). Free radicals in the physiological control of cell function. *Physiol. Rev., 82*, 47–95.

Ferlay, J., Soerjomataram, I., Dikshit, R., Eser, S., Mathers, C., Rebelo, M., Parkin, D. M., et al., (2015). Cancer incidence and mortality worldwide: Sources, methods and major patterns in GLOBOCAN 2012. *Int. J. Cancer, 136*, 359–386.

Floyd, R. A., Watson, J. J., Wong, P. K., Altmiller, D. H., & Rickard, R. C., (1986). Hydroxyl free radical adduct of deoxyguanosine: Sensitive detection and mechanisms of formation. *Free Radic. Res. Commun., 1*, 163–172.

Galloway, E., Shin, T., Huber, N., Eismann, T., & Kuboki, S., (2008). Activation of hepatocytes by extracellular heat shock protein 72. *Am. J. Physiol. Cell Physiol., 295*, 514–520.

Genestra, M., (2007). Oxyl radicals, redox-sensitive signaling cascades and antioxidants. *Cell. Sign., 19*, 1807–1819.

Halliwell, B., (1998). Can oxidative DNA damage be used as a biomarker of cancer risk in humans? Problems, resolutions and preliminary results from nutritional supplementation studies. *Free Radic. Res., 29*, 469–486.

Halliwell, B., (2007). Biochemistry of oxidative stress. *Biochem. Soc. Trans., 35*, 1147–1150.

Hwang, E. S., & Bowen, P. E., (2007). DNA damage, a biomarker of carcinogenesis: Its measurement and modulation by diet and environment. *Crit. Rev. Food Sci. Nutr., 47*, 27–50.

Jarouliya, U., & Keservani, R. K., (2019). Pathways leading to child obesity. In: Debasis, B., (ed.), *Global Perspectives on Childhood Obesity: Current Status, Consequences and Prevention* (2nd edn., pp. 137–146). Academic Press, Elsevier, chapter 12. ISBN: 9780128128404.

Keservani, R. K., Sharma, A. K., & Kesharwani, R. K., (2020). *Nutraceuticals and Dietary Supplements: Applications in Health Improvement and Disease Management*. CRC Press. ISBN: 9781771888738.

Klaunig, J. E., & Kamendulis, L. M., (2007). Chapter 8: Chemical carcinogenesis. In: Klaassen, C. D., (ed.), *Casarett & Doull's Toxicology: The Basic Science of Poisons* (7th edn. pp. 329–380). McGraw-Hill, New York.

Konturek, P. C., Konturek, S. J., & Brzozowski, T., (2006). Gastric cancer and helicobacter pylori infection. *J. Physiol. Pharmacol., 57*, 51–65.

Kruk, J., & Aboul-Enein, H. Y., (2017). Reactive oxygen and nitrogen species in carcinogenesis: Implications of oxidative stress on the progression and development of several cancer types. *Mini. Rev. Med. Chem., 17*, 904–919.

Lobo, V., Patil, A., Phatak, A., & Chandra, N., (2010). Free radicals, antioxidants and functional foods: Impact on human health. *Pharmacogn. Rev., 4*, 118.

Lushchak, V. I., (2014). Free radicals, reactive oxygen species, oxidative stress and its classification. *Chem. Biol. Interact., 224*, 164–175.

Marengo, B., Nitti, M., Furfaro, A. L., Colla, R., Ciucis, C. D., Marinari, U. M., & Domenicotti, C., (2016). Redox homeostasis and cellular antioxidant systems: Crucial players in cancer growth and therapy. *Oxid. Med. Cell. Longev*.

Masella, R., Di Benedetto, R., Vari, R., Filesi, C., & Giovannini, C., (2005). Novel mechanisms of natural antioxidant compounds in biological systems: Involvement of glutathione and glutathione-related enzymes. *J. Nutr. Biochem., 16*, 577–586.

Mezzetti, A., Lapenna, D., Romano, F., Costantini, F., & Pierdomenico, S. D., (1996). Systemic oxidative stress and its relationship with age and illness. *J. Am. Geriatr. Soc., 44*, 823–827.

Molyneux, P., (2004). The use of the stable free radical diphenylpicrylhydrazyl (DPPH) for estimating antioxidant activity. *Songklanakarin. J. Sci. Technol., 26*, 211–219.

Morita, M., Naito, Y., Yoshikawa, T., & Niki, E., (2016). Plasma lipid oxidation induced by peroxynitrite, hypochlorite, lipoxygenase and peroxyl radicals and its inhibition by antioxidants as assessed by diphenyl-1-pyrenylphosphine. *Redox. Biology, 8*, 127–135.

Mosby, T. T., Cosgrove, M., Sarkardei, S., Platt, K. L., & Kaina, B., (2012). Nutrition in adult and childhood cancer: Role of carcinogens and anti-carcinogens. *Anticancer Res., 32*, 4171–4192.

Niizuma, H., Nakamura, Y., Ozaki, T., Nakanishi, H., & Ohira, M., (2006). Bcl-2 is a key regulator for the retinoic acid-induced apoptotic cell death in neuroblastoma. *Oncogene, 25*, 5046–5055.

Noda, N., & Wakasugi, H., (2001). Cancer and oxidative stress.*Japan Med. Assoc. J., 44*, 535–539.

Nordberg, J., & Arner, E. J., (2001). Reactive oxygen species, antioxidants, and the mammalian thioredoxin system. *Free Radic. Biol. Med., 31*, 1287–1312.

Nourazarian, A. R., Kangari, P., & Salmaninejad, A., (2014). Roles of oxidative stress in the development and progression of breast cancer. *Asian Pac. J. Cancer Prev., 15*, 4745–4751.

Pacher, P., Beckman, J. S., & Liaudet, L., (2007). Nitric oxide and peroxynitrite in health and disease. *Physiol. Rev., 87*, 315–424.

Pan, M. H., & Ho, C. T., (2008). Chemopreventive effects of natural dietary compounds on cancer development. *Chem. Soc. Rev., 37*, 2558–2574.

Phaniendra, A., Jestadi, D. B., & Periyasamy, L., (2015). Free radicals: Properties, sources, targets, and their implication in various diseases. *Indian J. Clin. Biochem., 30*, 11–26.

Pisoschi, A. M., & Pop, A., (2015). The role of antioxidants in the chemistry of oxidative stress: A review. *Eur. J. Med. Chem., 97*, 55–74.

Ranchoux, B., Meloche, J., Paulin, R., Boucherat, O., Provencher, S., & Bonnet, S., (2016). DNA damage and pulmonary hypertension. *Int. J. Mol. Sci., 17*, 990.

Rane, B. R., & Keservani, R., (2020). Introduction to nutraceuticals and dietary supplements. In: *Nutraceuticals and Dietary Supplements* (pp. 35, 56). Apple Academic Press. ISBN: 9781771888738.

Seril, D. N., Liao, J., Yang, G. Y., & Yang, C. S., (2003). Oxidative stress and ulcerative colitis-associated carcinogenesis: Studies in humans and animal models. *Carcinogenesis, 24*, 353–362.

Smith, J. A., Park, S., Krause, J. S., & Banik, N. L., (2013). Oxidative stress, DNA damage, and the telomeric complex as therapeutic targets in acute neurodegeneration. *Neurochem. Int., 62*, 764–775.

Torre, L. A., Bray, F., Siegel, R. L., Ferlay, J., Lortet-Tieulent, J., & Jemal, A., (2015). Global cancer statistics, 2012. *CA Cancer J. Clin., 65*, 87–108.

Troselj, K. G., Gueraud, F., Glavan, T. M., Pierre, F., & Zarkovic, N., (2016). A review on food-associated carcinogenesis. In: *Food Toxicology* (pp. 35–56). CRC Press: Boca Raton, FL, USA.

Valko, M., Leibfritz, D., Moncol, J., Cronin, M. T., Mazur, M., & Telser, J., (2007). Free radicals and antioxidants in normal physiological functions and human disease. *Int. J. Biochem. Cell Bio., 39*, 44–84.

Waris, G., & Ahsan, H., (2006). Reactive oxygen species: Role in the development of cancer and various chronic conditions. *J. Carcinog., 5*, 1–8.

CHAPTER 6

BREAST CANCER PREVENTION BY NUTRACEUTICALS

BUI THANH TUNG,[1] DANG KIM NGAN,[1] RAJ K. KESERVANI,[2] and BHUSHAN R. RANE[3]

[1]*VNU University of Medicine and Pharmacy, Vietnam National University, Hanoi, Vietnam*

[2]*Faculty of B. Pharmacy, CSM Group of Institutions, Prayagraj, Uttar Pradesh, India*

[3]*Department of Pharmaceutics, Shri D. D. Vispute College of Pharmacy & Research Center, Panvel, Dist Raigad, Maharashtra, India*

ABSTRACT

Breast cancer is not only the leading cancer in women but also one of the three most common cancers worldwide. Breast cancer shares major risk factors with some diseases, such as obesity, metabolic syndrome, and diabetes. Breast cancer initiation potentially involves inflammatory, diet-related pro-oxidative, and procarcinogenic processes, that interact through estrogen metabolism, combined lipid/fatty acid peroxidation, and related DNA- adduct/depurination/mutation formation. The nutritional contributions toward breast cancer prevention have enormous potential, which is reviewed and related to critical stages in the life cycle and their implications for carcinogenic as well as pathometabolic trajectories. In this chapter, we review about diverse nutraceuticals that are used to prevent breast cancer.

Nutraceuticals in Cancer Prevention, Management, and Treatment. Raj K. Keservani, Bui Thanh Tung, Sippy Singh, & Rajesh K. Kesharwani, PhD (Eds.)

6.1 INTRODUCTION

Breast cancer is increasing in prevalence among women worldwide, particularly the postmenopausal women, and in areas where the incidence had previously been low, such as Japan, China, and southern and eastern Europe (Fund and Research, 2007). This epidemiological pattern follows those of other western epidemics, and shares similar risk factors such as cardiovascular disease, obesity, and type 2 diabetes mellitus (T2DM). It is strongly suggested that it is part of the pathometabolic prevalence because it is closely related to western lifestyle patterns. Therefore, a nutritional approach may support to breast cancer prevention.

Among breast cancer cases, 90–95% were because of environmental and lifestyle factors such as diet and obesity contributing ~30–35 and 10–20%, with only 5–10% attributable to genetic defects, respectively (Anand et al., 2008). Many cases, among the 5–10% of genetically based breast cancer cases, were caused by inherited mutations in either the BRCA1 or the BRCA2 genes (Anderson and Badzioch, 1993, Blackwood and Weber, 1998). That is why breast cancer is a disease which can be prevented with major lifestyle changes (Kunnumakara et al., 2008). Over the recent decades, according to the number of cohorts, it showed a marked increase in penetration which possibly reflected increased western reproductive and lifestyle risk factors, including smoking, western diet, over-fatness, and low physical activity (Friebel et al., 2014; Pettapiece-Phillips et al., 2015).

It has been widely studied that nutraceuticals is as a leading factor in the prevention of breast cancer. In spite of the challenges in relating breast cancer risk to consumption of specific nutrients, particularly in the context of a total diet, valuable information has been contributed by many investigators. A wide variety of other dietary factors including total energy, dietary fiber, alcohol, micronutrients, phytochemicals (Keservani and Sharma, 2014), specific foods, and food constituents have been studied in relation to breast cancer. Results of epidemiological studies which related consumption of these dietary factors to breast cancer have increased the knowledge base to provide rationale for various nutritional strategies to contribute to breast cancer prevention (Duncan 2004; Keservani et al., 2010a, 2010b; Keservani and Sharma, 2014).

6.2 MEDICINAL PLANTS USING FOR BREAST CANCER PREVENTION

Nutraceuticals have been shown effective to prevent and reduce breast cancer incidence. Many studies presented the effect of total medicinal plant extracts on breast cancer and to isolate and find out the bioactive compounds. Many compounds are found, including carotenoids, flavonoids, stilbenes, sulfur-containing compounds, and other phenolic compounds (Gosslau and Chen, 2004). They were isolated from medicinal plants such as soya bean, garlic, ginger, and tea (Gosslau and Chen, 2004), particularly brassica vegetables like cauliflower, broccoli, and cabbage (Hanf et al., 2005). Below we summarize some medicinal plants and bioactive compounds are used for breast cancer prevention.

6.2.1 TOMATO

The tomato, a member of the genus *Lycopersicon*, is very important for not only consumption as a fresh crop but also inclusion as a major constituent in many prepared foods. Besides, red tomatoes contain numerous health-promoting ingredients, including antioxidative carotenoids (lycopene, β-carotene, lutein), anthocyanins, phenolic compounds (caffeic acid, chlorogenic acid), and flavonoids (kaempferol, naringenin, quercetin) as well as the vitamins A, B, and C (Dorais et al., 2008) and lectins (De Mejía et al., 2005). Recent epidemiologic studies have shown good correlation between dietary intake of tomato and reduced risk of cancer and cardiovascular diseases (Heber, 2000). Lycopene and β-carotene can induce apoptosis in malignant lymphoblast cells (Müller, Carpenter et al., 2002) as well as prostate cancer cells (Kotake-Nara et al., 2001) at a concentration range of 3 to 30 μM within 24 h. Tomatidine had a weak inhibitory effect on breast (MCF-7), liver (HepG2) cancer cell lines, and no effect on the other cell lines (Friedman et al., 2009). Moreover, preliminary *in vitro* evidence also indicates that cellular proliferation, induced by insulin-like growth factors being potent mitogens, in various cancer cell lines is reduced with lycopene (Levy et al., 1995).

6.2.2 TEA

Tea is known as one of the most popular beverages consumed worldwide, second only to water. It is prepared by pouring boiling or hot water over fresh or cured leaves of *Camellia sinensis*. In Chinese, drinking green tea has been recommended for the prevention of disease. The important naturally occurring compounds in fresh tea leaves are polyphenols, which account for unique flavor as well as its pungency. The four primary polyphenols which account for up to 30% of dry weight of the fresh tea leaves are epigallocatechin gallate (EGCG), epicatechin gallate, epicatechin, and epigallocatechin. Among these four polyphenols, EGG is the most abundant (Graham, 1992). Extensive in vitro research has shown that the green and black tea extracts are possible to prevent breast cancer. Multiple mechanisms which are suggested are involved, including induction of apoptosis (Vergote et al., 2002) and cell cycle arrest (Liang et al., 1999), inhibition of vascular endothelial growth factor (Sartippour et al., 2002), down-regulation of telomerase (Mittal, Pate et al., 2004), and suppression of aromatase activity (Way et al., 2004). Rodents after administration of chemical carcinogens are fed green tea extracts or catechins, which decreased multiplicity and the size of mammary tumors (Hirose et al., 1994, Tanaka et al., 1997). Besides, Black tea extract also has the ability to inhibit tumorigenesis in animal models, including skin (Javed et al., 1998), lung (Yang et al., 1997), colon (Weisburger et al., 1998), esophagus (Morse et al., 1997), and mammary gland (Rogers et al., 1998).

6.2.3 BRASSICA VEGETABLES

It was showed that a large number of potentially anticarcinogenic compounds are present in fruits and vegetables was showed, especially in those belonging to the genus *Brassica* such as turnips, kale, cauliflower, cabbage, and broccoli (Hocman and Biochemistry, 1989, Steinmetz et al., 1991, Block et al., 1992). These cruciferous plants contain high quantities of glucosinolates, and it was shown that hydrolytic products of glucosinolates could delay, prevent, or reverse carcinogenesis which is induced by various chemical compounds. (Fahey et al., 1997; Verhoeven et al., 1997; Conaway et al., 2002). Moreover, in the Brassica plants, dietary indoles present have been shown to be protective against several cancers (Steinmetz et al., 1991). Indole-3-carbinol, which is produced by the myrosinase-mediated hydrolysis of glucobrassicin present, exhibits protective activities in vitro and in vivo, particularly associated with mammary neoplasia (Bradlow et al., 1991; Tiwari et al., 1994; Cover et al., 1998; Rahman et al., 2000). For instance, female C3H/OuJ mice were fed a diet containing indole-3-carbinol, which resulted in a 50% reduction in both spontaneous mammary tumor incidence and multiplicity compared with the untreated control mice (Bradlow et al., 1991). Besides, indole-3-carbinol also inhibited the proliferation of estrogen-responsive (Tiwari et al., 1994) and estrogen-receptor deficient (Cover et al., 1998) human breast cancer cells..

6.2.4 SOY FOOD

For centuries, soy and its products have been a staple in the Asian diet. Soy is consumed in various forms, including dried or green soybeans, tofu (soybean curd), natto (fermented soybeans), miso (fermented soybean paste), okara (tofu lees), kinako (soy flour), soybean sprouts, soymilk, yuba (soy milk skin), and soy sauce. The predominant source of isoflavones is soybeans. Moreover, soy isoflavone compounds are genistein which was first isolated in 1899 (Perkin and Newbury 1899) and the isoflavone glycosides, including genistin and daidzin, which were isolated ≈ 40 years later (Walz, 1931, Walter, 1941). The recognized etiologic association between breast cancer risk and estrogen is the biological plausibility that dietary soy intake can have anticarcinogenic effect on the breast. Soy isoflavones may influence breast cancer development because a favored mechanism is via their affinity and competition with endogenous estrogens as well as other substrates in binding with estrogen receptors. It is shown that genistein was a specific inhibitor of tyrosine protein kinase which is an enzyme frequently overexpressed in cancer cells (Hunter and Cooper, 1985; Ogawara et al., 1986; Akiyama et al., 1987; Akiyama and Ogawara, 1991). Besides, it has also been shown that the antiproliferative, antioxidative, antiangiogenic, and anti-inflammatory properties of soy isoflavones may influence breast cancer risk (Gilani and Anderson 2002).

6.2.5 GARLIC

Garlic (*Allium sativum*) which is grown and consumed worldwide is a member of the *Liliaceae* family. The use of garlic for medicinal purposes can be traced back to ancient times. Among the various components of garlic, organic sulfur compounds (OSCs) are considered to be the main biologically active components. Garlic oil (GO) contains more than 30 OSCs (Wu et al., 2001). Garlic is well known for their anticancerous potential among the dietary products studied (Cooke et al., 2005); Tsubura et al., 2011). Components of garlic exhibit antidiabetic, immune boosting, cardioprotective, antioxidant, and anticancerous functions (Neil and Silagy, 1994; Borek, 2001, Kyo et al., 2001; Lamm and Riggs, 2001; Rowe et al., 2011; Tsubura et al., 2011). Besides, it has been shown that garlic can inhibit the growth of tumors in mice (Perchellet et al., 1990). Moreover, aged garlic extract not only reduced the risk of cancer but also prevented the decline of natural killer cells in patients with advanced cancer (Ishikawa et al., 2006; Tanaka et al., 2006).

Various derivatives of garlic and garlic constituents were shown to inhibit the growth of several cancer cell types (Hirsch et al., 2000; El-Bayoumy et al., 2006; Malki et al., 2009). The effect of various dietary products on morphological differentiation of the breast cancer cell line MCF7 is studied and it found that 2–3 hours of exposure to garlic extract (fresh but not boiled) was sufficient to alter the morphology and arrest the growth of MCF7 cells (Modem et al., 2012).

6.2.6 *GINGER*

Ginger (*Zingiber officinale* Roscoe) has been used as a condiment for centuries worldwide, especially in Asian countries. Ginger has also been used as a herbal medicine (Rane et al., 2020) because it can treat a wide range of disorders such as inflammation, nausea, dyspepsia, pain, vomiting, the common cold and diarrhea (Ali et al., 2008). The biologically active components of ginger are reportedly phenylpropanoid-derived compounds including shogaols and gingerols (Kundu et al., 2009). Shogaols, a dehydrated product of gingerols, are present in larger amounts in dried ginger but exist in fresh ginger at low levels (Jolad et al., 2005). It is studied that 6-shogaols may reduce gastric cancer viability by impairing tubulin polymerization (Ishiguro et al., 2007) and induce apoptosis via activation of caspase and the production of reactive oxygen species in human colorectal carcinoma cells (Pan et al., 2008). Moreover, 6-shogaols has also been reported inhibit effectively the expression of inflammatory mediators, inducible cyclooxygenase-2 and nitric oxide synthase induced by either lipopolysaccharide or phorbol 12-myristate 13-acetate (PMA) (Pan et al., 2008). With highly invasive characteristics, MDA-MB-231 cell line is known as an breast carcinoma cell line while 6- shogaols is the most potent among shogaols which were found to inhibit PMA-induced invasion of MDA-MB-231 cells by reducing MMP-9 activity (Ling et al., 2010).

6.2.7 *CURCUMA ZEDOARIA*

Curcuma zedoaria, a herb that belongs to the Zingiberaceae family. It is used widely, especially in Asia. Because in killing cancer, *Curcuma zedoaria* has active natural occurring compounds, it is used as an alternative medicine for cancer-related diseases (Awang et al., 2010; Hasima et al.,

2010). The mechanism of cell death that is exerted by some compounds of *Curcuma zedoaria* and the cytotoxic components of *Curcuma zedoaria* is reported (Matthes et al., 1980; Shiobara et al., 1985; Matsuda et al., 1998; Jang et al., 2004; Park et al., 2005; Oh et al., 2007; Lobo et al., 2009; Ahmed Hamdi et al., 2010; Widjastuti and Andriani, 2010; Lakshmi et al., 2011; Lu et al., 2012; Kimura et al., 2013; Rahman et al., 2013). Petroleum ether extracts of *Curcuma zedoaria* inhibited MDA-MB-231 cells (Gao et al., 2014). It's shown that *Curcuma zedoaria* can possess several compounds which have antiproliferative effect on four cancer cell lines, including MCF-7, PC-3, Ca Ski, and HT-29. Two compounds of *Curcuma zedoaria* which are curcumenone and curcumenol can induce apoptosis in MCF-7 cells because they can inhibit the proliferation of the cancer cells (Hamdi et al., 2014). In Indonesia, *Curcuma zedoaria* is consumed for the treatment of cervical and breast cancers in the form of "jamu" (Widjastuti and Andriani, 2010).

6.3 BIOACTIVE COMPOUNDS FROM THE MEDICINAL PLANT FOR BREAST CANCER PREVENTION

6.3.1 *LYCOPENE*

Lycopene is the precursor of β-carotene. Lycopene and beta-carotene widely distributed in fruits and vegetables are carotenoids with potential anticancer activity (Gloria et al., 2014). They can induce apoptosis in prostate cancer cells (Gosslau and Chen, 2004). Similarly, consumption of lycopene reducing the risk of breast cancer is suggested in several reports (Aune et al., 2012; Eliassen et al., 2012; Tanaka et al., 2012). It was investigated about the cellular and molecular mechanisms of lycopene against three human breast cancer cell lines by the growth-inhibitory activity (Takeshima et al., 2014). It was shown that cell proliferation in mcf-7 human breast cancer cells is inhibited by lycopene but in the mcf-10 mammary epithelial cells is not (Uppala et al., 2013; Figure 6.1).

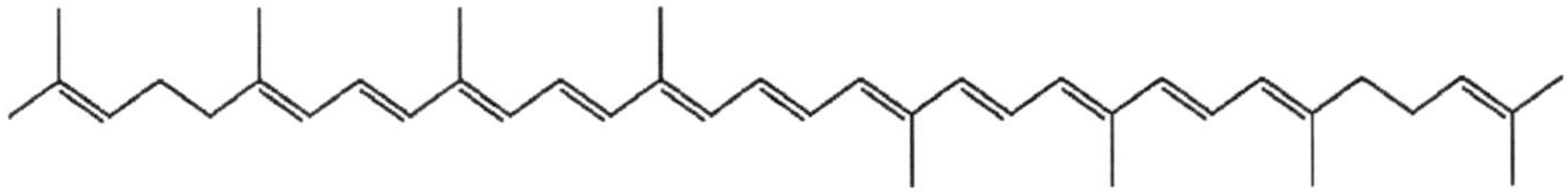

FIGURE 6.1 Structure of lycopenen.

6.3.2 FLAVONOIDS

Flavonoids are a group of many polyphenolic compounds which are naturally present in foods of plant origin. These compounds possess a common phenyl-benzopyrone structure (C6-C3-C6), and they are categorized according to the saturation level and opening of the central pyran ring, mainly into flavones, flavonols, isoflavones, flavonols, flavanone, and flavanonols (Yang et al., 2001). Recently, a case-control study from 2007 to 2018 which analyzed 1,522 breast cancer cases in Chinese women and 1547 matched control subjects shown an inverse correlation between the consumption of total flavonoids, proanthocyanidins, anthocyanidins, flavanones, flavones, flavonols, and isoflavones and the risk of breast cancer (Feng et al., 2019). Another case study in the USA, which used a total of 1434 breast cancer patients and 1440 control patients, demonstrated that the risk of breast cancer in postmenopausal women was reduced by the intake of all flavonoids except anthocyanidins, flavanones, and isoflavones (Fink et al., 2007). Besides, in a large meta-analysis, the dose of isoflavone is shown to be a critical factor for its effect in reducing breast cancer risk. This study indicated that breast cancer risk was decreased by 3% (95% CI 1–5%) by a higher amount of daily soy consumption, approximately 10 mg/day. Last but not least, another recent meta-analysis also shown that breast cancer mortality by 9% was reduced by a daily consumption of 10 mg/day of soy isoflavones (Nachvak et al., 2019; Figure 6.2).

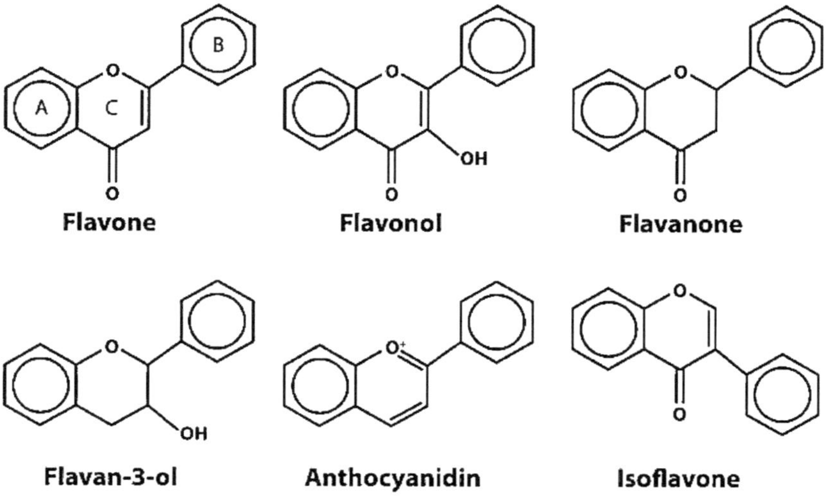

FIGURE 6.2 Structure of flavonoids.

6.3.3 RESVERATROL

Resveratrol (3,5,4-trihydroxy-trans-stilbene), a phytoalexin present in grapes, peanuts, and pines, has antioxidant and anti-inflammatory activities (Jeandet et al., 1991). Moreover, its potential as a cancer chemopreventive agent has been extensively reviewed recently (Gusman et al., 2001; Bhat and Pezzuto, 2002; Savouret et al., 2002; Aziz et al., 2003). *In vitro*, resveratrol induces apoptosis and inhibits the growth of various human tumor cells, including oral squamous carcinoma (Elattar and Virji, 1999), promyelocytic leukemia (Surh et al., 1999), human breast cancer cells (Lu and Serrero, 1999), prostate cancer cells (Hsieh and Wu, 1999; Narayanan et al., 2003), esophageal carcinoma cells (Zhou et al., 2003), pancreatic cancer cells (Ding and Adrian, 2002) and monocytic leukemia cells (Tsan et al., 2000). It has been shown that in human breast cancer cells, resveratrol has a crucial role in apoptosis induction (Pozo-Guisado et al., 2005; Alkhalaf et al., 2008; Figure 6.3).

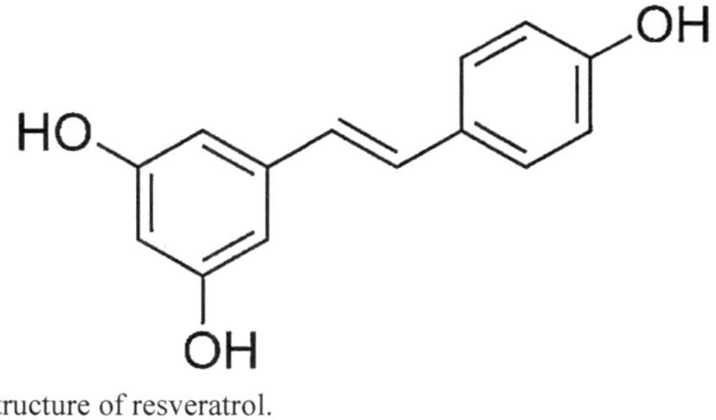

FIGURE 6.3 Structure of resveratrol.

6.3.4 SULFUR-CONTAINING COMPOUNDS

The allyl-sulfur compounds derived from garlic have significant antiproliferative activity against human cancers (Knowles and Milner, 2001; Pinto and Rivlin, 2001). Diallyl sulfide (DAS), diallyl trisulfide (DATS), and diallyl disulfide (DADS) induce apoptosis in non–small cell lung cancer cells (Hong et al., 2000) and in prostate cancer and breast cancer cells (Pinto and Rivlin, 2001). Another garlic component, Z-ajonene, also induces apoptosis of HL-60 cells (Li et al., 2002). Edible Brassica plants (e.g., broccoli and cauliflower) contain substantial amounts of glucosinolates, which are converted into isothiocyanates such as sulforaphane. Animal studies have suggested that isothiocyanates have cancer chemopreventive activity (Hecht, 1995). Whereas no significant effects of garlic as well as its constituents on estradiol metabolism have been reported, it has been observed that a synthetic estrogen known to increase mammary cancer in animal models. Diethylstilbestrol is able to increase lipid hydroperoxides in mammary tissue, which is a part of the effects of diethylstilbestrol on breast cancer risk. Recent studies have demonstrated that the reduction of reactive oxygen species related to a depression in DNA adducts and this increase in them can be attenuated by providing DAS in the diet (Green et al., 2003; Figure 6.4).

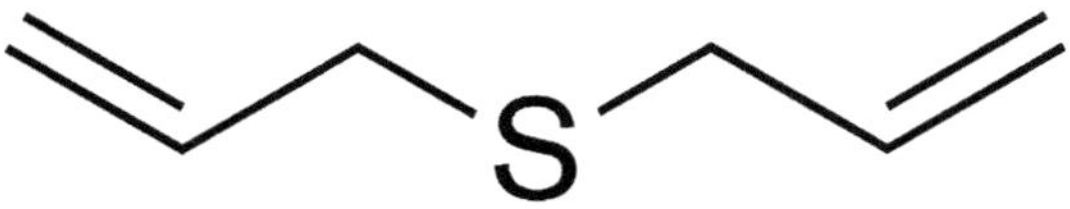

Diallyl sulfide

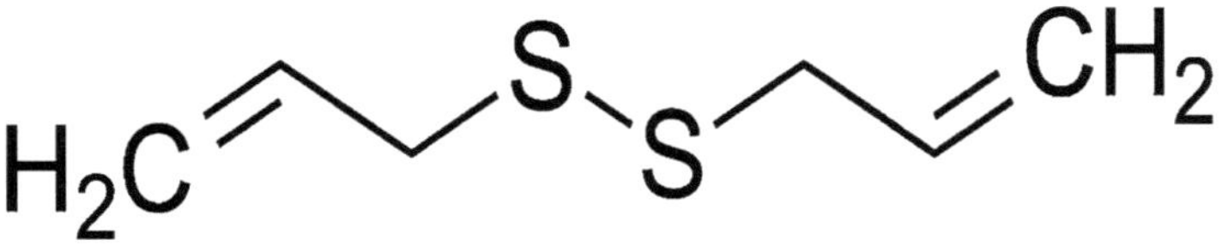

Diallyl disulfide

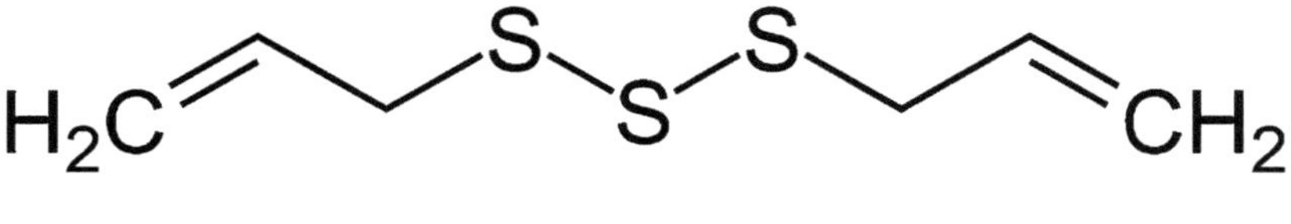

Diallyl trisulfide

FIGURE 6.4 Structure of sulfur-containing compounds.

6.3.5 CAFFEIC ACID PHENETHYL ESTER

Caffeic acid phenethyl ester is an active phenolic component extracted from honeybee propolis (Huang et al., 1996). The NF-κB nuclear factor in breast cancer has been shown its activation and consequent overexpression of anti-apoptotic genes (Bhat-Nakshatri et al., 2002; Lawrence, 2009; Scimeca et al., 2016). CAPE (phenethyl ester of caffeic acid) acts as a specific inhibitor of NF-κB in breast cancer cells (Natarajan et al., 1996; Watabe et al., 2004;

Onori et al., 2009). Moreover, research studies of breast cancer have shown MCF-7 and MDA-231 breast cancer cells was affected by CAPE but healthy cells was not while CAPE is known as an inhibitor of FGF-2 (fibroblasts growth factor type 2), which is a factor of tumor growth. (Wu et al., 2011; Rzepecka-Stojko et al., 2015; Figure 6.5).

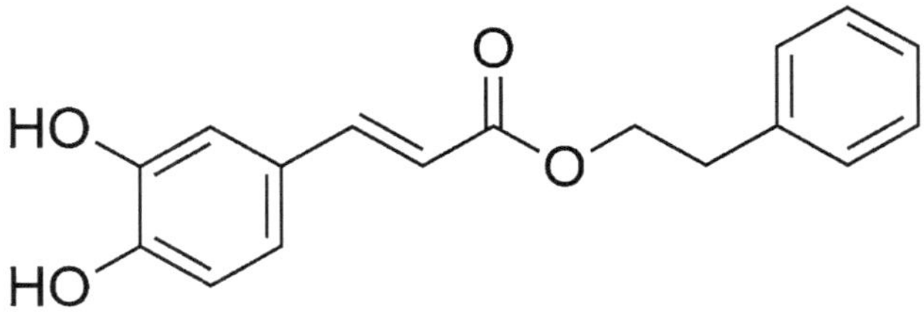

FIGURE 6.5 Structure of caffeic acid phenethyl ester.

6.3.6 *CURCUMIN*

Curcumin, a diferuloylmethane, is a major active polyphenolic component of the food flavor turmeric (Curcuma longa) (Huang et al., 1997). Curcumin could induce apoptosis in most, but not all, breast cancer cell lines by inducing changes in cell membrane potential (Karunagaran et al., 2005). It has been established that apoptosis in tumor cells via a p53-dependent pathway is induced by curcumin after using p53-null mutant or a stable transfectant whose p53 expression is under tight tetracycline control (Choudhuri et al., 2002). Moreover, curcumin may reverse the resistance of breast cancer stem cells to Mitomycin C. Thus, curcumin could improve the therapeutic effect of current breast cancer therapies because it can not only sensitize breast cancer cells but also provide a novel approach for cancer therapy (Zhou et al., 2015). Curcumin could inhibit tumor formation by BCSCs that have successfully migrated from breast tissues to reattach to other organs, such as the lungs, bones, or liver (Charpentier et al., 2014; Figure 6.6).

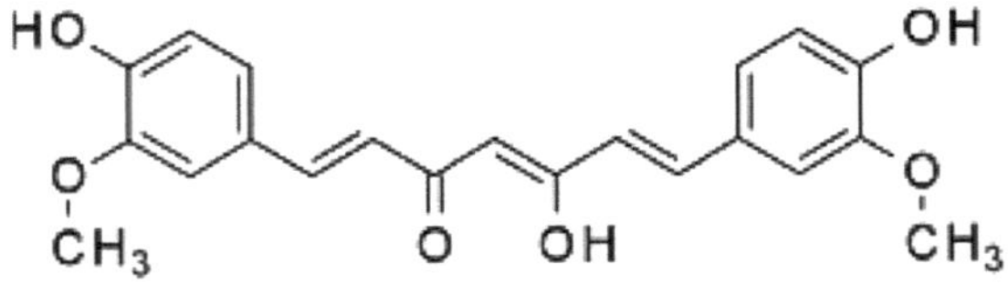

FIGURE 6.6 Structure of curcumin.

6.4 CONCLUSION

Many medicinal plants have been shown may be applied to reduce signals and towards the treatment of breast cancer. Currently, the use of nutraceuticals in breast cancer prevention is a potential and effective method with fewer side effects than other methods. Moreover, the source of herbs, as well as herbal compounds, is extremely abundant. That is why further research on breast cancer prevention by nutraceuticals is necessary.

KEYWORDS

- **tomato**
- **ginger**
- **tea**
- **soy food**
- **breast cancer**

REFERENCES

Ahmed, H. O., Awang, K., Hadi, A. H. A., Syamsir, D. R., & Ng, S. W. (2010). *Curcumenol from Curcuma Zedoaria: A Second Monoclinic Modification, 66*(11), o2844.

Akiyama, T., & Ogawara, H. (1991). *Use and Specificity of Genistein as Inhibitor of Protein-Tyrosine Kinases, 201,* 362–370.

Akiyama, T., Ishida, J., Nakagawa, S., Ogawara, H., Watanabe, S. I., Itoh, N., Shibuya, M., & Fukami, Y. (1987). *Genistein, a Specific Inhibitor of Tyrosine-Specific Protein Kinases, 262*(12), 5592–5595.

Ali, B. H., Blunden, G., Tanira, M. O., Nemmar, A., & Toxicology, J. (2008). *Some Phytochemical, Pharmacological and Toxicological Properties of Ginger (Zingiber officinale Roscoe): A Review of Recent Research, 46*(2), 409–420.

Alkhalaf, M., El-Mowafy, A., Renno, W., Rachid, O., Ali, A., & Al-Attyiah, R. J. (2008). *Resveratrol-Induced Apoptosis in Human Breast Cancer Cells is Mediated Primarily Through the Caspase-3-Dependent Pathway, 39*(2), 162–168.

Anand, P., Kunnumakara, A. B., Sundaram, C., Harikumar, K. B., Tharakan, S. T., Lai, O. S., Sung, B., & Aggarwal, B. B., (2008). *Cancer is a Preventable Disease that Requires Major Lifestyle Changes, 25*(9), 2097–2116.

Anderson, D. E., & Badzioch, M. D., (1993). *Familial Breast Cancer Risks. Effects of Prostate and Other Cancers, 72*(1), 114–119.

Aune, D., Chan, D., Vieira, A., Rosenblatt, D. N., Vieira, R., Greenwood, D., & Norat, T., (2012). *Fruits, Vegetables and Breast Cancer Risk: A Systematic Review and Meta-Analysis of Prospective Studies, 134*(2), 479–493.

Awang, K., Nurul, A. M. N., Lian, A. L. I., Nazif, A. A. N., H. Ibrahim, H., & Hasima, N. N., (2010). *The Apoptotic Effect of 1's-1'-Acetoxychavicol Acetate from Alpinia Conchigera on Human Cancer Cells, 15*(11), 8048–8059.

Aziz, M. H., Kumar, R., & Ahmad, N. J. (2003). *Cancer Chemoprevention by Resveratrol: In Vitro and In Vivo Studies and the Underlying Mechanisms, 23*(1), 17–28.

Bhat, K. P., & Pezzuto, J. M. (2002). *Cancer Chemopreventive Activity of Resveratrol, 957*(1), 210–229.

Bhat-Nakshatri, P., Sweeney, C. J., & Nakshatri, H. J. O., (2002). *Identification of Signal Transduction Pathways Involved in Constitutive NF-κB Activation in Breast Cancer Cells, 21*(13), 2066–2078.

Blackwood, M. A., & Weber, B. L. (1998). *BRCA1 and BRCA2: From Molecular Genetics to Clinical Medicine, 16*(5), 1969–1977.

Block, G., Patterson, B., Subar, A., & Cancer, J. N. (1992). *Fruit, Vegetables, and Cancer Prevention: A Review of the Epidemiological Evidence, 18*(1), 1–29.

Borek, C. (2001). *Antioxidant Health Effects of Aged Garlic Extract, 131*(3), 1010S–1015S.

Bradlow, H. L., Michnovicz, J. J., Telang, N. T., & Osborne, M. (1991). *Effects of Dietary Indole-3-Carbinol on Estradiol Metabolism and Spontaneous Mammary Tumors in Mice, 12*(9), 1571–1574.

Charpentier, M. S., Whipple, R. A., Vitolo, M. I., Boggs, A. E., Slovic, J., Thompson, K. N., Bhandary, L., & Martin, S. (2014). *Curcumin Targets Breast Cancer Stem–Like Cells with Microtentacles that Persist in Mammospheres and Promote Reattachment, 74*(4), 1250–1260.

Choudhuri, T., Pal, S., Agwarwal, M. L., Das, T., & Sa, G. (2002). *Curcumin Induces Apoptosis in Human Breast Cancer Cells Through p53-Dependent Bax Induction, 512*(1–3), 334–340.

Conaway, C., Yang, Y., & Chung, F. (2002). *Isothiocyanates as Cancer Chemopreventive Agents: Their Biological Activities and Metabolism in Rodents and Humans, 3*(3), 233–255.

Cooke, D., Steward, W. P., Gescher, A. J., & Marczylo, T. (2005). *Anthocyans from Fruits and Vegetables–Does Bright Color Signal Cancer Chemopreventive Activity? 41*(13), 1931–1940.

Cover, C. M., Hsieh, S. J., Tran, S. H., Hallden, G., Kim, G. S., Bjeldanes, L. F., & Firestone, G. (1998). *Indole-3-Carbinol Inhibits the Expression of Cyclin-Dependent Kinase-6 and Induces a G1 Cell Cycle Arrest of Human Breast Cancer Cells Independent of Estrogen Receptor Signaling, 273*(7), 3838–3847.

De Mejía, E. G., & Prisecaru, V. I., (2005). *Lectins as Bioactive Plant Proteins: A Potential in Cancer Treatment, 45*(6), 425–445.

Ding, X. Z., & Adrian, T. E., (2002). *Resveratrol Inhibits Proliferation and Induces Apoptosis in Human Pancreatic Cancer Cells, 25*(4), e71–e76.

Dorais, M., & Ehret, D. L., (2008). *Tomato (Solanum lycopersicum) Health Components: From the Seed to the Consumer, 7*(2), 231.

Duncan, A. M., (2004). *The Role of Nutrition in the Prevention of Breast Cancer, 15*(1), 119–135.

Elattar, T., & Virji, A., (1999). *The Effect of Red Wine and its Components on Growth and Proliferation of Human Oral Squamous Carcinoma Cells, 19*(6B), 5407–5414.

El-Bayoumy, K., Sinha, R., Pinto, J. T., & Rivlin, R. S., (2006). *Cancer Chemoprevention by Garlic and Garlic-Containing Sulfur and Selenium Compounds, 136*(3), 864S-869S.

Eliassen, A. H., Hendrickson, S. J., Brinton, L. A., Buring, J. E., Campos, H., Dai, Q., Dorgan, J. F., Franke, A. A., Gao, Y. T., & Goodman, M. T., (2012). *Circulating Carotenoids and Risk of Breast Cancer: Pooled Analysis of Eight Prospective Studies, 104*(24), 1905–1916.

Fahey, J. W., Zhang, Y., & Talalay, P., (1997). *Broccoli Sprouts: An Exceptionally Rich Source of Inducers of Enzymes That Protect Against Chemical Carcinogens, 94*(19), 10367–10372.

Feng, X. L., Ho, S. C., Mo, X. F., Lin, F. Y., Zhang, N.-Q., Luo, H., Zhang, X., & Zhang, C. X., (2019). *Association Between Flavonoids, Flavonoid Subclasses Intake and Breast Cancer Risk: A Case-Control Study in China, 29*(6), 493–500.

Fink, B. N., Steck, S. E., Wolff, M. S., Britton, J. A., Kabat, G. C., Schroeder, J. C., Teitelbaum, S. L., Neugut, A. I., & Gammon, M. D., (2007). *Dietary Flavonoid Intake and Breast Cancer Risk Among Women on Long Island, 165*(5), 514–523.

Friebel, T. M., Domchek, S. M., & Rebbeck, T. R., (2014). *Modifiers of Cancer Risk in BRCA1 and BRCA2 Mutation Carriers: A Systematic Review and Meta-Analysis, 106*(6), dju091.

Friedman, M., Levin, C. E., Lee, S. U., Kim, H. J., Lee, I. S., Byun, J. O., & Kozukue, N., (2009). *Tomatine-Containing Green Tomato Extracts Inhibit Growth of Human Breast, Colon, Liver, and Stomach Cancer Cells, 57*(13), 5727–5733.

Fund, W. C. R., (2007). *Food, Nutrition, Physical Activity, and the Prevention of Cancer: A Global Perspective.* Amer Inst for Cancer Research.

Gao, X. F., Li, Q. L., Li, H. L., Zhang, H. Y., Su, J. Y., Wang, B., Liu, P., & Zhang, A. Q., (2014). *Extracts from Curcuma Zedoaria Inhibit Proliferation of Human Breast Cancer Cell MDA-MB-231 in Vitro.*

Gilani, G. S., & Anderson, J. J., (2002). *Phytoestrogens and Health.* The American Oil Chemists Society.

Gloria, N. F., Soares, N., Brand, C., Oliveira, F. L., Borojevic, R., & Teodoro, A. J., (2014). *Lycopene and Beta-Carotene Induce Cell-Cycle Arrest and Apoptosis in Human Breast Cancer Cell Lines, 34*(3), 1377–1386.

Gosslau, A., & Chen, K. Y., (2004). *Nutraceuticals, Apoptosis, and Disease Prevention, 20*(1), 95.

Graham, H. N., (1992). *Green Tea Composition, Consumption, and Polyphenol Chemistry, 21*(3), 334–350.

Green, M., Thomas, R., Gued, L., & Sadrud-Din, S., (2003). *Inhibition of DES-Induced DNA Adducts by Diallyl Sulfide: Implications in Liver Cancer Prevention, 10*(3), 767–771.

Gusman, J., Malonne, H., & Atassi, G., (2001). *A Reappraisal of the Potential Chemopreventive and Chemotherapeutic Properties of Resveratrol, 22*(8), 1111–1117.

Hamdi, O. A. A., Rahman, S. N. S. A., Awang, K., Wahab, N. A., Looi, C. Y., Thomas, N. F., & Abd, M. S., (2014). *Cytotoxic Constituents from the Rhizomes of Curcuma Zedoaria.*

Hanf, V., & Gonder, U., (2005). *Nutrition and Primary Prevention of Breast Cancer: Foods, Nutrients and Breast Cancer Risk, 123*(2), 139–149.

Hasima, N., Aun, L. I. L., Azmi, M. N., Aziz, A. N., Thirthagiri, E., Ibrahim, H., & Awang, K., (2010). *1′ S-1′-Acetoxyeugenol Acetate: A New Chemotherapeutic Natural Compound Against MCF-7 Human Breast Cancer Cells, 17*(12), 935–939.

Heber, D., (2000). *Colorful Cancer Prevention: A-Carotene, Lycopene, and Lung Cancer.* Oxford University Press.

Hecht, S. S., (1995). *Chemoprevention by Isothiocyanates, 59*(S22), 195–209.

Hirose, M., Hoshiya, T., Akagi, K., Futakuchi, M., & Ito, N., (1994). Inhibition of mammary gland carcinogenesis by green tea catechins and other naturally occurring antioxidants in female sprague-dawley rats pretreated with 7, 12-dimethylbenz [a] *Anthracene, 83*(1, 2), 149–156.

Hirsch, K., Danilenko, M., Giat, J., Miron, T., Rabinkov, A., Wilchek, M., Mirelman, D., Levy, J., & Sharoni, Y., (2000). *Effect of Purified Allicin, the Major Ingredient of Freshly Crushed Garlic, on Cancer Cell Proliferation, 38*(2), 245–254.

Hocman, G. J. C. B., (1989). *Prevention of Cancer: Vegetables and Plants, 93*(2), 201–212.

Hong, Y. S., Ham, Y. A., Choi, J. H., & Kim, J., (2000). *Effects of Allyl Sulfur Compounds and Garlic Extract on the Expression of Bcl-2, Bax, and p53 in Non-Small Cell Lung Cancer Cell Lines, 32*(3), 127–134.

Hsieh, T. C., & Wu, J. M., (1999). *Differential Effects on Growth, Cell Cycle Arrest, and Induction of Apoptosis by Resveratrol in Human Prostate Cancer Cell Lines, 249*(1), 109–115.

Huang, M. T., Ma, W., Yen, P., Xie, J. G., Han, J., Frenkel, K., Grunberger, D., & Conney, A. H., (1996). *Inhibitory Effects of Caffeic Acid Phenethyl Ester (CAPE) on 12-O-Tetradecanoylphorbol-13-Acetate-Induced Tumor Promotion in Mouse Skin and the Synthesis of DNA, RNA and Protein in HeLa Cells.*

Huang, M. T., Newmark, H. L., & Frenkel, K., (1997). *Inhibitory Effects of Curcumin on Tumorigenesis in Mice, 67*(S27), 26–34.

Hunter, T., (1985). *Protein-Tyrosine Kinases, 54*(1), 897–930.

Ishiguro, K., Ando, T., Maeda, O., Ohmiya, N., Niwa, Y., Kadomatsu, K., & Goto, H. J. B., (2007). *Ginger Ingredients Reduce Viability of Gastric Cancer Cells Via Distinct Mechanisms, 362*(1), 218–223.

Ishikawa, H., Saeki, T., Otani, T., Suzuki, T., Shimozuma, K., Nishino, H., Fukuda, S., & Morimoto, K., (2006). *Aged Garlic Extract Prevents a Decline of NK Cell Number and Activity in Patients with Advanced Cancer, 136*(3), 816S–820S.

Jang, M. K., Lee, H. J., Kim, J. S., & Ryu, J. H., (2004). *A Curcuminoid and Two Sesquiterpenoids from Curcuma zedoaria as Inhibitors of Nitric Oxide Synthesis in Activated Macrophages, 27*(12), 1220–1225.

Javed, S., Mehrotra, N., & Shukla, Y., (1998). *Chemopreventive Effects of Black Tea Polyphenols in Mouse Skin Model of Carcinogenesis, 11*(4), 307–313.

Jeandet, P., & Bessis, R., (1991). *The Production of Resveratrol (3, 5, 4'-Trihydroxystilbene) by Grape Berries in Different Developmental Stages, 42*(1), 41–46.

Jolad, S. D., Lantz, R. C., Chen, G. J., Bates, R. B., & Timmermann, B. N., (2005). *Commercially Processed Dry Ginger (Zingiber Officinale): Composition and Effects on LPS-Stimulated PGE2 Production, 66*(13), 1614–1635.

Karunagaran, D., Rashmi, R., & Kumar, T., (2005). *Induction of Apoptosis by Curcumin and its Implications for Cancer Therapy, 5*(2), 117–129.

Keservani, R. K., & Sharma, A. K., (2014). Flavonoids: Emerging trends and potential health benefits. *Journal of Chinese Pharmaceutical Sciences, 23*(12), 815.

Keservani, R. K., Kesharwani, R. K., Sharma, A. K., Vyas, N., & Chadoker, A., (2010b). Nutritional supplements: An overview. *International Journal of Current Pharmaceutical Review and Research, 1*(1), 59–75.

Keservani, R. K., Kesharwani, R. K., Vyas, N., Jain, S., Raghuvanshi, R., & Sharma, A. K., (2010a). Nutraceutical and functional food as future food: A review. *Der Pharmacia Lettre, 2*(1), 106–116.

Kimura, Y., Sumiyoshi, M., & Tamaki, T. J. F., (2013). *Effects of the Extracts and an Active Compound Curcumenone Isolated from Curcuma Zedoaria Rhizomes on Alcohol-Induced Drunkenness in Mice, 84*, 163–169.

Knowles, L. M., & Milner, J. A., (2001). *Possible Mechanism by which Allyl Sulfides Suppress Neoplastic Cell Proliferation, 131*(3), 1061S–1066S.

Kotake-Nara, E., Kushiro, M., Zhang, H., Sugawara, T., Miyashita, K., & Nagao, A., (2001). *Carotenoids Affect Proliferation of Human Prostate Cancer Cells, 131*(12), 3303–3306.

Kundu, J. K., Na, H. K., & Surh, Y. J., (2009). *Ginger-Derived Phenolic Substances with Cancer Preventive and Therapeutic Potential, 61*, 182–192.

Kyo, E., Uda, N., Kasuga, S., & Itakura, Y., (2001). *Immunomodulatory Effects of Aged Garlic Extract, 131*(3), 1075S–1079S.

Lakshmi, S., Padmaja, G., & Remani, P., (2011). *Antitumor Effects of Isocurcumenol Isolated from Curcuma Zedoaria Rhizomes on Human and Murine Cancer Cells.*

Lamm, D. L., Riggs, D. R., & (2001). *Enhanced Immunocompetence by Garlic: Role in Bladder Cancer and Other Malignancies, 131*(3), 1067S–1070S.

Lawrence, T., (2009). *The Nuclear Factor NF-κB Pathway in Inflammation, 1*(6), a001651.

Levy, J., Bosin, E., Feldman, B., Giat, Y., Miinster, A., Danilenko, M., & Sharoni, Y., (1995). *Lycopene is a More Potent Inhibitor of Human Cancer Cell Proliferation Than Either α-Carotene or β-Carotene.*

Li, M., Min, J. M., Cui, J. R., Zhang, L. H., Wang, K., Valette, A., Davrinche, C., Wright, M., Leung-Tack, J., & J. N. and cancer, (2002). *Z-Ajoene Induces Apoptosis of HL-60 Cells: Involvement of Bcl-2 Cleavage, 42*(2), 241–247.

Liang, Y. C., Lin-Shiau, S. Y., Chen, C. F., & Lin, J. K., (1999). *Inhibition of Cyclin-Dependent Kinases 2 and 4 Activities as Well as Induction of Cdk Inhibitors p21 and p27 During Growth Arrest of Human Breast Carcinoma Cells by (−)-Epigallocatechin-3-Gallate, 75*(1), 1–12.

Ling, H., Yang, H., Tan, S. H., Chui, W. K., & Chew, E. H., (2010). *6-Shogaol, an Active Constituent of Ginger, Inhibits Breast Cancer Cell Invasion by Reducing Matrix Metalloproteinase-9 Expression via Blockade of Nuclear Factor-κB Activation, 161*(8), 1763–1777.

Lobo, R., Prabhu, K. S., Shirwaikar, A., & Shirwaikar, A., (2009). *Curcuma Zedoaria Rosc. (White Turmeric): A Review of its Chemical, Pharmacological and Ethnomedicinal Properties, 61*(1), 13–21.

Lu, J. J., Dang, Y. Y., Huang, M., Xu, W. S., Chen, X. P., & Wang, Y. T., (2012). *Anti-Cancer Properties of Terpenoids Isolated from Rhizoma Curcumae–A Review, 143*(2), 406–411.

Lu, R., & Serrero, G., (1999). *Resveratrol, a Natural Product Derived from Grape, Exhibits Antiestrogenic Activity and Inhibits the Growth of Human Breast Cancer Cells, 179*(3), 297–304.

Malki, A., El-Saadani, M., Sultan, A. S., (2009). *Garlic Constituent Diallyl Trisulfide Induced Apoptosis in MCF7 Human Breast Cancer Cells, 8*(22), 2174–2184.

Matsuda, H., Ninomiya, K., Morikawa, T., Yoshikawa, M., & Letters J. B., (1998). *Inhibitory Effect and Action MECHANISM of Sesquiterpenes from Zedoariae Rhizoma on D-Galactosamine/Lipopolysaccharide-Induced Liver Injury, 8*(4), 339–344.

Matthes, H., Luu, B., & Orison, G., (1980). *Cytotoxic Components of Zingiber Zerumbet, Curcuma Zedoaria and C Domestica, 19*(12), 2643–2650.

Mittal, A., Pate, M. S., Wylie, R. C., Tollefsbol, T. O., & Katiyar, S. K., (2004). *EGCG Down-Regulates Telomerase in Human Breast Carcinoma MCF-7 Cells, Leading to Suppression of Cell Viability and Induction of Apoptosis, 24*(3), 703–710.

Modem, S., & DiCarlo, S. E., (2012). Reddy and cancer. *Fresh Garlic Extract Induces Growth Arrest and Morphological Differentiation of MCF7 Breast Cancer Cells, 3*(2), 177–186.

Morse, M. A., Kresty, L. A., Steele, V. E., Kelloff, G. J., Boone, C. W., Balentine, D. A., Harbowy, M. E., & Stoner, G. D., (1997). *Effects of Theaflavins on N-Nitrosomethylbenzylamine-Induced Esophageal Tumorigenesis.*

Müller, K., Carpenter, K. L., Challis, I. R., Skepper, J. N., & Arends, M. J., (2002). *Carotenoids Induce Apoptosis in the T-Lymphoblast Cell Line Jurkat E6.1, 36*(7), 791–802.

Nachvak, S. M., Moradi, S., Anjom-Shoae, J., Rahmani, J., Nasiri, M., Maleki, V., & Sadeghi, O., (2019). *Soy, Soy Isoflavones, and Protein Intake in Relation to Mortality from All Causes, Cancers, and Cardiovascular Diseases: A Systematic Review and Dose–Response Meta-Analysis of Prospective Cohort Studies, 119*(9), 1483–1500. e1417.

Narayanan, B. A., Narayanan, N. K., Re, G. G., & Nixon, D. W., (2003). *Differential Expression of Genes Induced by Resveratrol in LNCaP Cells: P53-Mediated Molecular Targets, 104*(2), 204–212.

Natarajan, K., Singh, S., Burke, T. R., Grunberger, D., & Aggarwal, B. B., (1996). *Caffeic Acid Phenethyl Ester is a Potent and Specific Inhibitor of Activation of Nuclear Transcription Factor NF-Kappa B, 93*(17), 9090–9095.

Neil, A., & Silagy, C., (1994). *Garlic: Its Cardio-Protective Properties, 5*(1), 6–10.

Ogawara, H., Akiyama, T., Ishida, J., Watanabe, S. I., & Suzuki, K., (1986). *A Specific Inhibitor for Tyrosine Protein Kinase from Pseudomonas, 39*(4), 606–608.

Oh, O. J., Min, H. Y., & Lee, S. K., (2007). *Inhibition of Inducible Prostaglandin E2 Production and Cyclooxy-Genase-2 Expression by Curdione from Curcuma Zedoaria, 30*(10), 1236–1239.

Onori, P., DeMorrow, S., Gaudio, E., Franchitto, A., Mancinelli, R., Venter, J., Kopriva, S., Ueno, Y., Alvaro, D., & Savage, J., (2009). *Caffeic Acid Phenethyl Ester Decreases Cholangiocarcinoma Growth by Inhibition of NF-κB and Induction of Apoptosis, 125*(3), 565–576.

Pan, M. H., Hsieh, M. C., Hsu, P. C., Ho, S. Y., Lai, C. S., Wu, H., Sang, S., & Ho, C. T., (2008). *6-Shogaol Suppressed Lipopolysaccharide-Induced Up-Expression of iNOS and COX-2 in Murine Macrophages, 52*(12), 1467–1477.

Pan, M. H., Hsieh, M. C., Kuo, J. M., Lai, C. S., Wu, H., Sang, S., & Ho, C. T., *6-Shogaol Induces Apoptosis in Human Colorectal Carcinoma Cells via ROS Production, Caspase Activation, and GADD 153 Expression, 52*(5), 527–537.

Park, S. D., Jung, J. H., Lee, H. W., Kwon, Y. M., Chung, K. H., Kim, M. G., & Kim, C. H., (2005). *Zedoariae Rhizoma and Curcumin Inhibits Platelet-Derived Growth Factor-Induced Proliferation of Human Hepatic Myofibroblasts, 5*(3), 555–569.

Perchellet, J. P., Perchellet, E. M., & Belman, S., (1990). *Inhibition of DMBA-Induced Mouse Skin Tumorigenesis by Garlic Oil and Inhibition of Two Tumor-Promotion Stages by Garlic and Onion Oils.*

Perkin, A. G., & Newbury, F. G., (1899). *LXXIX.—The Coloring Matters Contained in Dyer's Broom (GENISTA TINCTORIA) and Heather (Calluna Vulgaris), 75*, 830–839.

Pettapiece-Phillips, R., Narod, S. A., & Kotsopoulos, J., (2015). *The Role of Body Size and Physical Activity on the Risk of Breast Cancer in BRCA Mutation Carriers, 26*(3), 333–344.

Pinto, J. T., & Rivlin, R. S., (2001). *Antiproliferative Effects of Allium Derivatives from Garlic, 131*(3), 1058S–1060S.

Pozo-Guisado, E., Merino, J., Mulero-Navarro, S., Lorenzo-Benayas, M., & Centeno, F., Varez-Barrientos, A., & Fernandez-Salguero, P. M., (2005). *Resveratrol-induced Apoptosis in MCF-7 Human Breast Cancer Cells Involves a Caspase-Independent Mechanism with Downregulation of Bcl-2 and NF-kappaB, 115*, 74–84.

Rahman, K. W., Aranha, O., Glazyrin, A., Chinni, S. R., & Sarkar, F. H., (2000). *Translocation of Bax to Mitochondria Induces Apoptotic Cell Death in Indole-3-Carbinol (I3C) Treated Breast Cancer Cells, 19*(50), 5764–5771.

Rahman, S., Wahab, N., & Abd, M. S., (2013). *In vitro* morphological assessment of apoptosis induced by antiproliferative constituents from the rhizomes of *Curcuma zedoaria*. *Evidence-Based Complementary Altern Med., 2013*. doi. org.

Rane, B. R., Patil, A. S., Keservani, R. K., & Jain, A. S., (2020a). Novel approaches in herbal formulation. In: Rajesh, K. K., Raj, K. K., & Anil, K. S., (eds.), *Enhancing the Therapeutic Efficacy of Herbal Formulations Through Novel Drug Delivery Systems* (pp. 43–68). IGI Global International Publisher, Pennsylvania, USA, Chapter 2. ISBN13: 9781799844532.

Rogers, A. E., Hafer, L. J., Iskander, Y. S., & Yang, S. J. C., (1998). *Black Tea and Mammary Gland Carcinogenesis by 7, 12-Dimethylbenz [a] Anthracene in Rats Fed Control or High Fat Diets, 19*(7), 1269–1273.

Rowe, C. A., Nantz, M. P., Nieves, Jr. C., West, R. L., & Percival, S. S., (2011). *Regular Consumption of Concord Grape Juice Benefits Human Immunity, 14*(1, 2), 69–78.

Rzepecka-Stojko, A., Kabała-Dzik, A., Moździerz, A., Kubina, R., Wojtyczka, R. D., Stojko, R., Dziedzic, A., Jastrzębska-Stojko, Z., Jurzak, M., & Buszman, E. J. M., (2015). *Caffeic Acid Phenethyl Ester and Ethanol Extract of Propolis Induce the Complementary Cytotoxic Effect on Triple-Negative Breast Cancer Cell Lines, 20*(5), 9242–9262.

Sartippour, M. R., Shao, Z. M., Heber, D., Beatty, P., Zhang, L., Liu, C., Ellis, L., Liu, W., Go, V. L., & Brooks, M. N., (2002). *Green Tea Inhibits Vascular Endothelial Growth Factor (VEGF) Induction in Human Breast Cancer Cells, 132*(8), 2307–2311.

Savouret, J. F., & Quesne, M., (2002). *Resveratrol and Cancer: A Review, 56*(2), 84–87.

Scimeca, M., Antonacci, C., Colombo, D., Bonfiglio, R., Buonomo, O. C., & Bonanno, E., (2016). *Emerging Prognostic Markers Related to Mesenchymal Characteristics of Poorly Differentiated Breast Cancers, 37*(4), 5427–5435.

Shiobara, Y., Asakawa, Y., Kodama, M., Yasuda, K., & Takemoto, T., (1985). *Curcumenone, Curcumanolide A and Curcumanolide B, Three Sesquiterpenoids from Curcuma Zedoaria, 24*(11), 2629–2633.

Steinmetz, K. A., & Potter, J. D., (1991). *Vegetables, Fruit, and Cancer. I. Epidemiology, 2*(5), 325–357.

Surh, Y. J., Hurh, Y. J., Kang, J. Y., Lee, E., Kong, G., & Lee, S. J., (1999). *Resveratrol, an Antioxidant Present in Red Wine, Induces Apoptosis in Human Promyelocytic Leukemia (HL-60) Cells, 140*(1, 2), 1–10.

Takeshima, M., Ono, M., Higuchi, T., Chen, C., Hara, T., & Nakano, S., (2014). *Anti-Proliferative and Apoptosis-Inducing Activity of Lycopene Against Three Subtypes of Human Breast Cancer Cell Lines, 105*(3), 252–257.

Tanaka, H., Hirose, M., Kawabe, M., Sano, M., Takesada, Y., Hagiwara, A., & Shirai, T., (1997). *Post-Initiation Inhibitory Effects of Green Tea Catechins on 7, 12-Dimethylbenz [a] Anthracene-Induced Mammary Gland Carcinogenesis in Female Sprague–Dawley Rats, 116*(1), 47–52.

Tanaka, S., Haruma, K., Yoshihara, M., Kajiyama, G., Kira, K., Amagase, H., & Chayama, K., (2006). *Aged Garlic Extract has Potential Suppressive Effect on Colorectal Adenomas in Humans, 136*(3), 821S–826S.

Tanaka, T., Shnimizu, M., & Moriwaki, H., (2012). *Cancer Chemoprevention by Carotenoids, 17*(3), 3202–3242.

Tiwari, R., Guo, L., Bradlow, H. L., Telang, N., & Osborne, M., (1994). *Selective Responsiveness of Human Breast Cancer Cells to Indole-3-Carbinol, a Chemopreventive Agent, 86*(2), 126–131.

Tsan, M. F., White, J. E., Maheshwari, J. G., Bremner, T. A., & Sacco, J., (2000). *Resveratrol Induces Fas Signaling-Independent Apoptosis in THP-1 Human Monocytic Leukemia Cells, 109*(2), 405–412.

Tsubura, A., Lai, Y. C., Kuwata, M., Uehara, N., & Yoshizawa, K., (2011). *Anticancer Effects of Garlic and Garlic-Derived Compounds for Breast Cancer Control, 11*(3), 249–253.

Uppala, P. T., Dissmore, T., Lau, B. H., Andacht, T., & Rajaram, S., (2013). *Selective Inhibition of Cell Proliferation by Lycopene in MCF-7 Breast Cancer Cells in Vitro: A Proteomic Analysis, 27*(4), 595–601.

Vergote, D., Cren-Olivé, C., Chopin, V., Toillon, R. A., Rolando, C., Hondermarck, H., & Le Bourhis, X., (2002). *(−)-Epigallocatechin (EGC) of Green Tea Induces Apoptosis of Human Breast Cancer Cells but Not of Their Normal Counterparts, 76*(3), 195–201.

Verhoeven, D. T., Verhagen, H., Goldbohm, R. A., Van, D. B. P. A., & Van, P. G., (1997). *A Review of Mechanisms Underlying Anti-carcinogenicity by Brassica Vegetables, 103*(2), 79–129.

Walter, E., (1941). *Genistin (an Isoflavone Glucoside) and Its Aglucone, Genistein, from Soybeans, 63*(12), 3273–3276.

Walz, E., (1931). *Isoflavon-Und Saponin-Glucoside in Soja Hispida, 489*(1), 118–155.

Watabe, M., Hishikawa, K., Takayanagi, A., Shimizu, N., & Nakaki, T., (2004). *Caffeic Acid Phenethyl Ester Induces Apoptosis by Inhibition of NFκB and Activation of Fas in Human Breast Cancer MCF-7 Cells, 279*(7), 6017–6026.

Way, T. D., Lee, H. H., Kao, M. C., & Lin, J. K (2004). *Black Tea Polyphenol Theaflavins Inhibit Aromatase Activity and Attenuate Tamoxifen Resistance in HER2/neu-Transfected Human Breast Cancer Cells Through Tyrosine Kinase Suppression, 40*(14), 2165–2174.

Weisburger, J. H., Rivenson, A., Reinhardt, J., Aliaga, C., Braley, J., Pittman, B., & Zang, E., (1998). *Effect of Black Tea on Azoxymethane-Induced Colon Cancer, 19*(1), 229–232.

Widjastuti, T., & Andriani, L., (2010). *The Use of Curcuma Zedoaria, Rosc Meal to Reduce Abdominal Fat and Meat Cholesterol in Broiler, 53*, 126–129.

Wu, C., Sheen, L., Chen, H. W., Tsai, S. J., & Lii, C. K., (2001). *Effects of Organosulfur Compounds from Garlic Oil on the Antioxidation System in Rat Liver and Red Blood Cells, 39*(6), 563–569.

Wu, J., Omene, C., Karkoszka, J., Bosland, M., Eckard, J., Klein, C. B., & Frenkel, K., (2011). *Caffeic Acid Phenethyl Ester (CAPE), Derived from a Honeybee Product Propolis, Exhibits a Diversity of Anti-Tumor Effects in Pre-Clinical Models of Human Breast Cancer, 308*(1), 43–53.

Yang, C. S., Landau, J. M., Huang, M. T., & Newmark, H. L., (2001). *Inhibition of Carcinogenesis by Dietary Polyphenolic Compounds, 21*(1), 381–406.

Yang, G. Y., Liu, Z., Seril, D. N., Liao, J., Ding, W., Kim, S., Bondoc, F., & Yang, C. S., (1997). *Black Tea Constituents, Theaflavins, Inhibit 4-(Methylnitrosamino)-1-(3-Pyridyl)-1-Butanone (NNK)-Induced Lung Tumorigenesis in A/J Mice, 18*(12), 2361–2365.

Zhou, H. B., Yan, Y., Sun, Y. N., & Zhu, J. R., (2003). *Resveratrol Induces Apoptosis in Human Esophageal Carcinoma Cells, 9*(3), 408.

Zhou, Q., Ye, M., Lu, Y., Zhang, H., Chen, Q., Huang, S., & Su, S., (2015). *Curcumin Improves the Tumoricidal Effect of Mitomycin C by Suppressing ABCG2 Expression in Stem Cell-Like Breast Cancer Cells, 10*(8), e0136694.

CHAPTER 7

PROSTATE CANCER PREVENTION BY NUTRACEUTICALS

ASHWINI V. SHELKE,[1] SWATI G. TALELE,[2] and ANIL G. JADHAV[3]

[1]*Department of Pharmaceutical Chemistry, Sandip Institute of Pharmaceutical Sciences, Savitribai Phule Pune University, Nashik, Maharashtra, India*

[2]*Department of Pharmaceutics, Sandip Institute of Pharmaceutical Sciences, Savitribai Phule Pune University, Nashik, Maharashtra, India*

[3]*Department of Pharmacognosy, Sandip Institute of Pharmaceutical Sciences, Savitribai Phule Pune University, Nashik, Maharashtra, India*

ABSTRACT

A "nutraceutical" is a substance that can be regarded as a food or a component of a food that has medical or health advantages, including illness prevention and treatment. It is a broad term that refers to any product generated from food sources that provide additional health advantages beyond the fundamental nutritional content present in foods. Prostate cancer begins in the prostate gland and spreads to other parts of the body. In the United States, it is the second greatest origin of cancer mortality in men. Australia, northern Europe, the Caribbean islands, and North America have the highest rates of prostate cancer. In South America, Central America, Asia, and Africa, it is less frequent. Prostate cancer takes a long time to develop and is more common in men over 50. Prostate cancer screening, diagnosis, therapy, and palliative care are all expensive and contribute to an increased economic burden. Prostate cancer will become a significant health problem in the coming years as the older population in the US and many other countries grow. Even

Nutraceuticals in Cancer Prevention, Management, and Treatment. Raj K. Keservani, Bui Thanh Tung, Sippy Singh, & Rajesh K. Kesharwani, PhD (Eds.)

though today's therapies are quite powerful and successful, some factors like disease resistance, metastatic progression, therapy-associated toxicities, and efficacy-related difficulties arise with time in various populations, to address these fundamental hurdles in the clinical treatment and management of prostate cancer, nontoxic and effective therapeutic techniques are required. As a result, numerous naturally generated dietary components have been investigated in an attempt to develop a natural preventative medication for prostate cancer.

Foods having compounds with anticancer qualities can be included in diets to prevent precancerous lesions from forming in chemopreventive techniques. The balance and availability of dietary chemopreventive substances can be influenced by changing one's diet to include more beneficial phytochemicals. Vitamin D, Vitamin E, GREEN TEA, GREEN TEA polyphenols, zinc, silbinin, grape seed extract (GSE), grape skin extract, and resveratrol are some examples of nutrients. Fish and fish oil, Omega-3 fatty acids, cruciferous vegetables, isothiocyanates and sulforaphane (SFN), soy isoflavones and genistein, quercetin, tomatoes, and lycopene are just a few of the nutraceuticals that have been investigated in human studies for the prevention of prostate cancer. In this chapter, we will emphasize to discuss benefit all possibly promising nutraceutical-based agents.

7.1 INTRODUCTION

Cancer is frequently a slow-growing disease, and the risk of having cancer rises with age (Saldanha et al., 2012). Prostate cancer is rare in men below the age of 40, but it grows more common after that. Prostate cancer affects approximately 60% of males after the age of 65. Prostate cancer strikes African–American men and Caribbean men of African origin more frequently than other races. While it does develop in these males, it usually happens when they are younger. Prostate cancer is less common among Asian-American and Hispanic/Latino men than in non-Hispanic white men. The causes of these racial and ethnic disparities remain unknown (Society, 2013). Prostate cancer has also been reported to occur in some families, suggesting that there may be a hereditary or genetic factor in some cases. Despite this, the majority of prostate cancers occur in men who have no family background of the disease (Cheng et al., 2019). The epidemiology of this disease is markedly affected by factors such as diet and lifestyle. The finest example is a Japanese immigrant to North America who adopts local food and lifestyle and, as a result, has a higher prostate cancer risk than men in his country of origin (Shimizu et al., 1991). Prostate cancer's genetic processes for initiation, development, and progression are not completely known but it appears to be a multistep process, according to emerging evidence (Figure 7.1). High-grade prostatic intraepithelial neoplasia (HGPIN), which is an origin to prostate cancer, is thought to be caused by inflammation of the prostate gland (prostatitis) and proliferative inflammatory atrophy (PIA) (Nelson et al., 2003; De Marzo et al., 2007). There is always long period between conversion of localized lesion into invasive cancer thus it is possible to interfere into all these steps before development of metastatic cancer (Parnes et al., 2013).

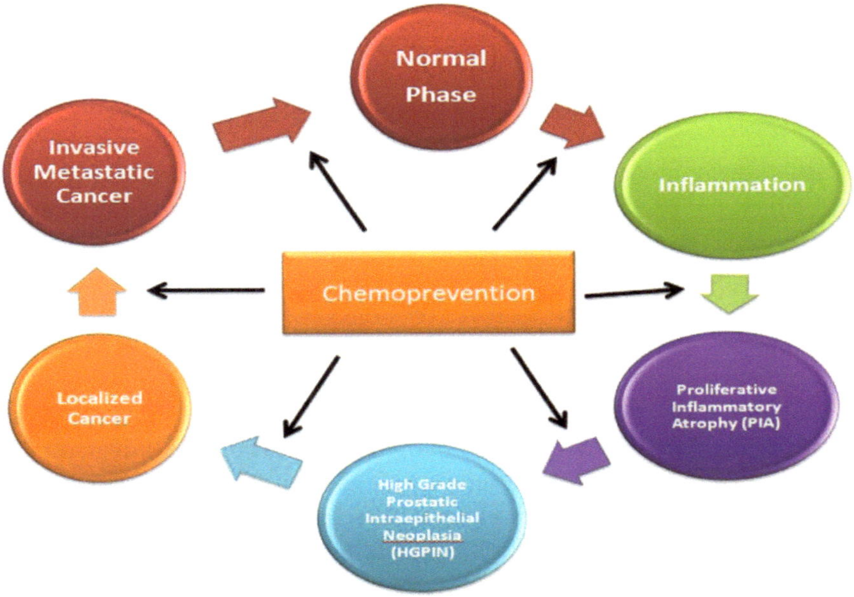

FIGURE 7.1 Prostate cancer's multistep genetic processes.

Almost every facet of a patient's life can be targeted with prevention techniques. Dietary alteration is an obvious focus and might include changes to a patient's usual intake along with the addition of anticancer foods or supplements. The term 'nutraceutical,' which was coined in 1989, refers to natural foods or supplements that have therapeutic properties. These investigations have been referred to as 'dietary agents,' 'natural products,' and 'nutritional factors,' among other terms. Dr. Stephen DeFelice invented the term nutraceutical in 1989, combining the words "nutrition" and "pharmaceutical" (Keservani et al., 2010a, 2010b; Kalra, 2003). The Food Directorate of Health Canada's Bureau of Nutritional Sciences has defined 'nutraceuticals' as "A product isolated or purified from foods that is generally sold in medicinal forms not usually associated with the food. A nutraceutical is demonstrated to have a physiological benefit or provide protection against chronic disease" (Health Canada, 2009).

Because between 43% (Lippert et al., 1999) and 80% (Nam et al., 1999) prostate cancer patients are receiving alternative treatment, the use of nutraceuticals in the prevention of prostate cancer is a growing field of investigation. These people include those who have a significant family history of prostate cancer, those who are on active surveillance, and those who have failed active prostate cancer treatments or are on androgen deprivation and are looking for natural ways to slow disease progression. Surgery, adjuvant chemotherapy, hormonal therapy (i.e., androgen deprivation), and/or radiation for advanced PCa are the most common treatments. Despite the fact that these therapeutic choices are extremely robust and effective, disease resistance, development to the stage of metastasis, therapy-related toxicities, and efficacy-related difficulties have developed throughout time in various populations. To address these fundamental hurdles in the clinical treatment and management of Prostate Cancer, effective and nontoxic therapeutic techniques are required. Nutraceutical drugs (Keservani et al., 2015, 2016) have been identified as a viable and nontoxic option for tumor prevention and enhancement of the therapeutic response to pre-existing anticancer treatments in previous and ongoing chemoprevention/intervention studies (Key et al., 2015). Due to significant epidemiological, preclinical, and pilot clinical research, a variety of nutraceuticals are having the possibility for development as prostate cancer chemopreventive medications. Their modes of action could include the capacity to target various molecular pathways involved in carcinogenesis while causing no harmful side effects. One of the main paradigms for designing and developing nontoxic treatment techniques that operate synergistically with existing clinical anticancer drugs is precision medicine employing a nutraceutical approach. Precision medicine techniques take into account the complex interactions of genetic, regional, and socioeconomic factors and include treatments that account for individual differences in pharmacogenomic responses to cancer medications as well as important Prostate Cancer risk factors Figure 7.2 (such as age, family history, race, and genetic predisposition) (Dominique et al., 2017).

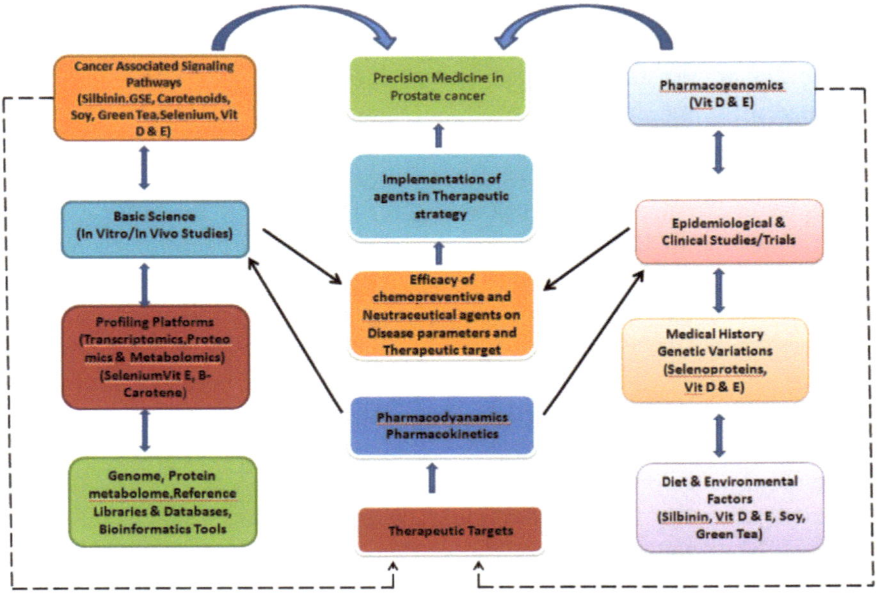

FIGURE 7.2 Precision medicine techniques in prostate cancer.

7.2 VITAMIN D

Vitamin D is found to be the powerful biological agent that plays a vital role in the body, including mineral metabolism. It is a fat-soluble nutraceutical that can be present in dairy, fermented foods, and fortified foods (Bandera et al., 2017). It has five isoforms, which include ergocalciferol with lumisterol (D1), ergocalciferol (D2), cholecalci-ferol (D3), 22-dihydroergocalciferol (D4), and sitocalciferol (D5). Two hydroxylation cycles (liver and kidney) of vitamin D3 (cholecalciferol), which is generated in skin under the action of ultraviolet B radiation, producing the active form of vitamin D, 1,25(OH)2D; calcitriol (Schwartz et al., 2005). The name "vitamin" is deceptive because cholecalciferol is a pro-peptide hormone to calcitriol, which regulates its physiological activities through the vitamin D3 receptor (VDR), which is found in cell nuclei (Schwartz et al., 2005). Calcitriol regulates cell differentiation and proliferation in a number of tumor cells, in addition to the typical physiological functions of vitamin D (calcium homeostasis and bone metabolism) (Hanchette et al., 1992). Interestingly vitamin D synthesis has been observed in non-kidney tissues, including prostate cells (Schwartz et al., 2005; Hanchette et al., 1992). Vitamin D receptors are found in benign and malignant prostate cells and prostate cancer cell lines of humans respond to vitamin D by growth restriction (Hanchette et al., 1992). In western countries, sun exposure is the predominant origin of vitamin D, while just a small amount received through diet. In contrast, vitamin D-rich diets can be obtained in other regions of the world, for example, in Japan Vit D level is extremely high in diet may be because of high fish consumption (Schwartz et al., 2005). The factors which lead to lower vitamin D content in some population include less sun exposure, thinner epidermis, people with darker skin has less ultraviolet B penetration power and people who are not physically active also has less sun exposure along with catabolic bone metabolism.

The association between vitamin D and prostate cancer was first proposed in 1990 by Shwartz and Hulka (Schwartz, 1990) who suggested that vitamin D is required to control differentiation of prostate cell. Hence vitamin D deficiency results into development of early pre-cancerous lesions into cancers. Multiple studies have shown that increasing regional UV radiation is attributed to a lower incidence and fatality of prostate cancer (Kafadar, 1997; Grant, 2002; Schwartz et al., 2006; Di Silverio et al., 1982; John et al., 2004; John et al., 2005).

7.3 GREEN TEA AND GREEN TEA POLYPHENOLS

Green tea, its constituent polyphenols, i.e., catechins, or the most prevalent polyphenol, (-)epigallocatechin-3-gallate EGCG, have demonstrated promising preventative and therapeutic effects on prostate cancer. Green tea polyphenols inhibit a number of prostate cancer-causing pathways (Yang et al., 2013; Yang et al., 2009). Antioxidant properties, inhibition of inflammatory pathways nuclear factor-kappaB (NF-kB) and cyclooxygenase 2 (COX-2), insulin-like growth factor (IGF), numerous kinases, and androgen blockade are some of the actions of EGCG. Topoisomerase inhibitors have been discovered in EGCG and other tea polyphenols, are similar to several chemotherapy agents and may be important for the anticancer effects (Suzuki et al., 2001). Although green tea has anticancer properties in animal models and cell culture, human studies reveal that it is more beneficial as a chemopreventive agent than as a treatment for individuals with advanced prostate cancer (Bemis et al., 2006). Moreover, green tea polyphenols (Keservani and Sharma 2014) are also limited in clinical use due to their low absorption and conversion to inactive methylated metabolites.

7.4 VITAMIN E

Vitamin E's preventive impact in PCa has been extensively explored in published publications and clinical trials (Key et al., 2015). Tocopherols (α, γ, and δ) are the most researched vitamin E bioactive elements in Prostate Cancer because they have vitamin E activity. Fat-soluble vitamin E that is found in a number of foods such nuts, seeds, and vegetable oil. Tocopherols are prominent in both European and Western diets. α-tocopherol is commonly found in European diets, whereas γ-tocopherol is commonly found in Western diets. Men's Prostate Cancer sensitivity has been discovered to influence by vitamin E intervention, supplementation, and associated genetic variations (Major et al., 2014; Martinez et al., 2014; Mondul et al., 2015; Bauer et al., 2013).

7.5 ZINC

When compared to any other soft tissue inside the body, normal prostatic tissue has the highest quantities of mineral zinc. Dietary zinc has previously been shown to have a protective effect in people with severe Prostate Cancer susceptibility in epidemiologic investigations (Sapota et al., 2014). Some reports, on the other side, contradict the protective impact of dietary zinc and add to the mixed findings on the link between zinc consumption and Prostate Cancer risk. Long-term dietary zinc from multivitamins or other supplements resulted in a non-significant two-times increase in Prostate Cancer risk in individuals in the US hospital-based Case-Control Surveillance Study (Zhang et al., 2009).

7.6 SILBININ

Silibinin (flavanolignan from milk thistle "Silybum marianum" seeds) has shown remarkable anti-carcinogenic activity against a variety of cancers, including Prostate Cancer, over the past decades (Ting et al., 2014; Bijak, 2017). Because of the significant anticancer efficacy of silibinin in preclinical animal models of Prostate Cancer, it was moved into a phase II clinical trial to assess its bioavailability in patients with localized Prostate Cancer illness (Flaig et al., 2010). Although patients' serum prostate-specific antigen (PSA) concentration did not respond to silibinin treatment in a partial or total way, disease stability was retained in several cases. Larger clinical trials using a more bio-available form of silibinin are mostly needed to prove its biological efficiency as a nutraceutical agent for the treatment of localized or advanced types of prostate cancer.

7.7 GRAPE SEED EXTRACT (GSE)

Extract of grape seed, known as proanthocyanidins, are a complex mixture of polyphenols containing procyanidins and their gallate derivatives. In various preclinical models, it has shown anticancer efficacy against PCa development and progression (Nassiri-Asl et al., 2009; Kaur et al., 2009).

7.8 GRAPE SKIN EXTRACTS AND RESVERATROL

Resveratrol (3,5,4-trihydroxy-trans-stilbene) is a polyphenolic phytoalexin found in berries, red grapes, and peanuts, among other natural plants. Resveratrol offers a wide range of health benefits, including anti-infective, antioxidant, and cardioprotective properties, and its possible cancer-prevention effect has been actively researched in recent years (Huang et al., 2011; Khan et al., 2010). The underlying mechanisms for resveratrol's chemoprevention effect have also been thoroughly investigated, and a number of pathways have been identified, including anti-oxidation, anti-inflammation, cell cycle modulation, modulating the expression or function of the androgen receptor, and epigenetic regulation (Aggarwal et al., 2004). However, due to significant glucuronidation and sulfation, as well as processing by gut bacterial enzymes, pharmacokinetic investigations of resveratrol have revealed a low bioavailability (only 1%) (Scott et al., 2012).

7.9 FISH, FISH OIL, AND OMEGA-3 FATTY ACIDS

Omega-3 polyunsaturated fatty acids have been extensively explored since the late 1980s because of their anti-inflammatory properties. Because of the link between chronic prostatic inflammation and cancer, omega-3 fatty acids are a possible agent for prostate cancer prevention (Laviano et al., 2013; Chua et al., 2012). Omega-3 fatty acids are found mostly in fish and differ from omega-6 fatty acids, which are found primarily in animal fats and vegetable oils. The ratio of omega-6 to omega-3 fatty acids in the diet has been shown to slow the development and progression of prostate cancer (Berquin et al.,

2007; Kobayashi et al., 2006). The omega-3 fatty acids like eicosapentaenoic acid (EPA), alpha-linolenic acid (ALA), and docosahexaenoic acid (DHA) have clinically meaningful effects on cancer (DHA) (Laviano et al., 2013). Although not all epidemiological research has found a link between fish diet and prostate cancer incidence, the findings are consistent. A Swedish study found a relationship between fish consumption and the progression of prostate cancer. The research revealed that men who don't consume fish had a two to three times increased prostate cancer risk over the course of 30 years compared to men who ate more fish (Terry et al., 2001). In a clinical setting, Aronson et al. (2001) conducted a prospective research in males with untreated prostate cancer to assess the role of a low-fat, fish oil-supplemented diet. The research discovered that following a low-fat, fish oil-supplemented diet for three months results in a considerable increase in the omega-3/omega-6 fatty acid ratios in plasma and adipose tissue.

Dietary omega-3 fatty acid consumption and prostate cancer risk have been explored in various ways. Men with high blood levels of long-chain omega-3 fatty acids have an increased risk of prostate cancer, according to certain research (Brasky et al., 2013). As a result, recommendations to increase fish oil or omega-3 fatty acid consumption should take into account the potential risks involved.

7.10 CRUCIFEROUS VEGETABLES, ISOTHIOCYANATES, AND SULFORAPHANE (SFN)

Isothiocyanates, which are made from glucosinolates present in cruciferous vegetables like broccoli and cauliflower, are another type of chemopreventive dietary agent. SFN and indole-3-carbinol (I3C) are two important and well-studied isothiocyanates. SFN has been researched extensively for its chemopreventive impact in a wide variety of in vivo-in vitro animal models, with promising results. SFN has been found to suppress cancer development by stimulating Phase II enzymes which detoxify carcinogens, while blocking Phase I enzymes which activate carcinogens (Clarke et al., 2008). SFN can slow the progression of cancer once it has been initiated. The nuclear factor (erythroid-derived 2)-like 2 (Nrf2) cytoprotective pathway, which boosts cell defense against oxidative damage and accelerates the elimination of carcinogens, was thought to be the chemopreventive mechanism of SFN (Juge et al., 2007). Other mechanisms, including as apoptosis induction, cell cycle suppression, angiogenesis inhibition, and anti-inflammatory effects, may possibly play a role in its action. More recently, it was shown that SFN metabolites block HDAC, which may be found more related to SFN chemoprevention, generating cytotoxic effects that are selective to cancer cells but not normal cells, which may be more important to SFN chemoprevention (Ho et al., 2011). In epidemiological studies, cruciferous vegetables like broccoli and cauliflower have been related to a decreased risk of prostate cancer (Kolonel et al., 2000; Cohen et al.).

7.11 SOY ISOFLAVONES AND GENISTEIN

Isoflavones have been demonstrated to have anticancer and chemopreventive properties through mechanisms such as estrogen receptor modulation, tyrosine protein kinase inhibition, anti-oxidative, anti-angiogenesis, and inhibition of 5a-reductases. The most studied isoflavones are genistein and daidzein. Isoflavones or genistein have been extensively studied for their potential in prostate cancer chemoprevention (Bemis et al., 2006; Van Poppel et al., 2011; Ahonen et al., 2000).

7.12 QUERCETIN

Anti-inflammatory and anti-oxidant properties of quercetin are well-known. Quercetin is a flavonoid generated from plants that can be obtained in a wide variety of fruits and vegetables, including onions, broccoli, apples, grapes (red wine), and soybeans. It has been shown in some research to have powerful antiproliferative effects against a variety of cancers. This impact is thought to be linked to the induction of cell death in cancer cells via several mechanisms. Quercetin has also been proven to lower the probability of prostate cancer metastasis, most likely by downregulating matrix metalloproteinases (Cimino et al., 2012).

7.13 TOMATO AND LYCOPENE

Lycopene is a red-colored carotenoid pigment seen in tomatoes, strawberries, and watermelons that lacks the beta-ionone ring and lacks vitamin A action. It is one of the most actively researched natural compounds capable of preventing or slowing carcinogenesis progression (Konijeti et al., 2010). Lycopene consumption has been demonstrated to lower the prostate cancer risk, probably due to its powerful antioxidant properties (De Souza et al., 2010; Society AC, 2013; Cazzaniga et al., 2012). In vitro studies indicated that, in addition to its antioxidant properties, lycopene has other targets. The HMG-CoA reductase, the RAS oncogene, and the NF-kB pathway are all molecular targets of lycopene (Palozza et al., 2010). Lycopene has been shown to increase the activity of Nrf2-regulated enzymes such as glutathione transferases (Qiu et al., 2013). Lycopene has also been demonstrated to prevent androgen signaling, deactivate the MAPK pathway, and reduce TNF-α signaling (Shen et al., 2010). For the prevention of prostate cancer, there is strong evidence for lycopene's cancer-preventive effect (Henderson et al., 2005). Consumption of tomatoes and tomato derivatives was first linked to a lower risk of prostate cancer, according to epidemiological studies (De Marzo et al., 2007; Boyd et al., 2012). Later investigations found that lycopene or its metabolites are the active ingredients in tomatoes that have a chemopreventive effect. Hence, lycopene has been employed in preclinical efficacy and mechanism research (Sporn et al., 2013).

7.14 CONCLUSION

In an effort to find natural preventative therapy for prostate cancer, several naturally derived dietary components have been examined. The most promising nutraceuticals for prostate cancer protection are vitamin D, vitamin E, green tea and green tea polyphenols, zinc, silibinin, grape seed extract (GSE), grape skin extract, and resveratrol, fish and fish oil, Omega-3-fatty acid, cruciferous vegetables, isothiocyanates and sulforaphane (SFN), soy isoflavones, and genistein, quercetin, tomato and lycopene. Recent results from significant trials on nutraceuticals and prostate cancer prevention has been generally abysmal. However, we should be cautious about excluding many nutraceuticals because the evidence against their usage is weak, and most randomized controlled trials are inadequate to identify favorable effects. Natural, nontoxic nutraceuticals have shown promise as powerful anti-prostate cancer therapies in preclinical and population-based efficacy investigations. as a result, the use of nutraceuticals and genetic study in a wide variety of populations could contribute to the creation and design of targeted therapy approaches to lessen the burden of chemotherapy-related toxicities, lower disease resistance, and cure both localized and progressed prostate cancer. As a result, larger, more comprehensive clinical trials are needed to thoroughly investigate the efficacy and treatment limits of these medicines in prostate cancer.

KEYWORDS

- **grape seed extract**
- **nutraceutical**
- **prostate cancer**
- **silibinin**

REFERENCES

Aggarwal, B. B., Bhardwaj, A., Aggarwal, R. S., et al., (2004). Role of resveratrol in prevention and therapy of cancer: Preclinical and clinical studies. *Anticancer Res., 24*, 2783–2840.

Ahonen, M. H., Tenkanen, L., Teppo, L., et al., (2000). Prostate cancer risk and prediagnostic serum 25-hydroxyvitamin d levels (Finland). *Cancer Causes Control, 11*, 847–852.

Aronson, W. J., Glaspy, J. A., Reddy, S. T., et al., (2001). Modulation of omega-3/omega-6 polyunsaturated ratios with dietary fish oils in men with prostate cancer. *Urology, 58*, 283–288.

Bandera, M. B., Morcillo, S., Martin, N. G., Tinahones, F. J., & Macias, G. M., (2017). The role of vitamin D and VDR in carcinogenesis: Through epidemiology and basic sciences. *J. Steroid Biochem. Mol. Biol., 167*, 203–218.

Bauer, S. R., Richman, E. L., Sosa, E., et al., (2013). Antioxidant and vitamin E transport genes and risk of high – grade prostate cancer and prostate cancer recurrence. *Prostate, 73*, 1786–1795.

Bemis, D. L., Katz, A. E., & Buttyan, R., (2006). Clinical trials of natural products as chemopreventive agents for prostate cancer. *Expert Opin. Investig. Drugs, 15*, 1191–1200.

Bemis, D. L., Katz, A. E., & Buttyan, R., (2006). Clinical trials of natural products as chemopreventive agents for prostate cancer. *Expert. Opin. Investig. Drugs, 15*, 1191–1200.

Berquin, I. M., Min, Y., Wu, R., et al., (2007). Modulation of prostate cancer genetic risk by omega-3 and omega-6 fatty acids. *J. Clin. Invest., 117*, 1866–1875.

Bijak, M., (2017). Silybin, a major bioactive component of milk thistle (Silybum marianum L. Gaernt.)-chemistry, bioavailability, and metabolism. *Molecules, 22*(11), 1942.

Boyd, L. K., Mao, X., & Lu, Y. J., (2012). The complexity of prostate cancer: Genomic alterations and heterogeneity. *Nat. Rev. Urol., 9*, 652–664.

Brasky, T. M., Darke, A. K., Song, X., et al., (2013). Plasma phospholipid fatty acids and prostate cancer risk in the select trial. *J Natl Cancer Inst., 105*(15), 1132–1141.

Cazzaniga, M., & Bonanni, B., (2012). Breast cancer chemoprevention: Old and new approaches. *J. Biomed. Biotechnol.*, 985620.

Cheng, H. H., & Nelson, P. S. (2022). *Genetic Risk Factors for Prostate Cancer*. (medilib.ir).

Chua, M. E., Sio, M. C., Sorongon, M. C., et al., (2012). Relationship of dietary intake of omega-3 and omega-6 fatty acids with risk of prostate cancer development: A meta-analysis of prospective studies and review of literature. *Prostate Cancer*, 826254.

Cimino, S., Sortino, G., Favilla, V., et al., (2012). Polyphenols: Key issues involved in chemoprevention of prostate cancer. *Oxid Med. Cell Longev*., 632959.

Clarke, J. D., Dashwood, R. H., & Ho, E., (2008). Multi-targeted prevention of cancer by sulforaphane. *Cancer Lett., 269*, 291–304.

Cohen, J. H., Kristal, A. R., & Stanford, J. L., (2000). Fruit and vegetable intakes and prostate cancer risk. *J Natl Cancer Inst., 92*, 61–68.

De Marzo, A. M., Platz, E. A., & Sutcliffe, S., (2007). Inflammation in prostate carcinogenesis. *Nat. Rev. Cancer, 7*, 256–269.

De Souza, P. L., Russell, P. J., Kearsley, J. H., et al., (2010). Clinical pharmacology of isoflavones and its relevance for potential prevention of prostate cancer. *Nutr Rev., 68*, 542–555.

Di Silverio, F., La Pera, G., & Tenaglia, R., (1982). Age adjusted mortality rate and regional distribution for prostatic carcinoma in Italy between 1969 and 1978. *Prostate, 3*(6), 631–636.

Dominique, R., Komal, R., & Rajesh, A., (2018). Nutraceuticals in prostate cancer therapeutic strategies and their neo-adjuvant use in diverse populations. *Precision Oncology, 2*, 15.

Flaig, T. W., et al., (2010). A study of high-dose oral silybin-phytosome followed by prostatectomy in patients with localized prostate cancer. *Prostate, 70*, 848–855.

Grant, W., (2002). An estimate of premature cancer mortality in the U. *S.* due to inadequate doses of solar ultraviolet-B radiation. *Cancer, 94*, 1867–1875.

Hanchette, C., & Schwartz, G., (1992). Geographic patterns of prostate cancer mortality. Evidence for a protective effect of ultraviolet radiation. *Cancer, 70*, 2861–2869.

Health Canada, (2013). *Nutraceuticals/Functional Foods and Healthclaims on Foods* (pp. 1–30). Policy Paper [Online] https://www.hc-sc.gc.ca/fn-an/label-etiquet/claims-reclam/nutra-functfoods-nutra-fonct (accessed on 05 February 2023).

Henderson, C. J., & Wolf, C. R., (2005). Disruption of the glutathione transferase pi class genes. *Methods Enzymol., 401*, 116–135.

Ho, E., Beaver, L. M., Williams, D. E., et al., (2011). Dietary factors and epigenetic regulation for prostate cancer prevention. *Adv. Nutr., 2*, 497–510.

https://www.cancer.org/cancer/prostate-cancer/causes-risks-prevention/risk-factors.html (accessed on 04 February 2023).

Huang, J., Plass, C., & Gerhauser, C., (2011). Cancer chemoprevention by targeting the epigenome. *Curr. Drug Targets., 12*, 1925–1956.

John, E., Dreon, D., Koo, J., & Schwartz, G., (2004). Residential sunlight exposure is associated with a decreased risk of prostate cancer. *J. Steroid Biochem. Mol. Biol., 89, 90*, 549–552.

John, E., Schwartz, G., Koo, J., Van, D. B. D., & Ingles, S., (2005). Sun exposure, vitamin D receptor gene polymorphisms, and risk of advanced prostate cancer. *Cancer Res., 65*, 5470–5479.

Juge, N., Mithen, R. F., & Traka, M., (2007). Molecular basis for chemoprevention by sulforaphane: A comprehensive review. *Cell Mol. Life Sci., 64*, 1105–1127.

Kafadar, K., (1997). Geographic trends in prostate cancer mortality: An application of spatial smoothers and the need for adjustment. *Ann. Epidemiol., 7*, 35–45.

Kalra, E. K., (2003). Nutraceutical-definition and introduction. *AAPS PharmSci., 5*(3), 27, 28.

Kaur, M., Agarwal, C., & Agarwal, R., (2009). Anticancer and cancer chemopreventive potential of grape seed extract and other grape-based products. *J. Nutr., 139*, 1806S–1812S.

Keservani, R. K., & Sharma, A. K., (2014). Flavonoids: Emerging trends and potential health benefits. *Journal of Chinese Pharmaceutical Sciences, 23*(12), 815.

Keservani, R. K., Kesharwani, R. K., Sharma, A. K., & Jarouliya, U., (2015). Dietary supplements, nutraceutical and functional foods in immune response (immunomodulators). In: Debasis, B., Harry, G. P., & Anand, S., (eds.), *Nutraceutical and Functional Foods in Human Life and Disease Prevention* (pp. 343–358). Boca Raton, Fl. Taylor and Francis, Chapter 20. ISBN: 9781482237214.

Keservani, R. K., Kesharwani, R. K., Sharma, A. K., Vyas, N., & Chadoker, A., (2010b). Nutritional supplements: An overview. *International Journal of Current Pharmaceutical Review and Research, 1*(1), 59–75.

Keservani, R. K., Kesharwani, R. K., Vyas, N., Jain, S., Raghuvanshi, R., & Sharma, A. K., (2010a). Nutraceutical and functional food as future food: A review. *Der Pharmacia Lettre, 2*(1), 106–116.

Keservani, R. K., Sharma, A. K., & Kesharwani, R. K., (2016). Medicinal effect of nutraceutical fruits for the cognition and brain health. *Scientifica*, 10. Article ID 3109254. doi: 10.1155/2016/3109254.

Key, T. J., Appleby, P. N., Travis, R. C., et al., (2015). Carotenoids, retinol, tocopherols, and prostate cancer risk: Pooled analysis of 15 studies. *Am. J. Clin. Nutr., 102*, 1142–1157.

Khan, N., Adhami, V. M., & Mukhtar, H., (2010). Apoptosis by dietary agents for prevention and treatment of prostate cancer. *Endocr. Relat. Cancer, 17*(1), R39–52.

Kobayashi, N., Barnard, R. J., Henning, S. M., et al., (2006). Effect of altering dietary omega-6/omega-3 fatty acid ratios on prostate cancer membrane composition, cyclooxygenase-2, and prostaglandin E2. *Clin. Cancer Res., 12*, 4662–4670.

Kolonel, L. N., Hankin, J. H., Whittemore, A. S., et al., (2000). Vegetables, fruits, legumes and prostate cancer: A multiethnic case-control study. *Cancer Epidemiol Biomarkers Prev., 9*, 795–804.

Konijeti, R., Henning, S., Moro, A., et al., (2010). Chemoprevention of prostate cancer with lycopene in the tramp model. *Prostate., 70*, 1547–1554.

Laviano, A., Rianda, S., Molfino, A., et al., (2013). Omega-3 fatty acids in cancer. *Curr. Opin. Clin. Nutr. Metab. Care, 16*, 156–161.

Lippert, M. C., McClain, R., Boyd, J. C., & Theodorescu, D., (1999). Alternative medicine use in patients with localized prostate carcinoma treated with curative intent. *Cancer, 86*, 2642–2648.

Major, J. M., et al., (2014). Genetic variants reflecting higher vitamin E status in men are associated with reduced risk of prostate cancer. *J. Nutr., 144*, 729–733.

Martinez, E. E., et al., (2014). A functional variant in NKX $_{3.1}$ associated with prostate cancer risk in the selenium and vitamin E cancer prevention trial (SELECT). *Cancer Prev. Res., 7*, 950–957.

Mondul, A. M., et al., (2015). Metabolomic analysis of prostate cancer risk in a prospective cohort: The alpha-tocolpherol, beta-carotene cancer prevention (ATBC) study. *Int. J. Cancer, 137*, 2124–2132.

Nam, R. K., Fleshner, N., Rakovitch, E., Klotz, L., et al., (1999). Prevalence and patterns of the use of complementary therapies among prostate cancer patients: An epidemiological analysis. *J. Urol., 161*, 1521–1524.

Nassiri-Asl, M., & Hosseinzadeh, H., (2009). Review of the pharmacological effects of *Vitis vinifera* (grape) and its bioactive compounds. *Phytother. Res., 23*, 1197–1204.

Nelson, W. G., De Marzo, A. M., & Isaacs, W. B., (2003). Prostate cancer. *N. Engl. J. Med., 349*, 366–381.

Palozza, P., Colangelo, M., Simone, R., et al., (2010). Lycopene induces cell growth inhibition by altering the mevalonate pathway and Ras signaling in cancer cell lines. *Carcinogenesis, 31*, 1813–1821.

Parnes, H. L., House, M. G., & Tangrea, J. A., (2013). Prostate cancer prevention: Strategies for agent development. *Curr. Opin. Oncol., 25*, 242–251.

Qiu, X., Yuan, Y., Vaishnav, A., et al., (2013). Effects of lycopene on protein expression in human primary prostatic epithelial cells. *Cancer Prev. Res. (Phila), 6*(5), 419–427.

Saldanha, S. N., & Tollefsbol, T. O., (2012). The role of nutraceuticals in chemoprevention and chemotherapy and their clinical outcomes. *J. Onc.*, Article ID 192464.

Sapota, A., et al., (2014). The bioavailability of different zinc compounds used as human dietary supplements in rat prostate: A comparative study. *Biometals, 27*, 495–505.

Schwartz, G. G., (2005). Vitamin D and the epidemiology of prostate cancer. *Semin. Dial., 18*, 276–289.

Schwartz, G., & Hanchette, C., (2006). UV, latitude, and spatial trends in prostate cancer mortality: all sunlight is not the same (United States). *Cancer Causes Control, 17*, 1091–1101.

Schwartz, G., & Hulka, B., (1990). Is vitamin D deficiency a risk factor for prostate cancer? (hypothesis). *Anticancer Res., 10*, 1307–1311.

Scott, E., Steward, W. P., Gescher, A. J., et al., (2012). Resveratrol in human cancer chemoprevention--choosing the 'right' dose. *Mol. Nutr. Food Res., 56*, 7–13.

Shen, J., Barrios, R. J., & Jaiswal, A. K., (2010). Inactivation of the quinone oxidoreductases nqo1 and nqo2 strongly elevates the incidence and multiplicity of chemically induced skin tumors. *Cancer Res., 70*, 1006–1014.

Shimizu, H., Ross, R. K., Bernstein, L., Yatani, R., Henderson, B. E., & Mack, T. M., (1991). Cancers of the prostate and breast among Japanese and white immigrants in Los Angeles County. *Br. J. Cancer, 63*, 963–966.

Society, A. C., (2013). *Cancer Facts and Figures.* American Cancer Society; Atlanta, GA.

Sporn, M. B., & Liby, K. T., (2013). Is lycopene an effective agent for preventing prostate cancer? *Cancer Prev. Res. (Phila), 6*, 384–386.

Suzuki, K., Yahara, S., Hashimoto, F., & Uyeda, M., (2001). Inhibitory activities of (-)-epigallocatechin-3-o-gallate against topoisomerases i and ii. *Biol. Pharm Bull., 24*, 1088–1090.

Terry, P., Lichtenstein, P., Feychting, M., et al., (2001). Fatty fish consumption and risk of prostate cancer. *Lancet, 357*, 1764–1766.

Ting, H., Deep, G., Agarwal, C., & Agarwal, R., (2014). The strategies to control prostate cancer by chemoprevention approaches. *Mutat. Res., 760*, 1–15.

Van, P. H., & Tombal, B., (2011). Chemoprevention of prostate cancer with nutrients and supplements. *Cancer Manag. Res., 3*, 91–100.

Yang, C. S., Li, G., & Yang, Z., (2013). Cancer prevention by tocopherols and tea polyphenols. *Cancer Lett., 334*(1), 79–85.

Yang, C. S., Wang, X., Lu, G., & Picinich, S. C., (2009). Cancer prevention by tea: Animal studies, molecular mechanisms and human relevance. *Nat Rev Cancer, 9*, 429–439.

Zhang, Y., Coogan, P., Palmer, J. R., Strom, B. L., & Rosenberg, L., (2009). Vitamin and mineral use and risk of prostate cancer: The case-control surveillance study. *Cancer Causes Control, 20*, 691–698.

CHAPTER 8

LUNG CANCER PREVENTION BY NUTRACEUTICALS

KHEMCHAND SURANA,[1] EKNATH D. AHIRE,[2] RITESH KHAIRNAR,[3] RITESH PAWAR,[4] SUNIL MAHAJAN,[5] SANJAY KSHIRSAGAR,[2] SWATI G. TALELE,[6] and BHAVANA AHIRE[7]

[1]*Department of Pharmaceutical Chemistry, Shreeshakti Shaikshanik Sanstha, Divine College of Pharmacy, Satana, Nashik, India*

[2]*Department of Pharmaceutics, MET's Institute of Pharmacy, Adgaon Nashik, India*

[3]*Department of Pharmaceutical Chemistry, St. John Institute of Pharmacy & Research, Palghar, Maharashtra, India*

[4]*Department of Pharmaceutical Chemistry, Poona College of Pharmacy, Pune, Maharashtra, India*

[5]*Department of Pharmaceutical Chemistry, MGV's Pharmacy College, Panchvati, Nashik, India*

[6]*Department of Pharmaceutics, Sandip Institute of Pharmaceutical Sciences, Affiliated to Savitribai Phule Pune University, Nashik, India*

[7]*Department of Quality Assurance Techniques, NDMVP's, College of Pharmacy, Nashik, India*

ABSTRACT

Lung cancer is another furthermost frequent disease worldwide and the main cause of cancer-related fatalities. In the United States, there were approximately 234,030 cases of lung cancer diagnosed in 2018, with approximately

Nutraceuticals in Cancer Prevention, Management, and Treatment. Raj K. Keservani, Bui Thanh Tung, Sippy Singh, & Rajesh K. Kesharwani, PhD (Eds.)

154,050 deaths. Most patients with lung cancer have an advanced-stage illness, for which palliative chemotherapy or radiation is the recommended treatment. Besides radiation and chemotherapy, nutraceuticals have been publicized to be operative at treating and preventing lung cancer. Nutraceuticals is a combination of the words "nutrition" and "pharmaceutical." Nutraceuticals, in general, are foods or parts of foods that have a substantial role in changing and sustaining normal physiological activity in humans. Nutraceuticals, which give health advantages and are an alternative to contemporary medicine, have gained popularity in recent years. Their ability to reduce cancer incidence in these studies is likely related to apoptosis. The ability of use of nutraceuticals as chemopreventive reagents has brought on a surge of in-vitro research on their organic results in cultured human cells. Chemoprevention uses small molecules, including nutritional or natural chemicals, to save you from cancers, instead of chemotherapeutics, wherein chemicals, in most cases synthetic, are used to dispose of or alleviate various cancers symptoms. Besides, they have a look at the organic results of those phytochemicals on the mobile stage gives the molecular foundation for their anti-tumor feature and allows them to set up the platform for producing stronger chemopreventive or even chemotherapeutic marketers. Nutraceutical-wealthy culmination and veggies are a crucial part of a balanced diet. The present demographic and health trends are the primary drivers of the nutraceutical market's global expansion. Dietary fiber, prebiotics, probiotics, polyunsaturated fatty acids, antioxidants, and other herbal/natural foods are examples of food products utilized as nutraceuticals.

8.1 INTRODUCTION

Stephen De Felice, MD, Founder, and Chairman of the Foundation for Innovation in Medicine (FIM), Cranford, NJ, invented the phrase "nutraceutical" in 1989, combining the words "nutrition" with "pharmaceutical." According to De Felice, nutraceuticals are "foods (or parts of foods) that give medicinal or health advantages, including disease prevention and/or therapy." A nutraceutical is a useful meal that assists withinside the prevention and/or remedy of disease(s) and/or disorder(s) aside from anemia (because maximum useful ingredients are anti-anemic in a few form, the exception to anemia is taken into consideration to offer a clean difference among the two words, useful meals and nutraceuticals). As a result, useful meals for one client is probably a nutraceutical for another. Fortified dairy products (consisting of milk) and citrus fruits (consisting of orange juice) are examples of nutraceuticals

(Kalra, 2003; Radhika et al., 2019; Keservani et al., 2010a, 2010b, 2020; Keservani and Sharma, 2014).

In Western Nations, lung cancer is the primary reason for cancers-associated fatalities. The mainstream of patients with lung cancer have an advanced-stage illness, for which palliative chemotherapy or radiation is the recommended treatment. Chemotherapy efficacy for advanced nonsmall cell lung cancer (NSCLC) is limited, with response rates of less than 30% reported in major studies of various chemotherapy combinations. Chemotherapy's effectiveness in advanced NSCLC has plateau, with minimal change in response rates, and it's been proposed that research should focus on new methodologies and unique therapies rather than alternative chemotherapy drug combinations (Rachel et al., 2019).

8.1.1 CONCEPT OF NUTRACEUTICALS

Clinical test findings for animal testing and research, as well as the verification of their therapeutic benefits, are required during the pharmaceutical development process. However, in the past, there was no technique for verifying the effectiveness of diets in avoiding illnesses. Food composition has been scientifically established to induce lifestyle-related disorders in recent years, and it has become a societal concern. The nutraceutical merchandise are diagnosed and convey fitness blessings like assuaging the chance of cancers and coronary heart disorder and additionally stopping or treating hypertension, excessive cholesterol, immoderate weight, osteoporosis, diabetes, arthritis, macular degeneration (main to irreversible blindness), cataracts, menopausal symptoms, insomnia, dwindled reminiscence and concentration, digestive upsets and constipation, now no longer to say headaches; different merchandise are touted as healing procedures for thinning hair, loss of confidence, bad complexion, varicose veins, alcoholism, depression, and lethargy (Radhika et al., 2019).

8.1.2 LUNG CANCER: A BRIEF OVERVIEW

Cancer is one of the most public reason of mortality worldwide. Lung cancer, in particular, is the most frequent disease worldwide and the main cause of cancer-related fatalities. In the United States, there were approximately 234,030 patients of lung cancer diagnosed in 2018, with almost 154,050 deaths (van Meerbeeck et al., 2011).

Non-small cell lung cancer (NSCLC) and small mobileular lung cancers (SCCLC) are the 2forms of lung cancers (SCLC). NSCLC debts for around 85% of all lung cancers. NSCLC is further split into adenocarcinoma, the most prevalent kind of NSCLC, squamous cell carcinoma, and big cell carcinoma, which is the most difficult to treat due to its proclivity for metastasizing. The second kind of lung cancer, SCLC, is believed to be more deadly due to its tendency to spread quickly (Peters et al., 1986). This form of cancer has a lot of risk factors. Smoking is the greatest powerful factor in lung cancer. About 85% of lung cancers are caused by smoking, while the other 15% are caused by secondhand smoke, air pollution, or other dangerous compounds such as asbestos, nickel, chromium, and arsenic (Behrouzian et al., 2003).

8.2 NUTRACEUTICALS IN AVOIDANCE OF LUNG CANCER

8.2.1 OMEGA-3 POLYUNSATURATED FATTY ACIDS

Fatty acids are biomolecules that have a carboxyl head attached to an aliphatic carbon chain covalently. They are usually separated into saturated fatty acids, which have solely alkyl sp^3hybridized carbons in the aliphatic chain, and unsaturated fatty acids, which have at least one carbon-carbon double bond (C=C) in the aliphatic chain. Saturated and unsaturated fatty acids may have an alkyl tail of even period commonly starting from 16 to 22 carbons, that's synthesized via way of means of elongate activity. Desaturases manufacture polyunsaturated fatty acids (PUFAs) from saturated fatty acids via an elimination process using a di-iron oxo catalyst (Owen et al., 2020). In recent years, researchers have looked into omega-3 polyunsaturated fatty acid (ω-3 PUFA) supplements for chemoinhibition of various cancers, including lung cancer. ω-3 PUFAs are immune nutrients that are often employed in cancer patients' nutritional treatment. ω-3 PUFAs have an significant function in cell signaling, cell shape, and membrane fluidity. They have a role in inflammation resolution and have anti-inflammatory properties. Complications of lung cancer include anorexia-cachexia syndrome, pain, and despair. The 2017 guidelines for cancer patients published by the European Society for Clinical Nutrition and Metabolism (ESPEN) exclusively cover the use of ω-3 PUFAs for cancer cachexia therapy, leaving out additional cancer-related problems that might benefit from ω-3 PUFAs. Furthermore, clinical investigations, data from cell lines, and animal models all point to ω-3 PUFAs having anticancer properties. The modulation of critical pathways underpinning the advancement of complications of lung cancer by ω-3 PUFAs and their metabolites has been indicated, representing that this is a potential field to investigate. More research is needed to determine the effects of ω-3 PUFAs as a supplement or as a pharmaceutical therapy for lung cancer (Ahire et al., 2020; Liu et al., 2001).

8.2.2 OMEGA-3 PUFAS

The important fatty acid alpha-linolenic acid (ALA) is the source of many ω-3 PUFAs. Humans can make the long-chain fatty acids eicosapentaenoic acid (EPA) and docosahexaenoic acid (DHA) from alpha-linolenic acid, which can be found in soy and some vegetables. EPA and DHA, on the other hand, are predominantly received from the food, principally through the consumption of fish oils, whereas ALA conversion accounts for just 2% to 10% of the total. All three PUFAs may be oxidized to oxylipins, which produce distinct signaling classes and molecules based on the saturation and length of the precursors. In addition to the percentage of PUFAs in the diet, several studies demonstrated that a high ω-3 to ω-6 PUFA ratio has been associated with several positive health factors. The omega-3 fatty acids EPA and DHA have also been accompanied with a lower risk of some malignancies. EPA and DHA have been shown to prevent tumor development generated by phorbol 12-tetradecanoate 13-acetate (TPA) and epidermal growth factor (EGF) (Kiss et al., 2014).

8.3 EVIDENCE OF THE EFFECT OF OMEGA-3 IN LUNG CANCER

Patients with nonsmall cell lung cancer may benefit from taking ω-3 during chemotherapy, particularly platinum-based chemotherapy, according to new research. Chemotherapy has caused esophagitis, nausea, and other side effects in individuals, affecting their nutritional condition and general well-being. Malnutrition has been linked to deprived reactions to chemotherapy and other cancer treatments in 45 to 69% of lung cancer patients, according to studies (Parthasarathy et al., 1990).

8.3.1 OMEGA-6 PUFAS

In recent times, a ω-6-rich diet is also linked to primarily unfavorable health outcomes. The oxidation of low-density lipoproteins has been shown to increase atherosclerosis in the arteries (Alnabulsi et al., 2017). In colorectal cancer, some metabolites of arachidonic acid (AA), the most important ω-6 fatty acid, have been linked to tumor development and metastasis via upregulating epidermal growth factor (EGF). AA is also a precursor to a range of pro-inflammatory mediators, including prostaglandins, which can enhance the inflammatory response (Geert et al., 2017).

8.3.2 VITAMINS

The prospect that a high administration of particular vitamins might protect against cancer has piqued researchers' curiosity since it could give a reasonably easy measure for cancer prevention in human populations (Virtamo, 1999). Diet has also been linked to the improvement of lung cancer. However, the exact nutrients involved are yet unknown. Antioxidant vitamins have gotten a lot of attention recently. In several prospective epidemiological investigations, β-carotene, the most effective provitamin A, was shown to be contrariwise linked with the incidence of lung cancer, particularly in studies evaluating blood β-carotene concentrations. The results of controlled studies, on the other hand, contradict the premise that β-carotene can prevent lung cancer, and instead imply that supplemental β-carotene increases the risk of lung cancer. Vitamin E appears to have no function in lung carcinogenesis, according to data from prospective studies and a controlled experiment. Although certain prospective epidemiological studies imply an adverse relationship between dietary vitamin C and the incidence of lung cancer, the independent contribution of dietary vitamin C is difficult to evaluate due to the significant correlation between dietary vitamin C and vegetable and fruit intake. No controlled trials of vitamin C on lung cancer have been published, and studies employing pre-diagnostic plasma concentrations of ascorbic acid do not support the role of vitamin C in lung carcinogenesis. As a result, antioxidant vitamin supplementation is not designated for lung cancer prevention (IARC, 1998).

8.3.3 VITAMIN A AND β-CAROTENE

High doses of retinoid have been shown to suppress carcinogenesis in the respiratory system in animal models, although b-carotene is ineffective (Mallesh 2021). In this study, milk and carrots contributed considerably to diet an intake, and every meals object become associated strongly and inversely to the threat of lung cancer. Early cohort research in Japan (Hirayama, 1979) discovered that daily eating of carotenoid-rich green or yellow vegetables was related to a lower incidence of lung cancer as compared to less frequent consumption. Abridged lung cancer risk was exclusively related to increasing carotene intake in the first cohort research examining the separate effects of dietary carotene and retinol (Peto et al., 1981) speculated that β-carotene, the maximum ample and successfully transformed of the provitamin carotenoids in veggies and fruits, may guard towards cancer, primarily based totally on the protecting consequences of accelerated vegetable and fruit intake in epidemiological research of lung and different cancers. Controlled clinical experiments to assess the potential of β-carotene in the inhibition of lung and other cancers were started in the 1980s based on the consistency of epidemiological data and evidence of tumor suppression in animal models (Keservani et al., 2010a, 2015; Anshul et al., 2017).

8.3.4 VITAMIN E

Only a few prospective studies have looked at the link between vitamin E intake and lung cancer, and the results have ranged from a modest negative connection to no association. Except for one study that originate an important opposite relationship between α-tocopherol serum concentrations and lung cancer. The impact of supplemental vitamin E (α-tocopherol) on the risk of lung cancer has only been studied in one controlled experiment. In the ATBC study, 14564 men got 50 mg/d α-tocopherol supplementation and 14 569 men did not get a-tocopherol supplementation for 5–8 (median 61) years, with no overall impact of a-tocopherol supplementation on lung cancer.

8.3.5 VITAMIN C

Six prospective studies investigated the association between vitamin C consumption from vegetables and fruits and lung cancer risk. The findings have ranged from an inverse to no association, but three of the most recent studies have initiated an important opposite relationship between dietary vitamin C and the risk of lung cancer. Two investigations found a link between plasma ascorbic acid concentration and lung cancer risk; in one, plasma ascorbic acid concentration was not predictive of eventual lung cancer mortality, while in the other, slight non-significant protection was shown. There have been no published skillful trials of vitamin C supplementation in connection to lung cancer (Anshul et al., 2017).

8.4 PROBIOTIC IN LUNG CANCER

Probiotics have been applied to treat a variety of diseases, counting those of the colon, blood, breast, rectum, cervical, prostate, skin, esophagus, liver, bladder, gall bladder, head, and neck. There is a link between oral illnesses and the risk of lung cancer. The biomarkers Capnocytophaga and Veillonella are the most common organisms in the saliva of lung cancer patients. Kefir, a fermented milk product containing the probiotic, has considerably enhanced T helper and cytotoxic T cells, as well as a significant reduction in lung and bone marrow metastases.

The occurrence of dysbiosis or malignancy in the lungs is linked to the dynamic interplay of several elements relating to the immune system, microbes, and the environment. Lung cancer cells (premalignant and senescent) produce IL-6 and IL-8, which are enhanced in inflammatory stress conditions in the lungs. Through their direct influence on boosting the NF-kB-1 pathway in lung epithelial cells, these circumstances cause lung cancer development. Kim et al., evaluated the effects of seven probiotic strains on lung cancer patients in 1991. Combination therapy has been demonstrated to have synergistic benefits in the treatment of cancer-induced animal models, with a 2–2.5-fold reduction in metastasis inhibition when compared to mice given only one vaccination.

Bacillus thetaiotaomicron or *Bacillus fragile* species can stimulate the immune response and improve the performance of CTLA-4 antibodies in a mouse model of sarcoma tumor development. At a concentration of 106 CFU/well, *L. casei* strain-fermented milk showed potential anticancer and anti-inflammatory effects, with substantial suppression of cancer growth. Treatment with cisplatin alone and in combination with probiotics has convincingly demonstrated probiotics' potential as anti-tumor agents. Aerosolization of antibiotics or probiotics modulates the pulmonary microbiome, according to Le Noci et al., in the lungs, slows the development of tumors. The chemical cyclophosphamide causes the elimination of bacteria. Immunomodulation has also been influenced by treatment owing to lower amounts of immune cells.

Although the significance of microbiota in lung cancer treatment has yet to be unwavering, research has yielded encouraging findings. For the research of the involvement of gut microbiota in lung cancer, several markers have been established. Oncomicrobiotics such as *Enterococcus hirae* and *Barnesiella intestinihominis* were proven to enhance the effectiveness of alkylating immunomodulatory agents. Na-Kyoung et al., investigated the effects of *L. lactis* (bacteria isolated from kimchi) on malignancies such as gastric carcinoma. Colon carcinoma, breast carcinoma, and lung carcinoma are all examples of cancers. This probiotic has exhibited intestinal adherence competition and prevented the attachment of six pathogens to the mucus layer. In addition to the potential anticancer action, it has been demonstrated to have a considerable antioxidant impact (Le Marchand et al., 2000).

8.5 PROBIOTICS PREVENTING RESPIRATORY-RELATED DISEASES

Probiotics are thought to have a protective mechanism linked to the increased working action of immune cells in the respiratory tract, such as natural killer (NK) cells and macrophages (alveolar system). Some probiotic bacterial species, such as Lactobacillus and Foley Bifidobacterium, have been shown to lower the pathogen burden in the respiratory system. Human NK cell function is decreased by cigarette smoking, which has been related to an increased risk of COPD and lung cancer. Asthma is one of the utmost communal childhood diseases, characterized by chronic pulmonary inflammation, airway hyper-reactivity, excessive mucus production, and respiratory obstruction. Chronic inflammation-induced generation of reactive oxygen/nitrogen species in the lungs was formerly thought to predispose people to lung cancer. A meta-analysis of the connection between lung cancer and asthma was recently published in a prestigious publication. The presence of inflammatory cells and mediators in the Bronchoalveolar lavage fluid (BALF) is used to assess pulmonary inflammation in mice that are sensitive to ovalbumin. Interleukin-4, IL-5, and IL-10 levels were lowered by Bifidobacterium M-16V, and allergic skin reactivity to OVA was reduced by *L. plantarum* NumRes8. *Lactobacillus gasseri* can decrease the Th17 pro-inflammatory response and prevent OVA-induced airway inflammation in mice, according to another research. A mouse model of asthma (21-dayovalbumin sensitization and challenge paradigm) was employed in this investigation, which was then followed with PM2.5 exposures. These findings suggest that probiotics can be beneficial in decreasing the prevalence of lung cancers in the ones who've asthma. The body's anomalous immune reaction may be avoided or handled with the management of useful probiotic bacterial strains. Probiotics showcase anti-cancers pastime and feature immunomodulatory results on cancers cells through herbal (Rane et al., 2020a, 2020b) killer (NK) cells, macrophages, T cells, elevated manufacturing of cytokines, antioxidants, and anti-angiogenic factors, and discount in cancers-particular proteins and seasoned carcinogenic enzymes.

8.6 EFFECT OF PROBIOTICS ON LUNG IMMUNITY

The human body is vulnerable to harmful substances that are either naturally occurring or generated industrially. Chemical carcinogens wreak havoc on a variety of metabolic pathways by disrupting genome integrity. Lung cancer is caused by benzopyrene, one of the most common mutagens in the air. It has been found that cell suspensions of several *Bifidobacterium* species had stronger antimutagenic properties than their supernatants when exposed to benzopyrene. Lung cancer is one of the foremost reasons of death, and it may be prevented by limiting the entry and exit of heavy metals into the body (Figure 8.1). Heavy metals could be bound by *Lactobacillus, Bifidobacterium longum, Lactobacillus rhamnosus*, and *Lactobacillus* plane *in vitro*. Pyridoxine rouses anticancer immune surveillance in the framework of cisplatin-based chemotherapy for non-small-cell lung cancer, according to a study (Hertog et al., 1995; Goldbohm et al., 1997).

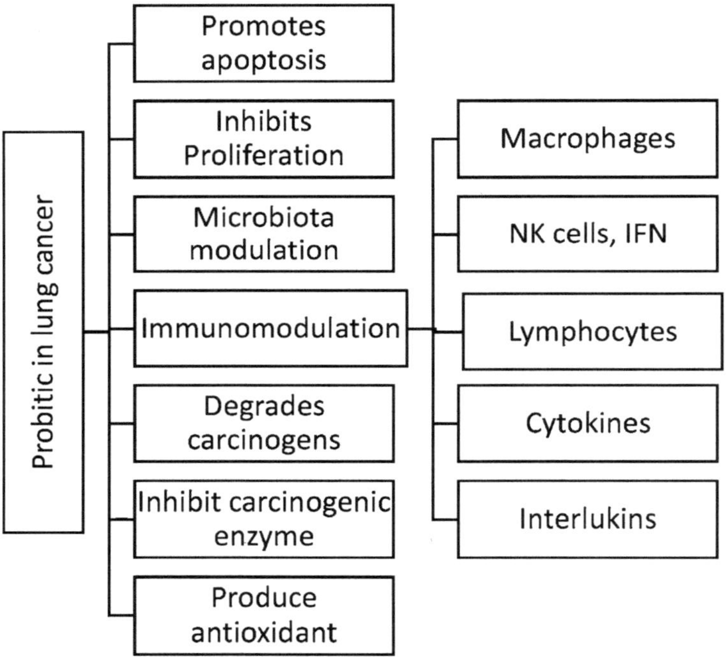

FIGURE 8.1 Role of prebiotic in lung cancer.

8.6.1 *FLAVONOIDS*

Numerous researches in recent years have revealed that polyphenolic flavonoids originate in fruits and vegetables may be cancer-protective. Knekt et al., looked studied a sample of approximately 10,000 cancer-free men and women who took part in a Finnish study between 1966 and 1975. The researchers discovered an inverse association between flavonoid consumption and cancer incidence using dietary history and flavonoid intake estimations (all sites combined). It was discovered that the link was predominantly with lung cancer and that the findings were independent of antioxidant vitamin E, C, and carotene consumption (Arts et al., 2001; Das et al., 1994). Following that, Le Marchand et al., in Hawaii, researchers conducted a population-based case-control study with over 500 smokers and 500 matched controls. After controlling for saturated fat and -carotene intakes, the researchers discovered an inverse relationship between flavonoids (quercetin and naringin) consumption and lung cancer risk. It's also value noticing that several well-designed research has found no link between flavonoid consumption and cancer incidence in different locations. No link was exposed between flavonoid ingesting and overall cancer death in four additional well-known studies (Middleton et al., 2000). It's also value noticing that indirect estimates of flavonoid consumption are frequently used in epidemiological, cohort, and case-control studies. Typically, just a small number of flavonoids from diverse meals are estimated (typically less than five or six out of thousands), with anthocyanins being excluded. Because of this flaw, determining the extent of any influence flavonoids, individually or collectively, may have on disease states in the general population is challenging. More controlled research on the links between flavonoid consumption and illness is needed. Das et al. (1994) and Middleton et al. (2000) provide comprehensive evaluations of flavonoids' antimutagenic effects (Surana et al., 2021a; Surana et al., 2021b).

8.7 CONCLUSION

Lung cancer is the foremost reason of cancer-related death in the world. Due to late diagnosis, tumor resistance, and a lack of effective treatments, the survival rate is low. In such an environment, Nutraceuticals are a revolutionary way to treat lung cancer that also has long-term advantages in the treatment of other respiratory illnesses. Rather than treating lung cancer, nutraceuticals are most effective at preventing it. Omega-3 polyunsaturated fatty acids, probiotics, flavonoids, and vitamins are some promising nutraceuticals in the inhibition of lung cancer. Some of these nutraceuticals can be used in chemoprevention, but further studies will be required to confirm this.

ACKNOWLEDGMENT

We thank MET, Institute of Pharmacy, BKC, affiliated with Savitribai Phule Pune University, Nashik, Divine College of Pharmacy Satana, and

Sandip Institute of Pharmaceutical Science for their constant support and for providing all facilities to complete this work. We are also thankful to the Ministry of Tribal Affairs Govt. of India for providing financial assistance in the form of fellowship (Award No: 202021-NFST-MAH-01235).

KEYWORDS

- **flavonoids**
- **lung cancer**
- **nutraceuticals**
- **omega-3 polyunsaturated fatty acids**
- **probiotics**
- **vitamin**

REFERENCES

Ahire, E. D., et al., (2020). Role of omega-3 fatty acids in different neurodegenerative disorders. *Applied Pharmaceutical Science and Microbiology* (pp. 173–194). Apple Academic Press.

Alnabulsi, A., Swan, R., Cash, B., Alnabulsi, A., & Murray, G. I., (2017). The differential expression of omega-3 and omega-6 fatty acid metabolizing enzymes in colorectal cancer and its prognostic significance. *Br. J. Cancer, 116*(12), 1612–1620. doi: 10.1038/bjc.2017.135.

Anshul, S., Buddolla, V., & Young-Seo, P., (2018). Role of probiotics in the management of lung cancer and related diseases: An update. *Journal of Functional Foods, 40*(2018), 625–633.

Arts, M. J., Haenen, G. R., Voss, H. P., & Bast, A., (2001). Masking of antioxidant capacity by the interaction of flavonoids with protein. *Food Chem. Toxicol., 39*(8), 787–791.

Behrouzian, B., & Buist, P. H., (2003). Mechanism of fatty acid desaturation: A bioorganic perspective. *Prostaglandins Leukotrienes and Essential Fatty Acids, 68*(2), 107–112. doi: 10.1016/S0952- 3278(02)00260-0.

Das, A., Wang, J. H., & Lien, E. J., (1994). Carcinogenicity, mutagenicity, and cancer-preventing activities of flavonoids: A structure-system-activity relationship (SSAR) analysis. *Prog. Drug Res., 42*, 133–166.

Geert, V. P., & Henk, V. D., B., (2017). *Vitamins and Cancer*. Nutrition and Food Research Institute, PO Box 360, 3700 AJ Z.&T, The Netherlands.

Goldbohm, R. A., Hertog, M. G. L., Brants, H. A. M., Van, P. G., & Van, D. B. P. A., (1997). Intake of flavonoids and cancer risk: A prospective cohort study. In: Armado, R., Anderson,

H., Bardóez, S., & Serra, F., (eds.), *Polyphenols in Food* (pp. 159–166). Luxembourg: Official Publications of the European Communities.

Hertog, M. G., Kromhout, D., Aravanis, C., Blackburn, H., Buzina, R., Fidanza, F., Giampaoli, S., et al., (1995). Flavonoid intake and long-term risk of coronary heart disease and cancer in the seven countries study. *Arch. Intern. Med., 155*(4), 381–386.

IARC Working Group on the Evaluation of Cancer Preventive Agents, (1998). *IARC Handbooks of Cancer Prevention: Carotenoids* (Vol. 2). Lyon, France: International Agency for Research on Cancer.

Kalra, E. K., (2003). Nutraceutical – definition and introduction. *AAPS PharmSci., 5*(3), Article 25.

Keservani, R. K., & Sharma, A. K., (2014). Flavonoids: Emerging trends and potential health benefits. *Journal of Chinese Pharmaceutical Sciences, 23*(12), 815.

Keservani, R. K., Kesharwani, R. K., Sharma, A. K., Vyas, N., & Chadoker, A., (2010b). Nutritional supplements: An overview. *International Journal of Current Pharmaceutical Review and Research, 1*(1), 59–75.

Keservani, R. K., Kesharwani, R. K., Vyas, N., Jain, S., Raghuvanshi, R., & Sharma, A. K., (2010a). Nutraceutical and functional food as future food: A review. *Der Pharmacia Lettre, 2*(1), 106–116.

Keservani, R. K., Sharma, A. K., & Kesharwani, R. K., (2020). *Nutraceuticals and Dietary Supplements: Applications in Health Improvement and Disease Management*. CRC Press. ISBN: 9781771888738.

Kiss, N. K., Krishnasamy, M., & Isenring, E. A., (2014). The effect of nutrition intervention in lung cancer patients undergoing chemotherapy and/or radiotherapy: A systematic review. *Nutrition Cancer, 66*(1), 47–56. doi: 10.1080/01635581.2014.847966.

Le Marchand, L., Murphy, S. P., Hankin, J. H., Wilkens, L. R., & Kolonel, L. N., (2000). Intake of flavonoids and lung cancer. *J. Natl. Cancer Inst., 92*(2), 154–160.

Liu, G., Bibus, D. M., Bode, A. M., Ma, W. Y., Holman, R. T., & Dong, Z., (2001). Omega 3 but not omega 6 fatty acids inhibit AP-1 activity and cell transformation in JB6 cells. *Proc. Natl. Acad. Sci. USA, 98*(13), 7510–7515. doi: 10.1073/pnas.131195198.

Mallesh, K., & Koteswara, R. G. S. N., (2021). Probiotics in lung cancer: An emerging field of multifarious potential and opportunities. *Probiotic Research in Therapeutics* (pp. 125–158) Springer Nature Singapore Pte Ltd.

Middleton, E. Jr., Kandaswami, C., & Theoharides, T. C., (2000). The effects of plant flavonoids on mammalian cells: Implications for inflammation, heart disease, and cancer. *Pharmacol. Rev., 52*(4), 673–751.

Murphy, R. A., Mourtzakis, M., Chu, Q. S., Baracos, V. E., Reiman, T., & Mazurak, V. C. (2011). Supplementation with fish oil increases first-line chemotherapy efficacy in patients with advanced nonsmall cell lung cancer. *Cancer, 117*(16), 3774–3780.

Owen, M. V., Shaheen, A., Zhen, T., Austin, T., & Huerta-Yepez, S., (2020). Omega-3 polyunsaturated fatty acids and lung cancer: Nutrition or pharmacology? *Nutrition and Cancer*. doi: 10.1080/01635581.2020.1761408.

Parthasarathy, S., Khoo, J. C., Miller, E., Barnett, J., Witztum, J. L., & Steinberg, D., (1990). Low-density lipoprotein rich in oleic acid is protected against oxidative modification: Implications for dietary prevention of atherosclerosis. *Proc. Natl. Acad. Sci USA, 87*(10), 3894–3898. doi: 10.1073/pnas.87.10.3894.

Peters, J. M., Thomas, D., Falk, H., Oberd€orster, G., & Smith, T. J., (1986). Contribution of metals to respiratory cancer. *Environ Health Perspect., 70*, 71–83. doi: 10.1289/ ehp.867071.

Radhika, P. R., Gowsalya, M., Kaviya, V., & Vigneshwari, M., (2019). Nutraceuticals: A review. *World Journal of Pharmaceutical Research, 8*(11), 1354–1374.

Rane, B. R., Bharath, M. S., Patil, R. R., Keservani, R. K., & Jain, A. S., (2020b). Novel approaches in nutraceuticals. In: Rajesh, K. K., Raj, K. K., & Anil, K. S., (eds.), *Enhancing the Therapeutic Efficacy of Herbal Formulations Through Novel Drug Delivery Systems* (pp. 241–266). IGI Global International Publisher, Pennsylvania, USA, Chapter 11. ISBN13: 9781799844532.

Rane, B. R., Patil, A. S., Keservani, R. K., & Jain, A. S., (2020a). Novel approaches in herbal formulation. In: Rajesh, K. K., Raj, K. K., & Anil, K. S., (eds.), *Enhancing the Therapeutic Efficacy of Herbal Formulations Through Novel Drug Delivery Systems* (pp. 43–68). IGI Global International Publisher, Pennsylvania, USA, Chapter 2. ISBN13: 9781799844532.

Surana, K. R., et al., (2021a). Informatics and methods in nutrition design and development. *Natural Food Products and Waste Recovery* (pp. 33–49). Apple Academic Press.

Surana, K. R., et al., (2021b). Biomolecular and molecular docking: A modern tool in drug discovery and virtual screening of natural products. *Applied Pharmaceutical Practice and Nutraceuticals* (pp. 209–223). Apple Academic Press.

Van M. J. P., Fennell, D. A., & De Ruysscher, D. K., (2011). Small-cell lung cancer. *Lancet. 378*(9804), 1741–1755. doi: 10.1016/S0140-6736(11)60165-7.

Virtamo, J., (1999). Vitamins and lung cancer. *Proceedings of the Nutrition Society, 58*(2), 329–333. doi: 10.1017/s0029665199000440.

CHAPTER 9

COLON CANCER PREVENTION BY MEDICINAL PLANTS

MADHURI VERMA,[1] EKNATH D. AHIRE,[2] and RAJ K. KESERVANI[3]

[1]*Naraina Group of Institutions of Pharmacy, Kanpur, Dr. APJ Abdul Kalam Technical University, India*

[2]*Department of Pharmaceutics, MET's Institute of Pharmacy, Affiliated to Savitribai Phule Pune University, BKC, Adgaon, Nashik, MH, India*

[3]*Faculty of B. Pharmacy, CSM Group of Institutions, Prayagraj, Uttar Pradesh, India*

ABSTRACT

Colon cancer is developed by factors like gender, lifestyle, age, diet, genetic predisposition, or inflammatory bowel disease. This malignancy was treated by surgical removal of cancer, radiotherapy, and chemotherapy. Chemoresistance and skin toxicities are developed in 80–90% of patients with monotherapy with drugs and other serious toxicities. Obesity, cigarette smoking, alcohol intake, intake of processed and red meat is the risk factor for colon cancer. Medicinal plants contain a mixture of various phytoconstituents which is a current concern of new research. They have the potential to prevent the occurrence or treat such cancerous conditions with no or lesser side effects. More than 1000 medicinal plants were reported to have an anticancer activity or prevent from risk factors. The rationale of this analysis is to present specific phytochemical, preclinical, and clinical studies related to colon cancer.

Nutraceuticals in Cancer Prevention, Management, and Treatment. Raj K. Keservani, Bui Thanh Tung, Sippy Singh, & Rajesh K. Kesharwani, PhD (Eds.)

9.1 INTRODUCTION

Colon cancer is the 3rd most ordinary cancer all over the globe. It is estimated that 52,980 deaths will be recognized to colorectal cancer this year (Colorectal Cancer, 2021). An enhance of 60% of this melanoma incidence is predictable by 2030 (Arnold, 2017). Colon cancer is frequently measured as one of the most preventable cancers because it often develops from polyps that can be detected and removed before cancer occurs. Several factors such as gender, age, genetic predisposition, lifestyle, diet, or complications from other ailments such as inflammatory bowel disease (IBD) (Bernstein, 2001) are closely associated with this malignancy. Men and women are aged 50 and over. More than 90% of people with this cancer are identified after the age of 50 (Selvanathan, 2020). Cancers of the colon appear from the colon's epithelial cells which line the organ's lumen (Markowitz, 2002, 2009). Hereditarily, colorectal cancer is classified into three types: sporadic (60%) relating to patients with no family the past, familial (30%) consist of patients with at least one blood relation with colorectal cancer or an adenoma, and inherited colorectal cancer (10%) ensuing from germline heritage of mutations (Kheirelseid, 2013). Approximately 8.5% of patient sufferers with CRC die from their cancer (Remmele, 1987; Johnson, 2013). The development of metastasis predominantly in the liver and lung are the deadly foremost reason of death and a severe obstruction to curative CRC. Lately, it has been exposed that Death-associated protein kinase 1 (DAPK1) might be a potential candidate adaptable metastasis in CRC. DAPK1as acting filament-associate calcium/calmodulin-regulated, stress-responsive serine/threonine kinase was account to be an tremendously pleiotropic molecule due to its unique multi-domain structure (Gozuacik, 2008) (Schneider-Stock, 2014; Johnson, 2013).

Treatment of colon cancer differs depending on the place of the tumor. One of the most common techniques for treating colon cancer involves the removal of tumors using surgical approaches combined with radiotherapy and chemotherapy. The most common chemotherapy regimens include the application of 5-fluoroarosyl and oxaliplatin (DeSantis, 2014). Despite the advent of new chemotherapeutic drugs, chemoresistance and excessive side effects have though been the biggest barrier to increasing the effectiveness of combined therapy (Wilhelm, 2016; Longley, 2003). In addition, cetuximab and panitumumab are two dissimilar monoclonal antibodies that intention and connect to the epidermal growth factor receptor (EGFR), thus reducing its activation and dimerization. Both promote the outcomes of metastatic colorectal cancer (MCRC) patients either in monotherapy or in amalgamation with chemotherapy (Garcia-Fonsilas, 2019). However, 80–95% of patients with MCRC reported skin toxicity by application of these monotherapies (Fakih, 2010).

9.2 RISK FACTORS

Other than genetic factors, some other risk factors contribute to colon cancer, such as obesity, cigarette smoking, alcohol intake, and consumption of processed and red meat (Johnson, 2013).

9.2.1 OBESITY

It has been established that the colorectal cancer threat amplified by 7% for each 2 kg/m2 increase in body mass index (Moghaddam, 2017). Lately examined 16 cohort investigation approved out among 1970 and 2014 and accomplished that fatness before the finding of colorectal cancer was linked with augmented colorectal cancer-specific death. It has been recommended that troubling the dynamic function of the adipocyte in energy homeostasis by fatness results in modification of adipokine (leptin and adiponectin) signaling (Lee, 2015). In accumulation, insulin resistance originated by fatness has been revealed to give to colorectal cancer expansion (Khandekar, 2011; Benarba, 2018).

9.2.2 CIGARETTE SMOKING

It has been demonstrated that nicotine is a major compound of tobacco smoke that has been promoted in vivo colon tumor development and angiogenesis by mounting COX-2 and PGE2 (Wong, 2007; Benares, 2018). Cigarette smoking encourages prostaglandin E2 (PGE2) synthesis, which is considered to be a high-risk cause for colon cancer (Useros, 2016; Benares, 2018) at high concentrations. This may be due to the establishment of an arachidonic cascade. Cyclooxygenase-2 (COX-2), a main enzyme in inflammation, exchange arachidonic acid to PGE2. The effects of COX-2 in colorectal carcinogenesis are mediated mainly through PGE2 inhibiting apoptosis and stimulating angiogenesis (Shrubsole, 2012) (Benaras, 2018).

9.2.3 CONSUMPTION OF PROCESSED MEAT AND RED MEAT

Epidemiological studies around the world have established a marked relationship between augmented colorectal cancer and elevated ingestion of red or developed meat have demonstrated a positive relationship between the intake of developed red meat and the risk of distal colon cancer in two large cohorts: The Nurses' Health Study (n = 87,108 women, 1980–2010) and follow health professional studies (n = 47,389 men, 1986–2010) (Bernstein, 2015). A large systematic review of fifteen cohort studies (Noret, 2010) found that red and processed meat intakes each contain 100 g/g/h. The daytime increase resulted in a summary relative risk of 1.16 for colorectal cancer. Similar findings have been reported at 120 g/h each in the first red and processed meat intake (Larsen, 2006; Bastid, 2011). Summaries of 1.28 for daytime growth were reported to show relative risk (Bastid, 2011) reviewed prospective cohort studies of heme intake reporting colon cancer (Santarelli, 2008; Benarba, 2018).

9.3 MEDICINAL PLANT EFFECTIVE IN COLON CANCER

9.3.1 ALOE

The *Aloe castellorum* and *Aloe pseudorubroviolacea* leaf extract were analyzed beside the human colon cancer cell line (HCT-116). The result have revealed that both plants extract have substantial cytotoxic activity, in the meantime, the methanolic extract of *Aloe castellorum* demonstrate advanced cytotoxic action than *Aloe pseudorubroviolacea* extract (Ahamed, 2020).

9.3.2 DATURA INOXIA

Rinoxia B (RB) was extracted from *Datura inoxia*, deliberate not in favor of human colon adenocarcinoma cells, HCT15. The cure shows an increase in cancer cell death. Additionally, the outcome of the comet, flow cytometry, and cell cycle study establish that most of the cells were found to have their S and G2/G2/S by blocking the mitotic spindle formation. M was arrested at the stage. In addition, RB also inhibits cell division by the expression of tumor suppressors (p53 and p21) and cell cycle regulatory proteins (Cyclins D1 and B1). Thus, the present finding concluded that baX/BX in RB HCT15 cells. Bcl2 may provide potential apoptotic effects by acting on the pathway, thus reducing colon cancer (Gajendran, 2019).

9.3.3 *BLEPHARIS PERSICA*

The treatment of hydrochloric extract of *Blepharis persica* and *Doxorubicin* was used separately as well as together on ASG and HT29 cell lines. The results have shown that *B. persica* extracts induced apoptosis in AGS and HT29 cells and its extract caused a dose-dependent rise in up-regulation of *BAX* level ($p < 0.05$) and down-regulation of *BCL2* ($p < 0.05$). *B. persica* exhibited a synergistic affect along with DOX on the HT29 cell line (Aghaabbasi, 2020).

9.3.4 *ARTEMISIA AUCHERI*

Artemisia aucheri extract in diverse doses of 0, 10, 100, 500, and 1000 μg/ml were subjected to study against human HT29 colon cancer cells at specified time intervals. In high dose 1000 μg/ml (80.63 ± 3.66) it shows maximum apoptosis. Furthermore, the survival rate of HT29 (IC50 = 57.88 μg/ml) and HEK (IC50 = 295 μg/ml) cancer cells decreased with increasing dose-dependently. Additionally, the induction of membrane lipid peroxidation was considerably more in HT29 evaluate with the control ($p < 0.001$). This exerted apoptotic effects against HT29 cells through the induction of membrane lipid peroxidation and apoptosis (Ali, 2021).

9.3.5 *CARLINA CURETUM*

The extracts were explored their ability to inhibit enzymes α-amylase, α-glucosidase, and lipase and evaluation of cytotoxic activity against HeLa and Colo-205 cells using standard biochemical and biotechnical methods. *C. curetum* 0.5 mg/g of acetone and hexane fractions. Ml had noticeable cytotoxic effects on the Colo-205 cancer cell line, and 0.625 mg/g of *C. curatedum* hexane fraction. This study showed that *C. curetum* has potentially α-amylase, α-glucosidase, porcine pancreatic lipase enzyme suppressive activity, and cytotoxic activity against HeLa and Colo-205 cancer cell lines (Jaradat, 2019).

9.3.6 MENTHA ARVENSIS

Nanoparticles of less than 100 mentha arvensis particle sizes are effective cytotoxic particles not in favor of HCT116 colon cancer cells, and ic50 is abridged to 1.7 μg/s was measured at ml. The annexin vapoptosis assay further confirmed that AgNPs persuade apoptosis in a dose-dependent approach. Experimental indication exposed that AgNPs capture the cell cycle and implicate a large number of cells in the sub-G1 phase, nest confirm the anticancer potential of AgNPs (Javed, 2020).

9.3.7 CITRUS FRUIT

Nobiletin (NOB), a polymethoxyflavone (PMF) extracted from citrus peel, and its derivatives were evaluated against HT-29 colon cancer cells. The learning resolute that the IC50 and IC90 of NOB alongside HT-29 cells were 4.7 μM and 13.9 μM, correspondingly, via the 3H-thymidine uptake assay (Stingl, 2011). As a product of autohydrolysis of NOB, 5-DMN was also estimated for its antiproliferative outcome alongside colon cancer cells. In-vitrostudies, NOB, and 5-DMN have exposed the cytotoxic properties towards colon cancer cells, predominantly by cell cycle arrest and initiation of apoptosis (Goh, 2019).

9.3.8 BETULA ETNENSIS

The methanolic extract of bark was explored against the human colon cancer cell line (CaCo2). The extract considerably abridged the cell feasibility of CaCo2, suggest necrotic cell death via dose-dependent manner. In accumulation, an augment in ROS levels and a reduction of RSH content devoid of variation in -GCS expression was spotted, with an increase in LOOH levels and a severe surge in HO-1 expression. These results advocate that the *B. etnensis* Raf. The extract promotes oxidative cellular microenvironment results in cancer cell demise by ferroptosis mediated by HO-1 hyperexpression (Malfa, 2019).

9.3.9 CARALLUMA FIMBRIATA

The *C. fimbriata* ethanolic leaf isolate exhibit the dose-dependent rise in cytotoxicity in COLO 320 human colon cancer cells. The current learning put on a show that the ethanolic leaf extract of *Caralluma fimbriata* is competent of declining cell broadcast by bringing to mind the cytotoxicity of COLO 320 cells (Ashwini, 2017).

9.3.10 SALVIA MILTIORRHIZA BUNGE

Patients identified as having malignant colon neoplasm during the catastrophic infection are included in the cohort. We use the Kaplan–Meier technique to approximate lung cancer cumulative incidences. After that, human colon cancers cells had been used to research the impact of dihydroisotanshinone I (DT) on the proliferation and apoptosis of human colon cancers cells and the fundamental mechanism. The *in-vivo* impact of DT remedy turned into investigated via a xenograft nude mouse model. Dihydroisotanshinone I (DT), a bioactive compound found in danshen, can restrain the propagation of colon cancer cells, HCT 116 cells, and HT-29 cells. Furthermore, DT triggered apoptosis of colorectal cancer cells. DT additionally reserved the protein appearance of Skp2 (S-Phase Kinase related Protein 2) and the mRNA. In addition, DT additionally blocked the colon cancer cells' recruitment cap potential of macrophage with the aid of using reducing CCL2 secretion in macrophages. DT remedy additionally considerably inhibited the very last tumor quantity in a xenograft nude mouse model (Lin, 2018).

9.3.11 MURRAYA KOENIGII

The pyranocarbazole alkaloids had been remoted from leaves of *Murraya koenigii* and their anti-cancers cappotential turned into investigated in one-of-a-kind cancer cell lines. Among all examined compounds, murrayazoline and O-methylmurrayamine A confirmed as an effective anticancer hobby in opposition to DLD-1 colon cancer cells with the IC50 values of 5.7 mM and 17.9 mM, respectively, with non-specific cytotoxicity in opposition to non-cancer HEK-293 and HaCaT cells. Research of natural compounds discovered that the anti-cancers hobby of compounds corresponds with altered cellular morphology, cellular cycle arrest in G2/M segment, reactive oxygen species stage, and mitochondrial membrane depolarization of colon cancer cells. In addition, those compounds activated caspase-three protein and upregulated Bax/Bcl-2 protein expression ratio main to induction of caspase-established apoptosis in DLD-1 cells. These occasions triggered with the aid of using carbazole alkaloids additionally coincide with downregulation of Akt/mTOR signifying downstream concentrated on of cellular survival pathway (Arun, 2017).

9.3.12 RUTIN AND SILIBININ

The gift look at objectives to recognize the cap potential healing performance of Rutin and Silibinin personally and in aggregate in colon cancer cells (HT-29) via concentrated on decisive molecular gamers of apoptosis, irritation, and mitogen-activated protein kinases (MAPK) pathways. The mechanism concerned withinside the cytotoxic impact turned into then scrutinized in terms of apoptosis the usage of comet assay, DNA fragmentation, and fluorescent microscopy examination. The apoptosis-related proteins viz; Caspase-3, 8, 9, Bax, Bcl-2, p53, irritation-related proteins viz; NFkB, IKK-a IKK-b, and MAPK pathway-related proteins viz; p38 and MK-2 had been decided with the aid of using western-blot and Real Time-PCR evaluation. Consequences recommend that Rutin and Silibinin produce anticancer outcomes thru induction of apoptosis in addition to amendable the expressions of genes associated with apoptosis, irritation, and MAPK pathway proteins greater successfully in aggregate than personally (Nafees, 2018).

9.3.13 DIOSCOREA ZINGIBERENSIS

The antitumor impact of dioscin in opposition to human colon cancer cells and assessed the molecular mechanism concerned on this process. The cellular of dioscin turned into characterized with the aid of using flow cytometry evaluation. Dioscin-triggered apoptosis turned into followed with the aid of using sustained phosphorylation of JNK, p38-MAPK. N-acetyl-L-cysteine, a scavenger of ROS, substantially reversed dioscin-triggered cellular loss of life and activation of JNK and p38. Collectively, the information suggests that the induction of apoptosis through dioscin is mediated via ROS proteins, which are essential upstream signals for JNK/p38-MAPK activation (Li, 2018).

9.3.14 CHINESE HAWTHORN (CRATAEGUS)

This look at established that a harmonized polysaccharide (HPS) isolated from Hawthorn exerted anticancer outcomes on colon cancer cells. Human colon cancer cell line HCT116 turned into treated 125–1000 μg/ml HPS for 12 h and next evaluation turned into execution on proliferation and signaling pathways. HPS downregulated the expression of Cyclin A1/D1/E1 and CDK-1/2. HPS triggered apoptosis on HCT116 cells via upregulation of caspase3, 7, 8, 9 and Fas, FADD, TNF-R1, TRADD, upregulation of caspase 3 protein turned into additionally observed. HPS has an anti-cancers cap potential withinside the remedy of human colon cancers which makes it a cap potential candidate in purposeful ingredients for cancers sufferers (Ma, 2020).

9.3.15 *ANGELICA DAHURICA*

It carries a phytochemical imperatorin, which examine for anticancer hobby the usage of HCT116, HeLa, and Hep3B cells. Major assays had been promoter-reporter gene assay, MTT, western blot evaluation, immunofluorescence assay, opposite transcription-PCR (RTPCR), glide cytometric evaluation, clonogenic assay, EdU labeling, immunofluorescence, xenografted assay, and VEGF ELISA. Results suggest the compound markedly reduced the hypoxia-caused accumulation of HIF-1α protein dose-dependently, while it did now no longer have an effect on the expressions of HIF-1β and topoisomerase-I (Topo-I). Further evaluation found out that imperatorin inhibited HIF-1α protein synthesis, without affecting the expression level of HIF-1α mRNA or degradation of HIF-1α protein. Furthermore, imperatorin averted the hypoxia-triggered expression of HIF-1 target genes, and flow cytometric evaluation indicate that imperatorin triggered G1 segment arrest withinside the human colon cancer cellular (HCT116). We determined that imperatorin management inhibits tumor boom and blocks tumor angiogenesis in a xenograft tumor model (Mi, 2017). Figure 9.1 elucidate the shape of imperatorin.

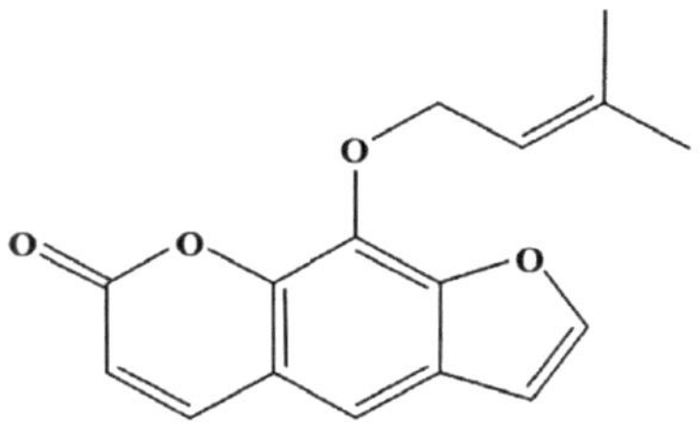

FIGURE 9.1 Structure of imperatorin.

9.3.16 *CASSIA ALATA*

In this examination, *C. alata* flower methanol extract (CME) has been applied to examine the antiproliferative and apoptosis properties in opposition to human colon cancer. In regular cells, including Vero cells and hMSCs, 0.2 mg/mL dose of CME showed the most effective 4% and 5% growth inhibition showed the HT-115 cellular-precise cytotoxic impact. This impact is probably because of the supply of phytoactive biomolecules in CME, which include cyclotrisiloxan, beta-sitosterol and alpha-tocopherol were shown with the aid of using GC–MS. Most fascinatingly, PI and AO/ErBr coloring of CME dealt with HT-115 cells proven early (25%), pro (17%), late (8%) apoptotic, and three% necrotic cells after 48 hrs. Treatment with CME extract confirmed a cap potential impact at the inhibition of protumorigenic inflammatory and oxidative strain genes. Protumorigenic COX-2/PGE-2 and TNF-a/NF-jB immune axis had been normalized after the CME remedy. Amounts of each apoptosis-associated mRNA p53, Bax, caspase three, and p21 genes had been upregulated, while it ended in a sizable discount withinside the anti-apoptotic marker mdm2 and Bcl-2 genes. In conclusion, bioactive compounds found in CME probably inhibit HT-115 colon cancer cell proliferation thru inhibition of the protumorigenic immune axis and stimulation of mitochondria established apoptotic pathway without necrotic impact (Salamatullah, 2021).

9.3.17 *ELEPHANTOPUS SCABER*

Ethanol and ethyl acetate isolates of *E. scaber* reserved the growth of HCT116 and HT-29 colorectal cancer cells. The *E. scaber* isolations induced apoptosis of colorectal cancer cells by activates the ROS-dependent mitochondrial pathway (loss of mitochondrial membrane potential, activation of caspase-3, cleavage of PARP, accumulation of ROS, upregulation of P53) (Chan, 2015). Recently, established that Deoxyelephantopin extracted from *E. scaber* was capable of inhibiting the HCT116 human colorectal carcinoma cells expansion. This cytotoxic outcome was come with by orientation of apoptosis and cell cycle detain at the S phase (Chan, 2016) (Benarba, 2018).

9.3.18 *ANDROGRAPHIS PANICULATE*

The T84 and COLO 205 cancer cell lines had been used to illustrate that andrographolide induces elevated ROS levels, corresponding anti-oxidant reaction molecules, and decreased mitochondrial membrane capability.

No will increase in ROS levels had been detected on top of things colon fibroblast cells. Andrographolide brought about cell demise, UPR signaling, and CHOP, Bax, and caspase 3 apoptosis factors had been all inhibited withinside the presence of the ROS scavenger NAC. Additionally, andrographolide-triggered suppression of cyclins B1 and D1 had been additionally reversed withinside the attendance of NAC. Finally, Akt phosphorylation and phospho-mTOR levels which might be commonly suppressed with the aid of using andrographolide have been additionally expressed at ordinary ranges withinside the absence of ROS. These statistics exhibit that andrographolide induces ER pressure leading to apoptosis thru the induction of ROS and that accelerated ROS additionally plays a crucial function in down-regulating mobileular cycle development and cell survival pathways as well (Salamatullah, 2021). The cytotoxic capability of andrographolide on HT-29 cells becomes decided with the aid of using MTT assay, trypan blue exclusion assay, colony formation assay, and morphological investigation; and apoptotic belongings with the aid of using DAPI and Hoechst staining, FITC-Annexin V assay, DNA fragmentation assay, and caspase-3 interest assay. To elucidate andrographolide motion, intracellular reactive oxygen species (ROS) stage becomes decided with the aid of using DCFDA dye; alternate in mitochondrial capability with the aid of using Rhodamine123 and Mito Tracker Red CMXRos dye, and cell cycle modulatory belongings with the aid of using go with the drift cytometric analysis. Results of the take a look at have proven that andrographolide reduced cell viability of HT-29 cells in a dose- and time-based manner. Furthermore, andrographolide brought about apoptosis in HT-29 cells, which appeared to be related to the augmented intracellular ROS stage and disruption of the mitochondrial membrane capability. Fascinatingly, andrographolide precipitated considerable molecular cycle arrest in the G2/M segment at decreased doses, but in G0/G1 segment at better doses. In review, our outcomes indicated that andrographolide showcase antiproliferative and apoptotic homes in opposition to colon cancers HT-29 cells (Banerjee, 2017).

9.3.19 *ALISMA ORIENTALE*

Alisol B 23-acetate (AB23A), a herbal triterpenoid from the rhizome of *Alisma orientale*, a Chinese medicinal herb, has a couple of physiological sports which includes anticancer. Autophagy additionally took place in AB23A-treated HCT116 cells, as evidenced by using the buildup of microtubule-related protein 1 mild chain three shape II (LC3-II) and degradation of SQSTM1/p62. An autophagy inhibitor, three-methyladenine (three-MA) was determined to reduce AB23A-mediated autophagy, apoptosis, and cell demise, representing that AB23A-triggered apoptotic reaction becomes dependent on the initiation of autophagy. In adding together, the treatment of HCT116 cells with AB23A resulted withinside the technology of reactive oxygen species (ROS) and phosphorylation of c-Jun N-terminal kinase (JNK). A ROS scavenger, N-acetylcysteine (NAC), and a JNK-particular inhibitor, SP600125 attenuated AB23A-triggered autophagy and apoptotic cell demise. Furthermore, NAC becomes capable of putting off AB23A-brought about JNK phosphorylation. This locating affords a unique mechanism of motion of AB23A in colon cancers HCT116 cells that AB23A induces autophagic-structured apoptotic cell demise in colon cancer cells, at the least in part, thru the buildup of intracellular ROS and next activation of JNK (Zhao, 2017). Figure 9.2 elucidate the shape of Alisol B-acetate.

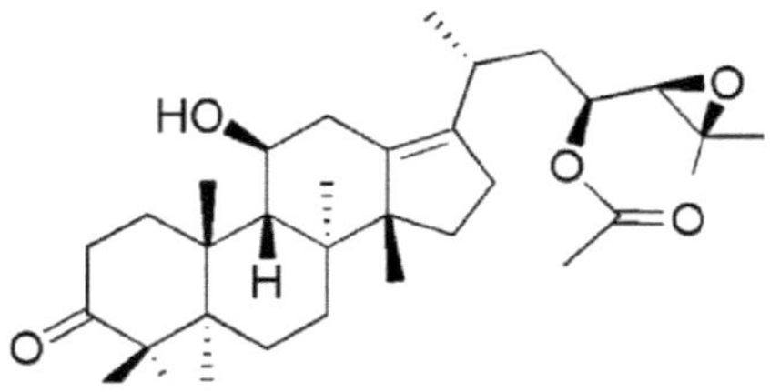

FIGURE 9.2 Structure of Alisol B 23-acetate.

9.3.20 *LITHOSPERMUM ERYTHRORHIZON*

Shikonin, a naphthoquinone consequent from the roots of the natural plant *Lithospermum erythrorhizon*, has been decided to be an amazing antitumor agent. The gift look aimed to locate the fundamental antitumor mechanism of shikonin in colon cancers. We observed that shikonin concealed the increase of colon cancer cells in a dose-established way in vitro and in vivo. Shikonin triggered mitochondria-mediated apoptosis, which became regulated via way of means of Bcl-2 family proteins. Shikonin improved the technology of intracellular ROS, which performed an upstream function in shikonin-brought on apoptosis. Our statistics indicated that technology of ROS, down-regulated expression of Bcl-2 and Bcl-xL, depolarization of the mitochondrial membrane capability, and activation of the caspase cascade have been additives of the programmed occasion of shikonin-brought on apoptosis in colon cancers cells. In addition, shikonin offered minimum toxicity to non-neoplastic colon cells and no liver damage in xenograft models, displaying protection withinside the management of the colon cancer cell increase in vitro and in vivo. Taken together, our findings propose that shikonin may function as a capability novel healing drug withinside the remedy for human colon cancer (Liang, 2017).

9.3.21 *BACOPA MONNIERI*

This examination came to similarly elucidate the antitumor capability of bacopaside II in colon cancers cells. Expression of AQP1 in HT-29, SW480, SW620, and HCT116 became decided via way of means of quantitative PCR and western immunoblot. Cells have been dealt with bacopaside II, and morphology, increase, autophagy, cell cycle, and apoptosis have been assessed via way of means of time-lapse microscopy, crystal violet, acridine orange, propidium iodide (PI), and annexin V/PI staining respectively. AQP1 expression became appreciably better in HT-29 than in SW480, SW620, and HCT116. Bacopaside II substantially decreased the increase at 20 μM for HT-29 and 15 μM for SW480, SW620, and HCT116. Inhibition of HT-29 at 20 μM became in most cases mediated via way of means of G0/G1 cell cycle arrest and at 30 μM via way of means of G2/M arrest and apoptosis. Inhibition of SW480, SW620, and HCT116 at 15 μM became mediated via way of means of G2/M arrest and apoptosis. These effects are the primary to expose that bacopaside II inhibits colon cancer cell increase via way of means of inducing cell cycle arrest and apoptosis (Smith, 2018).

9.3.22 *SCUTELLARIA BAICALENSIS*

Baicalin was isolated from the root part of *Scutellaria baicalensis* and is its major flavonoid (Keservani et al., 2010a, 2010b; Kesarwani and Sharma, 2014). The anticancer activity of baccalin has been evaluated in a variety of cancer types, particularly in CRC. in addition, our in vitro and in vivo learning demonstrate that baccalin suppressed oncomiR by reducing the expression of c-mic. Taken together, our study demonstrates a new method for the anticancer action of bekalin, that it induces apoptosis in colon cancer cells and suppresses tumor growth by falling the appearance of c-mic and oncomiR (Tao, 2018).

9.3.23 *ROSA CANINA*

The objective of the current investigation was to scrutinize the possible consequence of *R. canina* extract on cell feasibility, cell cycle, apoptosis, and appearance of telomerase in human colon cancer (WiDr) cells. The cytotoxic outcome of the extract was resolute by means of the MTT assay. The mechanisms involved in the cytotoxic effect of the extracts were then evaluated in terms of the cell cycle using apoptosis and flow cytometry. Mitochondrial membrane potential (MMP) was analyzed using the fluorometric method, and the expression levels of telomerase were designed by means of RT-PCR. *R. canina* extract displayed a selective cytotoxic effect on colon cancer cells compared with normal colon cells. Extract-induced cell cycle arrest and apoptosis in S-phase via reduced MMPs in WiDr cells. *R. canina* elicits significantly repressed telomerase expressions at the time of treatment of 48 and 72 h in WiDr cells. Our outcome recommend that *R. canina* may have significant possible for growth as a novel natural product based on Anticancer agents (Turan, 2018).

9.3.24 *CURCUMA KWANGSIENSIS*

Curcumol turned into dissolved in whole ethyl alcohol. The awareness of entire ethyl alcohol withinside the manipulated institution or experimental samples is continually 1/500 of the very last medium volume (v/v/ v) became. LoVo and SW480 cells have been dealt with distinctive concentrations of curcumol, And then the cell cycle of every institution became tested through float cytometry. Curcumol-caused mobileular cycle arrest withinside and Western blot facts confirmed that curcumol extended the expression of GSK3þ, P27, p21, and P16, and decreased. In addition, curcumol-caused reactive oxygen species (ROS) era in LoVo cells, and ROS scavenger N-acetylcysteine (NAC) considerably reversed curcumol-caused cell boom inhibition. In addition, curcumol additionally inhibited the boom of human colon cancers cells, which have been concerned withinside the nude mouse (Wang, 2018).

9.3.25 *GLYCYRRHIZA URALENSIS*

6,8-Diprenylorobol is a herbal compound determined specifically in *Glycyrrhiza uralensis* fisch. We with the purpose of comparing the antiproliferative consequences of 6,8diprenylorobol in LoVo and HCT15, sorts of human colon cancers cells. 6,8-Diprenylorobol inhibited the proliferation of LoVo and HCT15 cells in a dose-and-time-structured manner. The 40 μM of 6,8-diprenylorobol for 72 h decreased each cell viability by 50%. After the remedy of 6,8-diprenylorobol (forty and 60 μM) for 72 h, the past due apoptotic mobileular quantities in LoVo and HCT15 cells have been 24, 70%, and 13, 90%, respectively, which became shown through analyzing DNA fragmentation in each cell.

9.3.26 BRASSICACEAE MICROGREENS (BROCCOLI, KALE, MUSTARD, AND RADISH)

Their bioactivity became as compared with the digestion blank, whilst the colon cancers chemotherapeutic drug 5-fluorouracil became used as a nice manipulate. Cell viability (mitochondrial enzyme activity assay (MTT test) and Trypan blue test) and mechanisms associated with an antiproliferative hobby have been studied. All microgreen BFs extended ROS and reduced GSH, changing the redox reputation and inflicting mitochondrial membrane dissipation observed through a standard cell cycle arrest in G2/M and apoptotic cell dying through a Ca2+-unbiased mechanism. As a result, the antioxidant bioactive compounds gift withinside the semi-microgreen species decreased the proliferation of tumoral cells, displaying lesser consequences with broccoli microgreens, in keeping with their decreased ascorbic acid content material and general antioxidant capacity. Therefore, the day-by-day consumption of microgreens inside a balanced weight loss program might be a preventive dietary method to lessen a load of continual degenerative sicknesses together with colon cancers (Fuente, 2020).

9.3.27 MORUS NIGRA

The purpose of the prevailing take a look is to decide the anticancer impact of citrus black mulberry on the human colon cancers cells (HT-29). In the prevailing investigation, the entire phenol and flavonoids content material and antioxidant hobby of plant extracts have been quantified via way of means of the follin-siocalceau, AlC13, and DPPH methods, respectively. The anticancers consequences of *M. nigra* on HT-29 cells have been decided through cytotoxic, genotoxic, and molecular analysis. The plant extract considerably extended DNA harm and reduced cell viability. It became decided that the *M. nigra* software had made the Box/S. the Bcl-2 ranges brought about a growth and a lower in p53 and procasepase-three ranges. These outcomes imply that

M. nigra mediates cell demise in an unbiased pathway through lowering mutant p53 expression in HT-29 cells (Erden, 2021).

9.3.28 MEXICAN AVOCADO

In addition, the LEIS-induced loss of membrane mitochondrial capacity inhibited fatty acid oxidation and increased superoxide production and mitochondrial ROS. In addition, LEAS induced the secretion of cytokines IL-6 (~500%), IL-8 (~400%), and IL-10 (~150%); While IL-1þ secretion was subdued (~50%). The results suggest that LEAS induces apoptosis on Caco-2 cells, indicating that avocado reduces the risk for cancer development (Lara-Marquez, 2020).

9.3.29 MORINGA OLEIFERA

Moringa extract was collected of chlorogenic acid, quercetin glucoside, quercetin-malonyl-glucoside, and glucomoringin. IC50 values range from 0.17 to 3.17 mg/mL. were up to mL, suggesting that moringa leaf extracts displayed antiproliferative effects on colon cancer cells. GeH abridged the production of pro-inflammatory cytokines (TNF-α, IL-1 π). GEH (glucosinolates-enriched hydrolyzed extract) has produced HCT116 (IC50:0.55 mg/min) mL) increased apoptosis by 58.1% and increased apoptosis by HT-29 (IC50:0.59 mg/mL). mL) in up to 38%. GEH augmented ROS LDH activity, and induced the expression of markers of apoptosis such as Bax (HCT 116: 41%); HT-29: 52% and site C (HCT 116: 70%); HT-29:59% while reducing Bcl-2 (HCT 116:58%); HT-29: 43% contrast to unprocessed cells ($P < 0.05$). GEH can reduce colon cancer cell proliferation by upholding apoptosis by the ROS-mediated mitochondrial-dependent pathway (Cuellar-Núñez, 2020). Figure 9.3 elucidating the structure of glucosinolates.

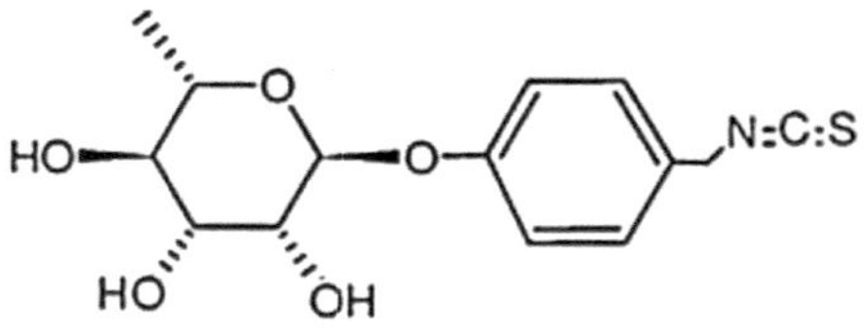

FIGURE 9.3 Structure of glucosinolates.

9.3.30 *OCIMUM SANCTUM*

Vicenin-2 is an apigenin form, 6,8-di-C-glucoside, isolated from *Ocimum sanctum*. The anti-proliferative consequence of Vicenin-2 on human colon cancer cells by inhibition of the Wnt/β-catenin signaling. Furthermore, immunoblot analysis exhibited that Vicenin-2 treatment boosted the expression of Cytochrome C, Bax, and caspase-3 whereas suppressed the Bcl-2 expression (Yang, 2018). Figure 9.4 elucidate the structure of Vicenin-2.

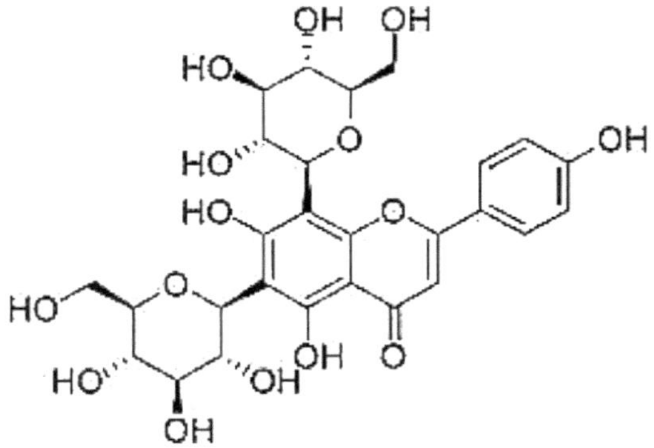

FIGURE 9.4 Structure of Vicenin-2.

9.3.31 HESPERIDIN LOADED ZN2+@ SA/PCT NANOCOMPOSITES

Additionally, immunoblotting analysis of cysteine proteases 3, 9, PARP, proapoptotic protein Bax, and antiapoptotic protein were performed. The outcome of the MTT assay authentically confirmed that the hesperidine nanocomposite inhibited HCT116 cell growth, and the results of fluorescent staining proved that the hesperidine nanocomposite induced apoptotic facilitating cell necrosis through promoting the expression of the apoptotic protein, leading to colon cancer (HCT116) cells (Yang, 2020) in persuaded apoptosis.

9.3.32 PROSOPIS FARCTA LOADED GOLD NANOPARTICLES

The cytotoxicity effect of Au-NPs was studied against a colon cancerous cell line via the MTT assay and the IC50 of Au-NPs was calculated to be 419.7 μg/mL. The results directed that the apoptotic effects were augmented on cells when the Au-NPs concentration reached 200 μg/mL. The Au-NPs were manufactured easily and with *P. farcta* extract (Miri, 2018).

9.3.33 BERBERINE

Berberine (BBR) was first isolated from the bark of the xanthoxylon Clava Hercules lin (Rutaceae). The anticancer mechanism of BBR was studied by connectivity map (CMAP) analysis. which found that 14 Hsp90, HDAC, PI3K, or mTOR protein inhibitors have similar functions with BBR. The study showed that BBR inhibited the proliferation of SW480 cells with ic50 of 3.436 lM, induced apoptosis, autophase, MMP depolarization, and arrested the G1 phase of the cell cycle at 1.0 lm. BBR dose-dependently up-regulated PTEN, while inhibiting Notch1, PI3K, Akt, and mTOR proteins at 1.0–9.0 LM ($p<0.05$). BBR also shows synergistic effects with Hsp90 and HDAC inhibitors (0.01 lM) in SW480 cells at 0.5 and 1.0 lm (Li, 2021). Figure 9.5 clarify the structure of berberine.

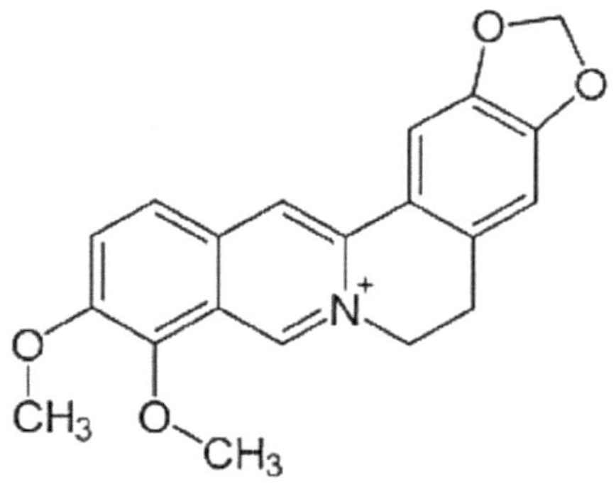

FIGURE 9.5 Structure of Berberine.

9.4 CLINICAL STUDIES

The clinical studies evaluating the preventive and therapeutic effects of phytoconstituents is shown in Table 9.1.

TABLE 9.1 Clinical Studies Evaluating the Preventive and Therapeutic Effects of Phytoconstituents (Afshari, 2019)

S. No.	Phytochemical name	Concomitant therapy	Intervention (duration, patient number, dosage)	Study design	Outcomes	References
1	Flavone acetic acid (FAA)	Sodium bicarbonate, intravenously, before FAA	23 patients with advanced colorectal carcinoma 4.8 g/m^2, 1-hr infusion, once weekly, 6 weeks	Clinical trial (Phase II)	No antitumor activity disease stabilization in 1 patient with CRC	Kaye et al., 1990
2	Flavone acetic acid (FAA)	-	19 patients with advanced colorectal carcinoma 8.6 g/m^2, 1-hr infusion, once-weekly, 6weeks	Clinical trial (Phase II)	No antitumor activity	Kerr et at., 1989
3	Curcumin and quercetin	-	Five familial adenomatous polyposis with previous colectomy curcumin 480 mg + quercetin 20 mg orally 3 times a day, a mean of 6 months	Observational study	↓ The number and size of adenomatous polyps	Cruz-Correa et al., 2006
4	Isorhamnetin Kaempferol Myricetin Quercetin	NSAID, hormone therapy	958 participants with colorectal adenoma within 6 months before the entry IL-6 at baseline, Year 1, and Year 3	Randomized, multicenter, nutritional interventional study	Flavonols especially of isorhamnetin, kaempferol, and quercetin are inversely associated with serum IL-6, and advanced adenoma recurrence Higher median flavonol → Equal or below median IL-6	Bobe et al., 2012
5	Quercetin	NSAID	1,163 cases, 1,501 controls, 45–80 years of age	Case-control study	Proximal colon cancer risk when fruit intake or healthy eating. The index score is high, or when tea intake is low ↑ distal colon cancer risk when total fruit intake is low	Djuric et al., 2012

TABLE 9.1 *(Continued)*

S. No.	Phytochemical name	Concomitant therapy	Intervention (duration, patient number, dosage)	Study design	Outcomes	References
6	Fisetin	CRC chemotherapy	37 CRC 100 mg fisetin/day (n = 18) or placebo (n = 19), 7consecutive weeks	Double-blind, randomized placebo-controlled clinical trial	↓ IL-8, hs-CRP, MMP-7	Farsad-Naeimi et al., 2018
7	Catechin	-	34,651 postmenopausal cancer-free women, 55–69 years of age Follow up: 12 years	Prospective cohort study	Inversely associated with rectal cancer Catechins from fruits, (+)-catechin and (−)-epicatechin, are inversely associated with upper GI tract cancer; catechins from tea are inversely associated with rectal cancer	Djuric et al., 2012
8	Proanthocyanidin		1,953 cases (1,225 colon cancers, 728 rectal cancers), 4,154 controls admitted for acute, non-neoplastic condition	Case-control study	↓ Risk of CRC with increasing intake of proanthocyanidins. The associations are stronger for rectal cancer	Rossi et al., 2010
9	Epigallocatechin gallate (EGCG)		2,534 patients with a history of polypectomy supplementation group: n = 1,267,150 mg, two times daily, 3 years control group: n = 1,267, placebo, 3years	Randomized placebo-controlled, multicenter clinical trial	Prevents from CRC	Stingl et al., 2011

TABLE 9.1 *(Continued)*

S. No.	Phytochemical name	Concomitant therapy	Intervention (duration, patient number, dosage)	Study design	Outcomes	References
10	Green tea	-	38,540participants (14,783 men, mean age = 52.8 years; 23,667 women, mean age = 56.8 years)	Prospective cohort study	No association between green tea consumption and CRC	Nagano et al., 2001
11	Green tea	Regular green tea drinking	136 patients with a history of polypectomy and 1 year of clean colon supplementation group: n = 71, 1.5g/day green tea extract, 12 months control group: n = 65	Randomized clinical trial	↓ Incidence of metachronous adenoma, size of the relapsed adenoma	Shimizu et al., 2008
12	Green tea	-	176 patients with a history of polypectomy supplementation group: n = 88, 0.9 g/day green tea extract, 12 months control group: n = 88	Randomized clinical trial	↓ Incidence of metachronous adenoma, number of relapsed adenomas no difference in body mass index, dietary intakes, serum lipid profiles, fasting serum glucose, and serum.	Shin et al., 2018
13	Resveratrol	-	20 patients with colorectal Adenocarcinoma, age,>18 years, daily for 8 d at 0.5 or 1.0 g, n=10	Clinical trial (Phase II)	Prevents from CRC	Patel et al., 2010

Source: Adapted with permission from Afshari et al. (2019)

9.5 CHALLENGES AND PROSPECTS

More preclinical and clinical studies on phytochemicals are required to establish their safety and efficacy for human use. Future studies may develop a relationship between phytochemicals and colon cancer and develop a robust technique to deliver phytochemical to colon cancer cells. The bioactive properties of many phytochemicals are yet to be explored in this area.

9.6 CONCLUSION

The various phytochemicals isolated from various medicinal plants show activity against cancer cells by inhibiting various pathways of colon cancer mechanism, which was evaluated by in-vivo and in vitro experiments. Nanoparticles of phytochemicals help to target cancer cells. Preclinical and clinical studies are exploring the relevance of the effectiveness and safety of phytochemicals.

KEYWORDS

- **aloe**
- **cigarette smoking**
- **colorectal cancer**
- ***Datura inoxia***
- **obesity**

REFERENCES

Afshari, K., Haddadi, N. S., Haj-Mirzaian, A., Farzaei, M. H., Rohani, M. M., Akramian, F., Naseri, R., et al., (2019). Natural flavonoids for the prevention of colon cancer: A comprehensive review of preclinical and clinical studies. *J. Cell Physiol., 234*(12), 21519–21546.

Aghaabbasi, K., Askari, N., Hassani, K. H., Torkzadeh-Mahani, M., & Ramzani-Ghara, A., (2020). The *Blepharis persica* seed hydroalcoholic extract synergistically enhances the apoptotic effect of doxorubicin in human colon cancer and gastric cancer cells. *Mol. Biol. Rep., 47*(2), 843–853.

Ahamed, A., et al., (2020). Molecular perspective and anticancer activity of medicinal plants. *Saudi Journal of Biological Sciences, 27*, 666–675.

Ali, A. N. M., Saeed, N. A. A. A. H., & Omear, H. A., (2021). The anticancer properties of *Artemisia aucheri* boiss extract on HT29 colon cancer cells. *J. Gastrointest. Cancer, 52*(1), 113–119.

Arnold, M., Sierra, M. S., Seorjomaram, I., Jemal, A., & Bray, F., (2017). Global patterns and trends in colorectal cancer incidence and mortality. *Gut., 66*, 683–691.

Arun, A., Patel, O. P. S., Saini, D., Yadav, P. P., & Konwar, R., (2017). Anti-colon cancer activity of *Murraya koenigii* leaves is due to constituent murrayazoline and O-methylmurrayamine A induced mTOR/AKT downregulation and mitochondrial apoptosis. *Biomed Pharmacother., 93*, 510–521.

Ashwini, S., Ezhilarasan, D., & Anitha, R., (2017). Cytotoxic effect of *Caralluma fimbriata* against human colon cancer. *Pharmacogn. J., 9*, 204–207.

Banerjee, A., Banerjee, V., Czinn, S., & Blanchard, T., (2017). Increased reactive oxygen species levels cause ER stress and cytotoxicity in andrographolide treated colon cancer cells. *Oncotarget., 8*(16), 26142–26153.

Bastide, N. M., Pierre, F. H. F., & Corpet, D. E., (2011). Heme iron from meat and risk of colorectal cancer: A meta-analysis and a review of the mechanisms involved. *Cancer Prev. Res., 4*, 177–184.

Benarba, B., & Pandiella, A., (2018). Colorectal cancer and medicinal plants: Principle findings from recent studies. *Biomed Pharmacother., 107*, 408–423.

Bernstein, A. M., Song, M., Zhang, X., Pan, A., Wang, M., Fuchs, C. S., Le, N., et al., (2015). Processed and unprocessed red meat and risk of colorectal cancer: Analysis by tumor location and modification by time. *PLoS One, 10*, e0135959.

Bernstein, C. N., Blanchard, J. F., Kliewer, E., & Wajda, A., (2001). Cancer risk in patients with inflammatory bowel disease: A population-based study. *Cancer, 91*, 854–862.

Bobe, G., Albert, P. S., Sansbury, L. B., Lanza, E., Schatzkin, A., Colburn, N. H., & Cross, A. J., (2010). Interleukin-6 as a potential indicator for prevention of high-risk adenoma recurrence by dietary flavonols in the polyp prevention trial. *Cancer Prev. Res. (Phila)., 3*(6), 764–775.

Chan, C. K., Chan, G., Awang, K., & Kadir, H. A., (2016). Deoxyelephantopin from *Elephantopus scaber* inhibits HCT116 human colorectal carcinoma cell growth through apoptosis and cell cycle arrest. *Molecules, 385*, 1–14.

Chan, C. K., Supriady, H., Goh, B. H., & Abdul, K. H., (2015). *Elephantopus scaber* induces apoptosis through ROS-dependent mitochondrial signaling pathway in HCT116 human colorectal carcinoma cells. *J. Ethnopharmacol., 168*, 291–304.

Choi, Y. J., Lee, J., Ha, S. H., Lee, H. K., Lim, H. M., Yu, S. H., Lee, C. M., et al., (2021). 6,8-Diprenylorobol induces apoptosis in human colon cancer cells via activation of intracellular reactive oxygen species and p53. *Environ. Toxicol., 36*(5), 914–925.

Colorectal Cancer: Statistics. Cancer.Net. *Oncologist Approved Cancer Information from the ASCO*. https://www.cancer.net/cancer-types/colorectal-cancer/statistics (accessed on 04 February 2023).

Cruz-Correa, M., Shoskes, D. A., Sanchez, P., Zhao, R., Hylind, L. M., Wexner, S. D., & Giardiello, F. M., (2006). Combination treatment with curcumin and quercetin of adenomas in familial adenomatous polyposis. *Clin. Gastroenterol Hepatol., 4*(8), 1035–1038.

Cuellar-Núñez, M. L., Loarca-Piña, G., Berhow, M., & Gonzalez De, M. E., (2020). Glucosinolate-rich hydrolyzed extract from *Moringa oleifera* leaves decreased the production of TNF-α and IL-1β cytokines and induced ROS and apoptosis in human colon cancer cells. *Journal of Functional Foods, 75*, 104270.

De Santis, C. E., Lin, C. C., Mariotto, A. B., Siegel, R. L., Stein, K. D., Kramer, J. L., et al., (2014). Cancer treatment and survivorship statistics 2014. *CA Cancer J. Clin., 64*(4), 252–271.

Djuric, Z., Severson, R. K., & Kato, I., (2012). Association of dietary quercetin with reduced risk of proximal colon cancer. *Nutr. Cancer, 64*(3), 351–360.

Erden, Y., (2021). Sour black mulberry (*Morus nigra* L.) causes cell death by decreasing mutant p53 expression in HT-29 human colon cancer cells. *Food Biosci., 42*, 101113.

Fakih, M., & Vincent, M., (2010). Adverse events associated with anti-EGFR therapies for the treatment of metastatic colorectal cancer. *Curr. Oncol., 17,* S18–30.

Farsad-Naeimi, A., Alizadeh, M., Esfahani, A., & Darvish, A. E., (2018). Effect of fisetin supplementation on inflammatory factors and matrix metalloproteinase enzymes in colorectal cancer patients. *Food Funct., 9*(4), 2025–2031.

Fuente, B., López-García, G., Máñez, V., Alegría, A., Barberá, R., & Cilla, A., (2020). Antiproliferative effect of bioaccessible fractions of four *Brassicaceae* microgreens on human colon cancer cells linked to their phytochemical composition. *Antioxidants (Basel), 9*(5), 368.

Gajendran, B., Durai, P., Madhu, V. K., & Chinnasamy, A., (2019). A novel phytosterol isolated from *Datura inoxia*, RinoxiaB is a potential cure colon cancer agent by targeting BAX/Bcl2 pathway. *Bioorganic & Medicinal Chemistry*. [Online].

García-Foncillas, J., Sunakawa, Y., Aderka, D., Wainberg, Z., Ronga, P., Witzler, P., & Stintzing, S., (2019). Distinguishing features of cetuximab and panitumumab in colorectal cancer and other solid tumors. *Front Oncol., 9*, 849.

Goh, J. X. H., Tan, L. T., Goh, J. K., Chan, K. G., Pusparajah, P., Lee, L. H., & Goh, B. H., (2019). Nobiletin and derivatives: Functional compounds from citrus fruit peel for colon cancer chemoprevention. *Cancers (Basel), 11*(6), 867.

Gozuacik, D., et al., (2008). DAP-kinase is a mediator of endoplasmic reticulum stress-induced caspase activation and autophagic cell death. *Cell Death Differ., 15*, 1875–1886.

Jaradat, N. A., Al-lahham, S., Zaid, A. N., & Hussein, F., (2019). *Carlina curetum* plant phytoconstituents, enzymes inhibitory and cytotoxic activity on cervical epithelial carcinoma and colon cancer cell lines. *European Journal of Integrative Medicine, 30*, 100933.

Javed, B., & Mashwani, Z. U., (2020). Synergistic effects of physicochemical parameters on bio-fabrication of mint silver nanoparticles: Structural evaluation and action against HCT116 colon cancer cells. *Int. J. Nanomedicine, 15*, 3621–3637.

Johnson, C. M., Wei, C., Ensor, J. E., Smolenski, D. J., Amos, C. I., Levin, B., & Berry, D. A., (2013). Meta-analyses of colorectal cancer risk factors. *Cancer Causes Control: CCC., 24*, 1207–1222.

Kaye, S. B., Clavel, M., Dodion, P., Monfardini, S., Bokkel-Huinink, W., Wagener, D. T., Gundersen, S., Stoter, G., Smith, J., Renard, J., et al., (1990). Phase II trials with flavone acetic acid (NCS. 347512, LM975) in patients with advanced carcinoma of the breast, colon, head and neck and melanoma. *Invest. New Drugs, 8*(1), S95–99.

Kerr, D. J., Maughan, T., Newlands, E., Rustin, G., Bleehen, N. M., Lewis, C., & Kaye, S. B., (1989). Phase II trials of flavone acetic acid in advanced malignant melanoma and colorectal carcinoma. *Br. J. Cancer., 60*(1), 104–106.

Keservani, R. K., & Sharma, A. K., (2014). Flavonoids: Emerging trends and potential health benefits. *Journal of Chinese Pharmaceutical Sciences, 23*(12), 815.

Keservani, R. K., Kesharwani, R. K., Sharma, A. K., Vyas, N., & Chadoker, A., (2010b). Nutritional supplements: An overview. *International Journal of Current Pharmaceutical Review and Research, 1*(1), 59–75.

Keservani, R. K., Kesharwani, R. K., Vyas, N., Jain, S., Raghuvanshi, R., & Sharma, A. K., (2010a). Nutraceutical and functional food as future food: A review. *Der Pharmacia Lettre, 2*(1), 106–116.

Khandekar, M. J., Cohen, P., & Spiegelman, B. M., (2011). Molecular mechanisms of cancer development in obesity. *Nat. Rev. Can., 11*, 886–895.

Kheirelseid, A. H., Miller, N., & Kerin, M. J., (2013). Molecular biology of colorectal cancer: Review of the literature. *Am. J. Mol. Biol., 3*, 72–80.

Lara-Márquez, M., Báez-Magaña, M., Raymundo-Ramos, C., Spagnuolo, P. A., Macías-Rodríguez, L., Salgado-Garciglia, R., Ochoa-Zarzosa, A., & López-Meza, J. E., (2020). Lipid-rich extract from Mexican avocado (*Persea americana* var. drymifolia) induces apoptosis and modulates the inflammatory response in Caco-2 human colon cancer cells. *Journal of Functional Foods, 64*, 103658.

Larsson, S. C., & Wolk, A., (2006). Meat consumption and risk of colorectal cancer: A meta-analysis of prospective studies. *Int. J. Cancer., 119*, 2657–2664.

Lee, J., Meyerhardt, J. A., Giovannucci, E., & Jeon, J. Y., (2015). Association between body mass index and prognosis of colorectal cancer: A meta-analysis of prospective cohort studies. *PLoS One, 10*, 1–25.

Li, G., Zhang, C., Liang, W., Zhang, Y., Shen, Y., & Tian, X., (2021). Berberine regulates the Notch1/PTEN/PI3K/AKT/mTOR pathway and acts synergistically with 17-AAG and SAHA in SW480 colon cancer cells. *Pharm. Biol., 59*(1), 21–30.

Li, S., Cheng, B., Hou, L., Huang, L., Cui, Y., Xu, D., Shen, X., & Li, S., (2018). Dioscin inhibits colon cancer cells' growth by reactive oxygen species-mediated mitochondrial dysfunction and p38 and JNK pathways. *Anticancer Drugs, 29*(3), 234–242.

Liang, W., Cui, J., Zhang, K., Xi, H., Cai, A., Li, J., Gao, Y., et al., (2017). Shikonin induces ROS-based mitochondria-mediated apoptosis in colon cancer. *Oncotarget., 8*(65), 109094–109106.

Lin, Y. Y., Lee, I. Y., Huang, W. S., Lin, Y. S., Kuan, F. C., Shu, L. H., Cheng, Y. C., et al., (2018). Corrigendum to danshen improves survival of patients with colon cancer and dihydroisotanshinone I inhibit the proliferation of colon cancer cells via apoptosis and skp2 signaling pathway. *J. Ethnopharmacol., 213*, 446.

Longley, D. B., Harkin, D. P., & Johnston, P. G., (2003). 5-fluorouracil: Mechanisms of action and clinical strategies. *Nat. Rev. Cancer, 3*, 330–338.

Ma, L., Xu, G. B., Tang, X., Zhang, C., Zhao, W., Wang, J., & Chen, H., (2020). Anticancer potential of polysaccharide extracted from hawthorn (*Crataegus*.) on human colon cancer cell line HCT116 via cell cycle arrest and apoptosis. *Journal of Functional Foods, 64*, 103677.

Malfa, G. A., Tomasello, B., Acquaviva, R., Genovese, C., La Mantia, A., Cammarata, F. P., Ragusa, M., et al., (2019). *Betula etnensis* Raf. (*Betulaceae*) extract induced HO-1 expression and ferroptosis cell death in human colon cancer cells. *Int. J. Mol. Sci., 20*(11), 2723.

Markowitz, S. D., & Bertagnolli, M. M., (2009). Molecular basis of colorectal cancer. *N. Engl. J. Med., 361*, 2449–2460.

Markowitz, S. D., Dawson, D. M., Willis, J., & Willson, J. K., (2002). Focus on colon cancer. *Cancer Cell, 1,* 233–236.

Mi, C., Ma, J., Wang, K. S., Zuo, H. X., Wang, Z., Li, M. Y., et al., (2017). Imperatorin suppresses proliferation and angiogenesis of human colon cancer cells by targeting HIF-1α via the mTOR/p70S6K/4E-BP1 and MAPK pathways. *J. Ethnopharmacol., 203,* 27–38.

Miri, A., Darroudi, M., Entezari, R., et al., (2018). Biosynthesis of gold nanoparticles using *Prosopis farcta* extract and its *in vitro* toxicity on colon cancer cells. *Res. Chem. Intermed., 44,* 3169–3177.

Moghaddam, A. A., Woodward, M., & Huxley, R., (2007). Obesity and risk of colorectal cancer: A meta-analysis of 31 studies with 70,000 events. *Can. Epidemiol. Biomarkers Prev., 16,* 533–2547.

Nafees, S., Mehdi, S. H., Zafaryab, M., Zeya, B., Sarwar, T., & Rizvi, M. A., (2018). Synergistic interaction of rutin and silibinin on human colon cancer cell line. *Arch Med Res., 49*(4), 226–234.

Nagano, J., Kono, S., Preston, D. L., & Mabuchi, K., (2001). A prospective study of green tea consumption and cancer incidence, Hiroshima and Nagasaki (Japan). *Cancer Causes Control, 12*(6), 501–508.

Norat, T., Chan, D., Lau, R., Aune, D., & Vieira, R., (2010). WCRF/AICR Systematic Literature Review Continuous Update Project Report: The Associations between Food, Nutrition and Physical Activity and the Risk of Colorectal Cancer Imperial College, London.

Patel, K. R., Brown, V. A., Jones, D. J., Britton, R. G., Hemingway, D., Miller, A. S., West, K. P., et al., (2010). Clinical pharmacology of resveratrol and its metabolites in colorectal cancer patients. *Cancer Res., 70*(19), 7392–7399.

Remmele, W., & Stegner, H. E., (1987). [Recommendation for uniform definition of an immunoreactive score (IRS) for immunohistochemical estrogen receptor detection (ERICA) in breast cancer tissue. *Pathologe., 8,* 138–140.

Rossi, M., Negri, E., Parpinel, M., Lagiou, P., Bosetti, C., Talamini, R., Montella, M., et al., (2010). Proanthocyanidins and the risk of colorectal cancer in Italy. *Cancer Causes Control, 21*(2), 243–250.

Salamatullah, A. M., Subash-Babu, P., Nassrallah, A., Alshatwi, A. A., & Alkaltham, M. S., (2021). Cyclotrisiloxan and β-Sitosterol rich *Cassia alata* (L.) flower inhibits HT-115 human colon cancer cell growth via mitochondrial dependent apoptotic stimulation. *Saudi J Biol Sci., 28*(10), 6009–6016.

Santarelli, R. L., Pierre, F., & Corpet, D. E., (2008). Processed meat and colorectal cancer. *Nutr. Cancer, 60,* 131–144.

Schneider-Stock, R., (2014). Death-associated kinase (DAPK): A cancer gene chameleon. *Apoptosis, 19,* 285.

Selvanathan, J., & Sundaresan, S., (2020). Cytotoxicity effects on negative breast and colon cancer cell lines of *Chromolaena odorata. A J. Comp. Theo., 13*(1), 223–243.

Shimizu, M., Fukutomi, Y., Ninomiya, M., Nagura, K., Kato, T., Araki, H., Suganuma, M., et al., (2008). Green tea extracts for the prevention of metachronous colorectal adenomas: A pilot study. *Cancer Epidemiol Biomarkers Prev., 17*(11), 3020–3025.

Shin, C. M., Lee, D. H., Seo, A. Y., Lee, H. J., Kim, S. B., Son, W. C., Kim, Y. K., et al., (2018). Green tea extracts for the prevention of metachronous colorectal polyps among patients who underwent endoscopic removal of colorectal adenomas: A randomized clinical trial. *Clin Nutr., 37*(2), 452–458.

Shrubsole, M. J., Cai, Q., Wen, W., Milne, G., Smalley, W. E., Chen, Z., Ness, R. M., & Zheng, W., (2012). Urinary prostaglandin E2 metabolite and risk for colorectal adenoma. *Cancer Prev. Res. (Philadelphia, Pa).*, *5*, 336–342.

Smith, E., Palethorpe, H. M., Tomita, Y., Pei, J. V., Townsend, A. R., Price, T. J., Young, J. P., et al., (2018). The purified extract from the medicinal plant *Bacopa monnieri*, Bacopaside II, inhibits the growth of colon cancer cells *in vitro* by inducing cell cycle arrest and apoptosis. *Cells, 7*(7), 81.

Stingl, J. C., Ettrich, T., Muche, R., Wiedom, M., Brockmöller, J., Seeringer, A., & Seufferlein, T., (2011). Protocol for minimizing the risk of metachronous adenomas of the colorectum with green tea extract (MIRACLE): A randomized controlled trial of green tea extract versus placebo for nutriprevention of metachronous colon adenomas in the elderly population. *BMC Cancer, 11*(1), 360.

Tao, Y., Zhan, S., Wang, Y., Zhou, G., Liang, H., Chen, X., & Shen, H., (2018). Baicalin, the major component of traditional Chinese medicine *Scutellaria baicalensis* induces colon cancer cell apoptosis through inhibition of oncomiRNAs. *Sci Rep., 8*(1), 14477.

Turan, I., Demir, S., Kilinc, K., Yaman, S. O., Misir, S., Kara, H., Genc, B., et al., (2018). Cytotoxic effect of *Rosa canina* extract on human colon cancer cells through repression of telomerase expression. *J. Pharm. Anal., 8*(6), 394–399.

Useros, M., & Foncillas, G., (2016). Obesity and colorectal cancer: Molecular features of adipose tissue. *J. Transl. Med., 14*, 1–12.

Wang, J., Li, X. M., Bai, Z., Chi, B. X., Wei, Y., & Chen, X., (2018). Curcumol induces cell cycle arrest in colon cancer cells via reactive oxygen species and Akt/ GSK3β/cyclin D1 pathway. *J. Ethnopharmacol., 210*, 1–9.

Wilhelm, M., Mueller, L., Miller, M. C., Link, K., Holdenrieder, S., Bertsch, T., Kunzmann, V., Stoetzer, O. J., Suttmann, I., Braess, J., Birkmann, J., Roessler, M., Moritz, B., et al., (2016). Prospective, multicenter study of 5-fluorouracil therapeutic drug monitoring in metastatic colorectal cancer treated in routine clinical practice. *Clin/ Colorectal Cancer, 15*, 381–388.

Wong, H. P., Yu, L., Lam, E. K., Tai, E. K., Wu, W. K., & Cho, C. H., (2007). Nicotine promotes colon tumor growth and angiogenesis through b-adrenergic activation. *Toxicol. Sci., 97*, 279–287.

Yang, D., Zhang, X., Zhang, W., & Rengarajan, T., (2018). Vicenin-2 inhibits Wnt/β-catenin signaling and induces apoptosis in HT-29 human colon cancer cell line. *Drug Des. Devel. Ther., 12*, 1303–1310.

Yang, Z., Yang, H., Dong, X., Pu, M., & Ji, F., (2020). Hesperidin loaded Zn2+@ SA/PCT nanocomposites inhibit the proliferation and induces the apoptosis in colon cancer cells (HCT116) through the enhancement of pro-apoptotic protein expressions. *J. Photochem. Photobiol. B., 204*, 111767.

Zhao, Y., Li, E. T. S., & Wang, M., (2017). Alisol B 23-acetate induces autophagic-dependent apoptosis in human colon cancer cells via ROS generation and JNK activation. *Oncotarget, 8*(41), 70239–70249.

CHAPTER 10

SKIN CANCER PREVENTION BY NUTRACEUTICALS

MOHAMMAD MEHDIZADEH,[1,2] ZOLEIKHA MEHDIZADEH,[3] EMAD JAFARZADEH,[4] ATUN ROY CHOUDHURY,[5,6] ZEINAB HAGHI,[7] AREZOO MATIN,[8] ALIASHRAF BAGHERI[9] and ANAHITA OMIDI[10]

[1]*Department of Agronomy and Plant Breeding, Faculty of Agriculture and Natural Resources, University of Mohaghegh Ardabili, Ardabil, Iran*

[2]*Ilam Science and Technology Park, Ilam, Iran*

[3]*Department of Biology, Payame Noor University, Tehran, Iran*

[4]*Department of Toxicology and Pharmacology, Faculty of Pharmacy, Tehran University of Medical Sciences (TUMS), Tehran, Iran*

[5]*Manager (HoD), Fecal Sludge Management Division, Banka BioLoo Limited, India*

[6]*Scholar, Department of Biological Sciences, BITS Pilani Hyderabad Campus, India*

[7]*Department of Plant Protection, School of Agriculture, Shiraz University, Shiraz, Iran*

[8]*Public Health school, Bam University of Medical Sciences, Bam, Iran*

[9]*Department of Nuclear Engineering, Faculty of Sciences and Modern Technologies, Graduate University of Advanced Technology, Kerman, Iran*

[10]*Department of GIS and Remote Sensing, Faculty of Geography, University of Tehran, Tehran, Iran*

Nutraceuticals in Cancer Prevention, Management, and Treatment. Raj K. Keservani, Bui Thanh Tung, Sippy Singh, & Rajesh K. Kesharwani, PhD (Eds.)

ABSTRACT

Skin cancer is one of the most prevalent cancers worldwide. Some limited therapy methods, including surgery, radiation therapy, and chemotherapy, are performed for squamous cell carcinoma, basal cell carcinoma, and melanoma, as well-known skin cancers. The current treatment methods have a relatively low success rate and may leave different side effects during and after therapy. Therefore, finding alternative methods without side effects to treat skin cancer has always been interesting to oncology researchers. Thus, nutraceuticals and herbal medicines for skin cancer treatment have become particularly important in recent years. In this regard, the main classes of nutraceutical compounds with powerful anticancer potential discussed in this book chapter are included phenolic acids, flavonoids, carotenoids, vitamins, and terpenes.

10.1 INTRODUCTION

Human life and functioning rely on having a healthy body. On the other hand, health issues could influence every perspective of human life. However, humans are continually exposed to different diseases and illnesses during their lives. Cancer is one of the worst-known diseases that regularly leads to the death of many people worldwide and imposes high medical costs on different populations. In 2018 in the United States, the highest deaths from diseases were related to heart disease (23%) and cancer (21%) (Siegel et al., 2021). As the greatest organ in the human body, the skin is the first defense barrier against invasive agents. The skin has several functions in protection, storage of substances, and maintenance of body heat (Pereira, 2018). The layers of the skin include the outer layer or epidermis and the inner layers dermis and hypodermis. The epidermis comprises three layers of stem cells, squamous cells, and melanocytes, each of which can be the source of various skin cancers. Common skin cancers include squamous cell carcinoma and basal cell carcinoma, and a rare type of skin cancer may appear in the form of melanoma, which is one of the deadliest and most dangerous skin cancers (Celić et al., 2019). For each kind of skin cancer, particular therapy methods could be considered depending on the extent and severity of cancer. Common treatments currently available for patients with skin cancer include surgery, radiation therapy, and chemotherapy (Conforti et al., 2019). In all of these methods, the cancer cells will be destroyed. However, with the destruction of cancer cells, some healthy cells are also destroyed, and this event is the cause of the side effects of cancer treatment. Therefore, finding alternative methods without side effects to treat cancer has always been interesting to oncology researchers. Thus, dietary supplements and promising herbal medicines for cancer treatment have become particularly important in recent years.

Recent studies recommend that diet and food play an essential role in supporting health conditions (Sreedhar et al., 2018; Sakkas et al., 2020; Ali et al., 2021). Eating high-value foods and daily physical exercise is an absolute requirement for having a healthy, steady life. Physical inactivity is known as a significant worldwide epidemic and a severe risk factor for many diseases (Lippi and Sanchis-Gomar, 2020; Cunningham et al., 2020). Unbalanced food consumption and reduction of physical exercise are correlated with enhanced risk of stress, obesity, diabetes, and even cancer (Ruiz-Nunez et al., 2013). As a significant global threat, cancer is the world's second leading cause of death. Therefore, the requirement to scale up cancer medication is essential. With the expanding variety of experimentations, the application of alternative or unconventional medicine seems to be increasing (Michalczyk et al., 2021; Pandey et al., 2021). Eisenberg et al. (1993) reported that approximately 40 percent of adults in the United States used alternative medicine and dietary complements. This extensive use of nutritional supplements has brought awareness to the effect of diet and food in cancer pathogenesis.

Generally, during a multi-step process, normal cells in the human body are exposed to a series of changes and turn into cancer cells. Approximately two hundred different types of cancers are identified that have entirely different symptoms and mechanisms (Majima, 2018). The most prevalent cancers globally include breast, colon, skin, pancreatic, prostate, liver, kidney, and lung (Leong et al., 2021). One of the most common types of cancer is skin cancer. Prolonged exposure to direct sunlight and UV radiations can damage the DNA of skin cells, which changes the nature of skin cells into cancer cells (Patra et al., 2020).

Although notable advances have been made in recent years in the methods and technologies used in cancer treatment, the side effects and consequences of such methods as chemotherapy and radiation therapy can affect patients' life during treatment and even after treatment. Accordingly, proper diet and consumption of required nutrients are essential in human health and could play a significant role in improving the patients' condition and moderating the side effects caused by chemotherapy and radiation therapy (Marventano et al., 2013). Therefore, according to the side effects of common cancer treatment methods, alternative therapies and unconventional medicines for cancer treatment are of great importance. Various factors play a role in the prevalence of cancer. However, the role of genetic background and nutritional diet is undeniable (Anand et al., 2008). In Western countries, which usually use processed foods, fast foods, red meat, and high-fat foods, cancer incidence is much higher than in Asian countries, which have a healthier diet such as low-fat foods, whole-grain foods, vegetables, and fruits (Jemal et al., 2011). On the other hand, in some Asian countries, herbal and natural-based medicines are traditionally used to treat some diseases. Most of these natural remedies are from plant-derived foods and are known as nutraceuticals. Nutraceutical is a term derived from nutrition and pharmaceuticals and refers to any compounds derived from food sources with medicinal properties and inhibitory effects on some diseases (Keservani et al., 2010a, 2010b; Keservani and Sharma 2014; Al Ali et al., 2021). Nutraceuticals have been widely used to treat some diseases and improve patients' health conditions in recent years (Daliu et al., 2019; Corzo et al., 2020; Ghaffari and Roshanravan, 2020; Augimeri et al., 2021; Carvalho and Lerner, 2021; Mannucci et al., 2021). This book chapter's key objective is to evaluate the effect of different nutraceutical compounds as a potential treatment for skin cancer.

10.2 SKIN CANCER

As the most common type of cancer, skin cancer includes about 40% of reported cancers worldwide (Dong et al., 2018; Lai et al., 2018). The occurrence of skin cancer has risen significantly during the past three decades and is rapidly expanded comparing other cancers (Wolff et al., 2009). Skin cancer is directly associated with exposure to Ultraviolet radiation. The global health protection agencies, such as the center for disease control and prevention (CDC), categorized skin cancer as an epidemic carcinoma and a formidable threat to the public's health (Okhovat et al., 2018). Squamous cell carcinoma, basal cell carcinoma, and melanoma are three distinguished types of skin cancer, which are described below. In another classification, there are two types of skin cancer, including non-melanoma (squamous cell carcinoma and basal cell carcinoma) and melanoma skin cancer.

10.2.1 SQUAMOUS CELL CARCINOMA

Squamous cell carcinoma is a malignancy that originates from epithelial cells. Epithelial cells are present in various organs, and especially the skin. Non-melanoma skin cancer is an abundant well-known accruing squamous cell carcinoma globally (Marinkovich, 2007). Despite significant advances in diagnostic and treatment methods and technologies, the rate of mortality caused by this type of cancer is concerning and significant (Ong et al., 2021). Generally, several treatments methods are introduced for this carcinoma. However, the surgical removal technique is considered an appropriate treatment option. This type of skin cancer generally occurs in tissue cells exposed to sunlight and could be easily treated if the disease is diagnosed in the early stages (Kwiek and Schwartz, 2016). However, if cancer cells develop and the infection spreads to deep tissues, it could lead to severe situations and mortality.

10.2.2 BASAL CELL CARCINOMA

Basal cell carcinoma, as the most prevalent kind of skin cancer (Gandhi and Kampp, 2015), spreads gradually and could destroy nearby tissue. However, the mortality rate caused by this cancer is negligible (Fania et al., 2020). The leading causes of basal cell carcinoma include exposure to sunlight and UV radiation, having light clear skin, radiotherapy, prolonged exposure to arsenical compounds, as well as having a weak immune system (Gandhi and Kampp, 2015). Surgical excision is considered a regular treatment procedure for basal cell carcinoma. Other treatment methods include cryosurgery, curettage, local chemotherapy, and laser surgery (Nasr et al., 2021). Oh et al. (2021) updated the skin cancer incidence rates in China, Malaya, and Singapore from 1968 to 2016. They reported 65.9, 28.3, and 5.8% cases for basal cell carcinoma, squamous cell carcinoma, and melanoma, respectively. The early diagnosis for cases with basal cell carcinoma is usually very advantageous. These kinds of injuries develop slowly and rarely metastasize (Sevli, 2021).

10.2.3 MELANOMA

Melanoma, frequently known as malignant melanoma, is a severe kind of skin cancer originating from melanocytes, the pigment-producing cells (Strashilov and Yordanov, 2021). Like other skin cancers, the fundamental cause of melanoma is exposure to UV radiation, especially in those people with lower melanin pigment content in their skin (Boo, 2020). People that continuously exposed to ultraviolet light originated from sun or tanning machines for a long time are disposed to this type of cancer. Different risk factors for melanoma include UV radiation, smoking, arsenical compound exposure, a vulnerable immune system, inherited susceptibility, and a family history of melanoma (Srinivas et al., 2021). Melanoma has the lowest incidence among skin cancers; however, the mortality associated with melanoma is significantly higher than other skin cancers (Sacco et al., 2020).

10.3 CURRENT TREATMENTS FOR SKIN CANCER

Diagnosis of skin cancer in the early stages is of particular importance. Selecting a treatment method for skin cancer depends on the lesions' type, size, depth, and position. Surface skin cancers rarely develop and could be removed by simple surgery treatment. However, other skin cancers, such as squamous cell carcinoma and melanoma, required further tests to determine the cancer stage and then select appropriate treatment. Nonmelanoma skin cancers could be treated by electrodessication, curettage, surgery, laser therapy, and cryotherapy (Fania et al., 2021). There are various methods to skin cancer treatment include surgery (surgical process to cancer cells removal), radiation therapy (employing high power x-rays or different kinds of radiation to destroy cancer cells), chemotherapy (applying various medicines to stop the development of cancer cells), photodynamic therapy (involving particular medication and an appropriate type of light to destroy cancer cells), immunotherapy (strengthen the patients' immune system), targeted therapy (uses medicines to recognize and attack particular cancer cells), chemical peel and other drug therapy (Gamez et al., 2020; Todorova and Mandinova, 2020; Alimardani et al., 2021; Bakirtzi et al., 2021; Kaur and Kesharwani, 2021). Depending on the cancer type and the individual's physical condition, these treatments may have different side effects. The most common side effects associated with skin cancer treatments are bleeding, anemia, losing appetite, exhaustion, swelling, diarrhea, vomiting, constipation, infection, fertility problems in men and women, hair loss, memory issues, nerve issues, sexual issues in men and women, sleeping difficulties, etc. (Aggarwal et al., 2021; Brook, 2021; Sous et al., 2021).

10.4 NUTRACEUTICALS AS A POTENTIAL TREATMENT FOR SKIN CANCER

Recently the role of food consumption and nutraceuticals in the inhibition of various diseases has achieved general consideration. Chemical prevention using nutraceuticals has been the focus of various inhibition investigations during the last decade. Evaluating the effects of nutraceuticals in the development of natural-based medicines have been considered by researchers. Historically, these compounds have been an assuring source of pharmaceutical products with curative potential for different disorders, especially cancer. An increasing variety of scientific studies has confirmed the protecting impact of these natural-based compounds, particularly nutraceuticals, to preserve the skin from several disorders such as skin cancers. The evaluation of resources available at the PubMed database shows that 443 studies associated with skin cancer and nutraceuticals were conducted during 1997–2021 (Figure 10.1). Since nutraceuticals are reliable, safe, and have insignificant side effects, they could be considered an appropriate alternative for skin cancer treatment (Strickland et al., 2015; Khan et al., 2021). Table 10.1 represent the anticancer effects of various nutraceuticals on basal cell carcinoma, squamous cell carcinoma, and melanoma.

Nutraceuticals with antioxidant, anti-inflammatory, and immunomodulatory properties have the most significant potential to show inhibitory performance in skin cancers (Katiyar, 2011). Different efforts have been performed to discover the relationship between the antioxidant characteristics of nutraceuticals and their anti-carcinogenic potential. In this regard, the main classes of nutraceuticals compounds with powerful anticancer potential discussed in this book chapter are included phenolic acids, flavonoids, carotenoids, vitamins, and terpenes.

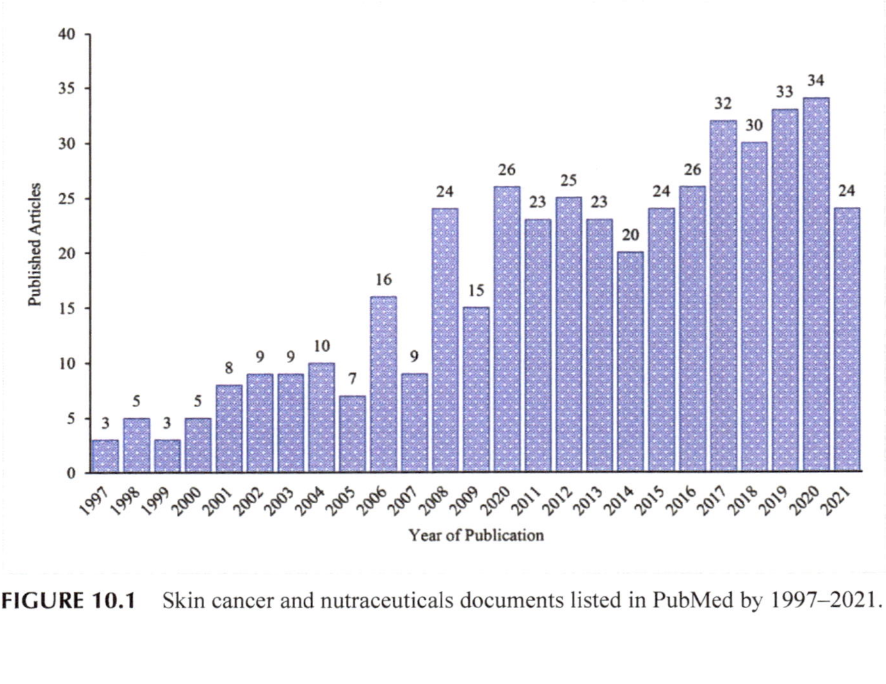

FIGURE 10.1 Skin cancer and nutraceuticals documents listed in PubMed by 1997–2021.

TABLE 10.1 Anticancer effects of nutraceuticals on different skin cancer.

Nutraceuticals	Skin cancer type	Results	Reference
Fisetin (a dietary flavonoid)	Melanoma and non-melanoma	Effective on management of melanoma by having anti-invasive and anti-metastatic properties	Pal et al., 2016
Epigallocatechin gallate (a polyphenols compound) originated from green tea (*Camellia sinensis*)	Melanoma	Significant inhibitory and anticancer effects of epigallocatechin gallate on melanoma skin cancer	Ravindranath et al., 2009
Epigallocatechin gallate (a polyphenols compound) originated from green tea (*Camellia sinensis*)	Melanoma	Inhibitory effect of epigallocatechin gallate on human melanoma cell invasion	Singh and Katiyar, 2011
Resveratrol (a polyphenolic phytoalexin stilbenoid)	Melanoma	enhances the sensitivity of melanoma cells to radiation by inhibiting proliferation and inducing apoptosis	Fang et al., 2013
Curcumin a polyphenolic, bioactive compound extracted from the rhizome of the dietary spice turmeric (*Curcuma longa*)	Melanoma	Curcumin has served as a potential in situ adjuvant for photothermal therapy of melanoma	Singh et al., 2018
Gossypetin (a flavonoids compound from the flowers of *Hibiscus sabdariffa*)	Basal cell carcinoma	Alleviate solar-UV-induced cutaneous basal cell carcinoma by blocking PDZ-binding kinase/T-LAK cell-originated protein kinase	Wang et al., 2019
Limonoids and tricyclic diterpenoids (from *Azadirachta indica*)	Melanoma	Exhibited melanogenesis inhibitory activities in α-MSH-stimulated B16 melanoma cells	Su et al., 2020
Anastatica hierochuntica extracts	Melanoma	Significant anti-inflammatory, hepatoprotective, and anti-melanogenic effects on melanoma cells	Gokce and Guler, 2021
Matrix metalloproteinases (a calcium-dependent zinc-containing endopeptidases)	Squamous cell carcinoma	Positive effects on invasion and proliferation of oral squamous cell carcinoma	Ricci et al., 2019
Combined plant extracts from *Arum palaestinum*, *Peganum harmala* and *Curcuma longa*	Squamous cell carcinoma	Significantly reduced in vitro assessments of Head and neck squamous cell carcinoma progression	Vishwakarma et al., 2018

TABLE 10.1 *(Continued)*

Nutraceuticals	Skin cancer type	Results	Reference
bitter melon (*Momordica charantia*) extract	Squamous cell carcinoma	An immunomodulatory effect on inhibition of head and neck squamous cell carcinoma growth	Bhattacharya et al., 2016
A combination of three nutrients, curcumin, resveratrol and epicatechin gallate	Squamous cell carcinoma	Anticancer therapeutic effects to manage the HPV-positive head and neck squamous cell carcinoma	Piao et al., 2017
Phytocannabinoids and terpenes originated from *Cannabis sativa*	Squamous cell carcinoma	Therapeutic and anticancer effects on squamous cell carcinoma	Kovalchuk et al., 2020
Terpenes compound from *Melaleuca alternifolia* (tea tree) oil	Melanoma	Inhibited the growth of aggressive, subcutaneous, chemo-resistant tumors	Greay et al., 2010
Berberine (a naturally occurring isoquino-line alkaloid)	Melanoma	Suppressed tumor growth in vitro and in vivo	Mittal et al., 2014
Quercetin (a flavonoid compound)	Melanoma	Inhibits the STAT3 signaling pathway, suggesting for prevention and treatment of melanoma	Cao et al., 2014
Proanthocyanidins (polyphenols compounds) originated from grape seeds	Melanoma	Inhibit melanoma cell invasion and migration	Vaid et al., 2011
Silymarin (a flavonolignans extracted from *Silybum marianum*)	Melanoma	Inhibits melanoma cell growth	Lee et al., 2013

10.4.1 PHENOLIC ACIDS

Phenolic acids have made significant interest due to their extensive biological and pharmacological characteristics, mainly their antioxidant, anti-inflammatory, anticarcinogenic, and antimutagenic activities. These compounds are a naturally generated subdivision of the phenolics class. Plants' phenolic acids have been correlated with different functions, including photosynthesis, protein synthesis, nutrient uptake, enzymatic activity, and allelopathic effects. Phenolic acids are essential elements of the human diet due to their possible antioxidant activity, their ability to reduce oxidative stress-induced tissue destruction following chronic disorders, and their probably critical anticancer activities (Harris et al., 2007). Ferulic acid, salicylic acid, cinnamic acids, 3-Hydroxybenzoic acid, gentisic acid, gallic acid, vanillic acid, sinapic acid, digallic acid, diferulic acids, rosmarinic acid are the most important plant-based phenolic acids (Saxena et al., 2012). Cichocki et al. (2010) evaluated the effects of phenolic acids on the inhibition of skin cancer in mice. They found that the inhibitory effects of phenolic acids, especially tannic acid, have become of great interest in preventing cancer. The inhibitory effects of caffeic acid on skin cancer and their protective impacts from UV variations are reported by Staniforth et al. (2006). Yang et al. (2014) reported the significant anticarcinogenic effects of caffeic acid as an effective phenolic acid compound. They suggested caffeic acid as a potential nutraceutical for the treatment of skin cancer. Caffeic acid and some of its derivatives could have antitumor activity toward colon carcinogenesis (Olthof et al., 2001). Kumar et al. (2019) reported the effectiveness of two phenolic acids (hydroxybenzoic and hydroxycinnamic acids) in preventing and treating cancer. As ultraviolet radiations are one of the significant factors affecting the development of skin cancer, ferulic acid could be considered a promising anticancer compound (Ambothi and Nagarajan, 2014).

10.4.2 FLAVONOIDS

Flavonoids have been shown to inhibit the invasion and proliferation of skin cancer cells significantly. Three important classes of flavonoids include flavons, flavonols, and isoflavonoids. Generally, flavonoids could be considered as a promising bioactive compound for treating melanoma. One of the primary flavonoid plant-based compounds is apigenin. Patel et al. (2007) reported antioxidant, anticarcinogenic, and anti-inflammatory effects for apigenin. As apigenin is an active compound identified from chamomile plants, using these plant extracts to treat dermatological diseases has a long story (Patel et al., 2007). The inhibitory effects of apigenin on tumor growth and the development of melanoma skin cancer have been reported in different studies (Caltagirone et al., 2000; Piantelli et al., 2006). Genistein is another flavonoids compound with anticancer properties; this compound, an isoflavone obtained from soybean crops with antioxidant impacts. The potential of genistein for the treatment of cancer and some other diseases is under investigation (Afaq and Katiyar, 2011; Danciu et al., 2013). Horibe et al. (2013) reported the melanogenesis and melanoma inhibition effects of luteolin, a flavonoid compound. Serafino et al. (2004) investigated the effect of cyanidin-3-O-beta-glucopyranoside (a flavonoid compound) on the proliferation and differentiation of human melanoma cells. They reported the effectiveness of cyanidin-3-O-beta-glucopyranoside on melanoma cell proliferation and suggested this compound as an appropriate molecule for melanoma treatment. Chen et al. (2012) studied the effectiveness of an active flavonoid compound (isoliquiritigenin) on mouse melanoma cells. They found the significant effect of isoliquiritigenin on melanoma cells inhibition. Zhang et al. (2005) suggested the use of quercetin as a potential flavonoid compound for treatment of murine melanoma cells.

10.4.3 CAROTENOIDS

Carotenoid compounds are a class of plant substances that give a brilliant color to various crops, including squash, carrots, and sweet potatoes. Carotenoids are classified into two main groups, including hydrocarbons, highly fat-soluble compounds, and xanthophylls, moderately polar compounds (Vainio and Rautalahti, 1998). Among so many identified carotenoids, there are 40 carotenoids involved in human dietary (Elvira-Torales et al., 2019). The most recognized carotenoids are beta-carotene, alpha-carotene, lycopene, fucoxanthin, and crocetin (Bhatt and Patel, 2020). Among them, beta-carotene is considered the most recognized carotenoid in the world. Different studies showed that carotenoids have a carcinogenesis effect with various proposed mechanisms (Black et al., 2020; Lim and Wang, 2020). The body could transform carotenoids to retinoids, suppressing carcinogenesis in multiple animal tumor patterns (Alizadeh et al., 2014). During the past decades, researchers have tried to confirm a correlation between nonmelanoma skin cancer and beta-carotene, which has been proposed to decrease the free radical destruction of DNA following UV exposure (Green et al., 1999; Van Dam et al., 2000). Heinen et al. (2007) evaluated the impact of two carotenoid compounds (lutein and zeaxanthin) on basal cell carcinoma and squamous cell carcinoma in the Australian population. They reported a positive correlation between intake of these bioactive substances and reduction in squamous cell carcinoma incidence in individuals with a history of skin cancer.

10.4.4 VITAMINS

Vitamins are groups of primary substances in foods. According to the literature, four kinds of vitamins (A, C, D, and E) have skin protection and anticancer effects. Due to antioxidant effects, Vitamin C proved to have therapeutic properties, especially in protecting skin from free radical destruction. Many fruits and vegetables, such as tomatoes, strawberries, and citrus plants have different vitamin C levels. The photoprotective impact of vitamin C is reported in different studies (Al-Niaimi and Chiang, 2017; Enescu et al., 2021). Also, vitamin E could preserve the cell membrane from peroxidation and destruction by free radicals (Paunović et al., 2017). The commonly used commercial form of vitamin E is alpha-tocopherol acetate which cosmetics manufacturers widely use. Kim et al. (2019) evaluated the effect of vitamin A on squamous cell carcinoma. They reported a significant protective effect of vitamin A on the development of this type of skin cancer. Retinoid is a well-known compound of vitamin A, which could originate from plants or animal food sources. Moreover, retinoids could be considered inhibitors of skin cancer tumors (Collins et al., 2019). Ottino and Duncan (1997) investigated the anti-proliferation effects of α-tocopherol and reported this compound's significant efficiency for melanoma skin cancer treatment. Several researchers studied the photoprotection efficiency of vitamin E compounds and their derivatives. Pedrelli et al. (2012) reported an appropriate photoprotective effect of tocopherols and tocotrienols. It was recommended that vitamin E was efficient in late-stage tumorigenesis, as it could influence tumor progress (Burns et al., 2013). The potential application of nano-formulation in developing vitamin E-based products for cancer therapy, combined with other anticancer factors, has been studied (Nicolas et al., 2014). Brozyna et al. (2011) reported the anti-skin cancer efficiency of vitamin D.

10.4.5 TERPENES

Terpenes compounds are one of the most extensive groups of naturally originated compounds primarily detected in plants. These compounds are categorized based on structure and the isoprene units number contained. Thermal protectant properties and pharmaceutical effects associated with terpenes are prominent for these compounds (Carsanba et al., 2021; Desaulniers Brousseau et al., 2021). There are many various plants containing terpenes and terpenoids compounds. Antimicrobial and antiparasitic, anticancer, and anti-inflammatory effects of cannabis plants are associated with the presence of terpenes compounds (Nuutinen, 2018). Various mushrooms, such as Ganoderma are some plants containing terpenoid compounds experimented with anti-melanoma properties (Lu et al., 2019). Harhaji et al. (2008) studied the effects of *Coriolus versicolor* extracts on melanoma skin cancer. They reported a significant reduction in cancer cells growth and tumor size by inhibiting cell reproduction and death. Valiahdi et al. (2013) extracted stylosin and tschimgine as two monoterpenes from *Ferula ovina* plants and found anti-melanoma effects of these compounds. Uddin et al. (2012) evaluated the impacts of terpenoid β-damascenone for skin protection from UV radiation in mice. According to their reports, applying 20 μL of this compound leads to UV protection and avoiding sunburn in mice. Greay et al. (2010) reported the inhibitory properties of oil extracted from tea tree (*Melaleuca alternifolia*) on melanoma cancer cell growth due to the presence of terpene components in the extracts.

10.5 FUTURE PROSPECTS

Further researches would be essential to stabilize accurate instructions for skin cancer patients. As the use of nutraceuticals in skin cancer therapy, it is required to determine particular guidelines for the patients, according to the skin cancer type and stage, patients' situations (age, gender, etc.), treatment methods, the compatibility of nutraceuticals compounds with other medicines, and the concentration of bioactive compounds. Nutraceutical science could be developed from numerous viewpoints. Genetic engineering, genome sequence, and genome-edition technologies can play a unique role in developing nutraceutical knowledge for cancer treatment and synthesizing novel nutraceuticals. Also, artificial intelligence and deep-learning technologies are essential for the industrialization and commercialization of nutraceuticals. Enhancing the bioavailability of these bioactive compounds should be considered. A promising method to increase nutraceuticals bioavailability is to promote more reliable delivery systems such as nano and microencapsulation of nutraceuticals to survive the stomach's acidic conditions.

10.6 CONCLUSION

Nutraceuticals represent an exciting experimentation area for identifying innovative health outputs with great potential for cancer treatment. This book chapter showed that nutraceuticals could be considered a key player and promising alternative method in future skin cancer therapy. This study has reviewed different nutraceuticals for their potential anti-carcinogenic properties. Nutraceuticals have been described to possess various health advantages, and continuing studies need to determine their physiological impacts. Growing studies and investigations in nutraceuticals suggest the high achievements of these compounds in skin cancer inhibition. Nutraceuticals are displaying popularity as they are safe and natural food components. Conventional application of nutraceuticals in skin cancer therapy is moderately economical compared to other treatment methods. Like synthetic medicines, plant-originated medicines could have toxicity effects in high concentrations that accumulate beyond the human body's acceptable level. However, numerous benefits are associated with medicinal plants; toxicological studies should be considered to avoid toxicity issues. Further investigations are required to explain the clinical trials' outcomes, which sometimes conflict with each other. Different researches have revealed that specific nutraceuticals could have synergy with various medicines, improving their efficiency. In this regard, phenolic acids, flavonoids, carotenoids, vitamins, and terpenes seem to be the assuring nutraceuticals for skin cancer therapy. Scientists have recognized that appropriate diet and nutraceuticals can impact various diseases. According to the literature, it is confirmed that nutraceuticals can promote well-being and inhibit particular disorders, and some of these compounds have shown similar efficiency as current medicines. Researchers reveal the defensive role of nutraceuticals in cancer therapy. Therefore, additional inclusive studies are required concerning their safety and effectiveness.

KEYWORDS

- **anticancer**
- **carotenoids**
- **flavonoids**
- **melanoma**
- **terpenes**

REFERENCES

Afaq, F., & Katiyar, S. K., (2011). Polyphenols: Skin photoprotection and inhibition of photocarcinogenesis. *Mini Reviews in Medicinal Chemistry, 11*(14), 1200–1215.https://doi.org/10.2174/138955751111091200.

Aggarwal, S., Verma, S. S., Aggarwal, S., & Gupta, S. C., (2021). Drug repurposing for breast cancer therapy: Old weapon for new battle. *Seminars in Cancer Biology, 68*, 8–20. http://dx.doi.org/10.1016/j.semcancer.2019.09.012.

AlAli, M., Alqubaisy, M., Aljaafari, M. N., Al-Ali, A. O., Baqais, L., Molouki, A., Abushelaibi, A., et al., (2021). Nutraceuticals: Transformation of conventional foods into health promoters/disease preventers and safety considerations. *Molecules, 26*, 2540. https://doi.org/10.3390/molecules26092540.

Ali, M. Y., Sina, A. A. I., Khandker, S. S., Neesa, L., Tanvir, E. M., Kabir, A., Khalil, M. I., & Gan, S. H., (2021). Nutritional composition and bioactive compounds in tomatoes and their impact on human health and disease: A review. *Foods, 10*, 45. https://doi.org/10.3390/foods10010045.

Alimardani, V., Abolmaali, S. S., Yousefi, G., Rahiminezhad, Z., Abedi, M., Tamaddon, A., & Ahadian, S., (2021). Microneedle arrays combined with nanomedicine approaches for transdermal delivery of therapeutics. *Journal of Clinical Medicine, 10*(2), 181. https://doi.org/10.3390/jcm10020181.

Alizadeh, F., Bolhassani, A., Khavari, A., Bathaie, S. Z., Naji, T., & Bidgoli, S. A., (2014). Retinoids and their biological effects against cancer. *International Immunopharmacology, 18*(1), 43–49.https://doi.org/10.1016/j.intimp.2013.10.027.

Al-Niaimi, F., & Chiang, N. Y. Z., (2017). Topical vitamin C and the skin: Mechanisms of action and clinical applications. *The Journal of Clinical and Aesthetic Dermatology, 10*(7), 14–17.

Ambothi, K., & Nagarajan, R. P., (2014). Ferulic acid prevents ultraviolet-B radiation induced oxidative DNA damage in human dermal fibroblasts. *International Journal of Nutrition, Pharmacology, Neurological Diseases, 4*, 203–213.https://doi.org/10.4103/2231-0738.139400.

Anand, P., Kunnumakara, A. B., Sundaram, C., Harikumar, K. B., Tharakan, S. T., Lai, O. S., Sung, B., & Aggarwal, B. B., (2008). Cancer is a preventable disease that requires major lifestyle changes. *Pharmaceutical Research, 25*(9), 2097–2116. https://doi.org/10.1007/s11095-008-9661–9.

Augimeri, G., Montalto, F. I., Giordano, C., Barone, I., Lanzino, M., Catalano, S., Andò, S., et al., (2021). Nutraceuticals in the Mediterranean diet: Potential avenues for breast cancer treatment. *Nutrients, 13,* 2557. https://doi.org/10.3390/nu13082557.

Bakirtzi, K., Papadimitriou, I., Andreadis, D., & Sotiriou, E., (2021). Treatment options and post-treatment malignant transformation rate of actinic cheilitis: A systematic review. *Cancers, 13*, 3354. https://doi.org/10.3390/cancers13133354.

Bhatt, T., & Patel, K., (2020). Carotenoids: Potent to prevent diseases review. *Natural Products and Bioprospecting, 10*, 109–117. https://doi.org/10.1007/s13659-020-00244-2.

Bhattacharya, S., Muhammad, N., Steele, R., Peng, G., & Ray, R. B., (2016). Immunomodulatory role of bitter melon extract in inhibition of head and neck squamous cell carcinoma growth. *Oncotarget, 7*(22), 33202–33209. https://doi.org/10.18632/oncotarget.8898.

Black, H. S., Boehm, F., Edge, R., & Truscott, T. G., (2020). The benefits and risks of certain dietary carotenoids that exhibit both anti-and pro-oxidative mechanisms-a comprehensive review. *Antioxidants, 9*, 264. https://doi.org/10.3390/antiox9030264.

Boo, Y. C., (2020). Emerging strategies to protect the skin from ultraviolet rays using plant-derived materials. *Antioxidants, 9*, 637. https://doi.org/10.3390/antiox9070637.

Brook, I., (2021). Early side effects of radiation treatment for head and neck cancer. *Cancer Radiotherapie, 25*(5), 507–513. https://doi.org/10.1016/j.canrad.2021.02.001.

Brozyna, A. A., Jozwicki, W., Janjetovic, Z. J., & Slominski, A. T., (2011). Original contribution: Expression of vitamin D receptor decreases during progression of pigmented skin lesions. *Human Pathology, 42*(5), 618–631.https://doi.org/10.1016/j.humpath.2010.09.014.

Burns, E. M., Tober, K. L., Riggenbach, J. A., Kusewitt, D. F., Young, G. S., & Oberyszyn, T. M., (2013). Differential effects of topical vitamin E and C E Ferulic® treatments on ultraviolet light B-induced cutaneous tumor development in Skh-1 mice. *PLoS One, 8*(5), e63809. https://doi.org/10.1371/journal.pone.0063809.

Caltagirone, S., Rossi, C., Poggi, A., Ranelletti, F. O., Natali, P. G., Brunetti, M., Aiello, F. B., & Piantelli, M., (2000). Flavonoids apigenin and quercetin inhibit melanoma growth and metastatic potential. *International Journal of Cancer, 87*(4), 595–600. https://doi.org/10.1002/1097-0215(20000815)87:4%3C595::aid-ijc21%3E3.0.co;2-5.

Cao, H. H., Tse, A. K. W., Kwan, H. Y., Yu, H., Cheng, C. Y., Su, T., Fong, W. F., & Yu, Z. L., (2014). Quercetin exerts anti-melanoma activities and inhibits STAT3 signaling. *Biochemical Pharmacology, 87*, 424–434.https://doi.org/10.1016/j.bcp.2013.11.008.

Carsanba, E., Pintado, M., & Oliveira, C., (2021). Fermentation strategies for production of pharmaceutical terpenoids in engineered yeast. *Pharmaceuticals, 14,* 295. https://doi.org/10.3390/ph14040295.

Carvalho, J. F., & Lerner, A., (2021). Fibromyalgia associated with chagas' disease treated with nutraceuticals. *Clinical Nutrition ESPEN, 42*, 212–214. https://doi.org/10.1016/j.clnesp.2021.01.037.

Celić, D., Lipozenčić, J., Kolarić, B., Ferenčak, G., Rajković, J. K., & Borlinić, T., (2019). Association between blood group and nonmelanoma skin cancers (basal cell carcinoma and squamous cell carcinoma). *International Journal of Environmental Research and Public Health, 16,* 2267. https://doi.org/10.3390/ijerph16132267.

Chen, X., Zhang, B., Yuan, X., Yang, F., Liu, J., Zhao, Z., Liu, L., et al., (2012). Isoliquiritigenin-induced differentiation in mouse melanoma B16F0 cell line. *Oxidative Medicine and Cellular Longevity, 534934*, 1–11. https://doi.org/10.1155/2012/534934.

Cichocki, M., Blumczyńska, J., & Baer-Dubowska, W., (2010). Naturally occurring phenolic acids inhibit 12-O-tetradecanoylphorbol-13-acetate induced NF-κB, iNOS and COX-2 activation in mouse epidermis. *Toxicology, 268*(1, 2), 118–124. https://doi.org/10.1016/j.tox.2009.12.013.

Collins, L., Asfour, L., Stephany, M., Lear, J. T., & Stasko, T., (2019). Management of non-melanoma skin cancer in transplant recipients. *Clinical Oncology, 31*(11), 779–788. https://doi.org/10.1016/j.clon.2019.08.005.

Conforti, C., Corneli, P., Harwood, C., & Zalaudek, I., (2019). Evolving role of systemic therapies in non-melanoma skin cancer. *Clinical Oncology, 31*(11), 759–768. https://doi.org/10.1016/j.clon.2019.08.011.

Corzo, L., Fernández-Novoa, L., Carrera, I., Martínez, O., Rodríguez, S., Alejo, R., & Cacabelos, R., (2020). Nutrition, health, and disease: Role of selected marine and vegetal nutraceuticals. *Nutrients, 12*, 747. https://doi.org/10.3390/nu12030747.

Cunningham, C., O'Sullivan, R., Caserotti, P., & Tully, M. A., (2020). Consequences of physical inactivity in older adults: A systematic review of reviews and meta-analyses. *Scandinavian Journal of Medicine & Science in Sports, 30*(5), 816–827. https://doi.org/10.1111/sms.13616.

Daliu, P., Santini, A., & Novellino, E., (2019). From pharmaceuticals to nutraceuticals: Bridging disease prevention and management. *Expert Review of Clinical Pharmacology, 12*(1), 1–7. https://doi.org/10.1080/17512433.2019.1552135.

Danciu, C., Borcan, F., Bojin, F., Zupko, I., & Dehelean, C., (2013). Effect of the isoflavone genistein on tumor size, metastasis potential and melanization in a B16 mouse model of murine melanoma. *Natural Product Communications, 8*(3), 343–346.http://dx.doi.org/10.1177/1934578X1300800318.

Desaulniers, B. V., Wu, B. S., MacPherson, S., Morello, V., & Lefsrud, M., (2021). Cannabinoids and terpenes: How production of photo-protectants can be manipulated to enhance *Cannabis sativa* L. phytochemistry. *Frontiers in Plant Science, 12*, 620021. https://doi.org/10.3389/fpls.2021.620021.

Dong, X., Han, Y., Sun, Z., & Xu, J., (2018). Actin gamma 1, a new skin cancer pathogenic gene, identified by the biological feature-based classification. *Journal of Cellular Biochemistry, 119*(2), 1406–1419. https://doi.org/10.1002/jcb.26301.

Eisenberg, D. M., Kessler, R. C., Foster, C., Norlock, F. E., Calkins, D. R., & Delbanco, T. L., (1993). Unconventional medicine in the United States: Prevalence, costs, and patterns of use. *The New England Journal of Medicine, 328*, 246–225. https://doi.org/10.1056/nejm199301283280406.

Elvira-Torales, L. I., García-Alonso, J., & Periago-Castón, M. J., (2019). Nutritional importance of carotenoids and their effect on liver health: A review. *Antioxidants, 8*, 229. https://doi.org/10.3390/antiox8070229.

Enescu, C. D., Bedford, L. M., Potts, G., & Fahs, F., (2021). A review of topical vitamin C derivatives and their efficacy. *Journal of Cosmetic Dermatology*. https://doi.org/10.1111/jocd.14465.

Fang, Y., Bradley, M. J., Cook, K. M., Herrick, E. J., & Nicholl, M. B., (2013). A potential role for resveratrol as a radiation sensitizer for melanoma treatment. *The Journal of Surgical Research, 183*(2), 645–653.https://doi.org/10.1016/j.jss.2013.02.037.

Fania, L., Didona, D., Morese, R., Campana, I., Coco, V., Di Pietro, F. R., Ricci, F., et al., (2020). Basal cell carcinoma: From pathophysiology to novel therapeutic approaches. *Biomedicines, 8*, 449. https://doi.org/10.3390/biomedicines8110449.

Fania, L., Samela, T., Moretta, G., Ricci, F., Dellambra, E., Mancini, M., Sampogna, F., et al., (2021). Attitudes among dermatologists regarding non-melanoma skin cancer treatment options. *Discover Oncology, 12*, 31. https://doi.org/10.1007/s12672–021–00421-w.

Gamez, M. E., Blakaj, A., Zoller, W., Bonomi, M., & Blakaj, D. M., (2020). Emerging concepts and novel strategies in radiation therapy for laryngeal cancer management. *Cancers, 12*, 1651. https://doi.org/10.3390/cancers12061651.

Gandhi, S. A., & Kampp, J., (2015). Skin cancer epidemiology, detection, and management. *The Medical Clinics of North America, 99*(6), 1323–1335. https://doi.org/10.1016/j.mcna.2015.06.002.

Ghaffari, S., & Roshanravan, N., (2020). The role of nutraceuticals in prevention and treatment of hypertension: An updated review of the literature. *Food Research International, 128*, 108749. https://doi.org/10.1016/j.foodres.2019.108749.

Gokce, M., & Guler, E. M., (2021). *A. hierchuntica* extract exacerbates genotoxic, cytotoxic, apoptotic and oxidant effects in B16F10 melanoma cells. *Toxicon, 198*, 73–79. https://doi.org/10.1016/j.toxicon.2021.04.026.

Greay, S. J., Ireland, D. J., Kissick, H. T., Heenan, P. J., Carson, C. F., Riley, T. V., & Beilharz, M. W., (2010). Inhibition of established subcutaneous murine tumor growth with topical *Melaleuca alternifolia* (tea tree) oil. *Cancer Chemotherapy and Pharmacology, 66*(6), 1095–1102.https://doi.org/10.1007/s00280-010-1267-3.

Green, A., Williams, G., Neale, R., Hart, V., Leslie, D., Parsons, P., Marks, G. C., et al., (1999). Daily sunscreen application and beta-carotene supplementation in prevention of basal-cell and squamous-cell carcinomas of the skin: A randomized controlled trial. *Lancet, 354*(9180), 723–729.https://doi.org/10.1016/s0140-6736(98)12168-2.

Harhaji, L. J., Mijatović, S., Maksimović-Ivanić, D., Stojanović, I., Momčilović, M., Maksimović, V., Tufegdžić, S., et al., (2008). Anti-tumor effect of *Coriolus versicolor* methanol extract against mouse B16 melanoma cells: *In vitro* and *in vivo* study. *Food and Chemical Toxicology, 46*, 1825–1833.https://doi.org/10.1016/j.fct.2008.01.027.

Harris, C. S., Mo, F., Migahed, L., Chepelev, L., Haddad, P. S., Wright, J. S., Willmore, W. G., et al., (2007). Plant phenolics regulate neoplastic cell growth and survival: A quantitative structure-activity and biochemical analysis. *Cancer Journal of Physiology and Pharmacology, 85*, 1124–1138. https://doi.org/10.1139/y07-101.

Heinen, M. M., Hughes, M. C., Ibiebele, T. I., Marks, G. C., Green, A. C., & Van, D. P. J. C., (2007). Intake of antioxidant nutrients and the risk of skin cancer. *European Journal of Cancer, 43*(18), 2707–2716. https://doi.org/10.1016/j.ejca.2007.09.005.

Horibe, I., Satoh, Y., Shiota, Y., Kumagai, A., Horike, N., Takemori, H., Uesato, S., et al., (2013). Induction of melanogenesis by 4'-O-methylated flavonoids in B16F10 melanoma cells. *Journal of Natural Medicines, 67*(4), 705–710. https://doi.org/10.1007/s11418-012-0727-y.

Jemal, A., Bray, F., Center, M. M., Ferlay, J., Ward, E., Forman, & and, D., (2011). Global cancer statistics. *CA: A Cancer Journal for Clinicians, 61*(2), 69–90. https://doi.org/10.3322/caac.20107.

Katiyar, S. K., (2011). Green tea prevents non-melanoma skin cancer by enhancing DNA repair. *Archives of Biochemistry and Biophysics, 508*(2), 152–158. https://doi.org/10.1016/j.abb.2010.11.015.

Kaur, H., & Kesharwani, P., (2021). Advanced nanomedicine approaches applied for treatment of skin carcinoma. *Journal of Controlled Release, 337*, 589–611. https://doi.org/10.1016/j.jconrel.2021.08.003.

Keservani, R. K., & Sharma, A. K., (2014). Flavonoids: Emerging trends and potential health benefits. *Journal of Chinese Pharmaceutical Sciences, 23*(12), 815.

Keservani, R. K., Kesharwani, R. K., Sharma, A. K., Vyas, N., & Chadoker, A., (2010b). Nutritional supplements: An overview. *International Journal of Current Pharmaceutical Review and Research, 1*(1), 59–75.

Keservani, R. K., Kesharwani, R. K., Vyas, N., Jain, S., Raghuvanshi, R., & Sharma, A. K., (2010a). Nutraceutical and functional food as future food: A review. *Der Pharmacia Lettre, 2*(1), 106–116.

Khan, H., Labanca, F., Ullah, H., Hussain, Y., Tzvetkov, N. T., Akkol, E. K., & Milella, L., (2021). Advances and challenges in cancer treatment and nutraceutical prevention: The possible role of dietary phenols in BRCA regulation. *Phytochemistry Reviews*. https://doi.org/10.1007/s11101-021-09771-3.

Kim, J., Park, M. K., Li, W. Q., Qureshi, A. A., & Cho, E., (2019). Association of vitamin A intake with cutaneous squamous cell carcinoma risk in the United States. *JAMA Dermatology, 155*(11), 1260–1268. https://doi.org/10.1001/jamadermatol.2019.1937.

Kovalchuk, O., Li, D., Rodriguez-Juarez, R., Golubov, A., Hudson, D., & Kovalchuk, I., (2020). The effect of cannabis dry flower irradiation on the level of cannabinoids, terpenes and anticancer properties of the extracts. *Biocatalysis and Agricultural Biotechnology, 29*, 101736. https://doi.org/10.1016/j.bcab.2020.101736.

Kumar, N., Gupta, S., Yadav, T. C., Pruthi, V., Varadwaj, P. K., & Goel, N., (2019). Extrapolation of phenolic compounds as multi-target agents against cancer and inflammation *Journal of Biomolecular Structure and Dynamics, 37*(9), 2355–2369. https://doi.org/10.1080/07391102.2018.1481457.

Kwiek, B., & Schwartz, R. A., (2016). Keratoacanthoma (KA): An update and review. *Journal of the American Academy of Dermatology, 74*(6), 1220–1233. https://doi.org/10.1016/j.jaad.2015.11.033.

Lai, V., Cranwell, W., & Sinclair, R., (2018). Epidemiology of skin cancer in the mature patient. *Clinics in Dermatology, 36*(2), 167–176. https://doi.org/10.1016/j.clindermatol.2017.10.008.

Lee, M. H., Huang, Z., Kim, D. J., Kim, S. H., Kim, M. O., Lee, S. Y., Xie, H., et al., (2013). Direct targeting of MEK1/2 and RSK2 by silybin induces cell-cycle arrest and inhibits melanoma cell growth. *Cancer Prevention Research, 6*(5), 455–465.https://doi.org/10.1158/1940-6207.capr-12-0425.

Leong, Y. Q., Lee, S. W. H., & Ng, K. Y., (2021). Cancer risk in Parkinson disease: An updated systematic review and meta-analysis. *European Journal of Neurology*. https://doi.org/10.1111/ene.15069.

Lim, J. Y., & Wang, X. D., (2020). Mechanistic understanding of β-cryptoxanthin and lycopene in cancer prevention in animal models. *Biochimica et Biophysica Acta (BBA) – Molecular and Cell Biology of Lipids, 1865*(11), 158652. https://doi.org/10.1016/j.bbalip.2020.158652.

Lippi, G., & Sanchis-Gomar, F., (2020). An estimation of the worldwide epidemiologic burden of physical inactivity-related ischemic heart disease. *Cardiovascular Drugs and Therapy, 34*, 133–137. https://doi.org/10.1007/s10557-019-06926-5.

Lu, C. T., Leong, P. Y., Hou, T. Y., Kang, Y. T., Chiang, Y. C., Hsu, C. T., Lin, Y. D., et al., (2019). Inhibition of proliferation and migration of melanoma cells by ketoconazole and *Ganoderma* immunomodulatory proteins. *Oncology Letters, 18*(1), 891–897. https://doi.org/10.3892/ol.2019.10355.

Majima, Y., (2018). SY25-5-Patients expectation for drug discovery development targeting rare cancers. *Annals of Oncology, 29*, vii36. https://doi.org/10.1093/annonc/mdy386.

Mannucci, C., Casciaro, M., Sorbara, E. E., Calapai, F., Di Salvo, E., Pioggia, G., Navarra, M., et al., (2021). Nutraceuticals against oxidative stress in autoimmune disorders. *Antioxidants, 10*, 261. https://doi.org/10.3390/antiox10020261.

Marinkovich, M. P., (2007). Laminin 332 in squamous-cell carcinoma. *Nature Reviews Cancer, 7*, 370–380. https://doi.org/10.1038/nrc2089.

Marventano, S., Forjaz, M., Grosso, G., Mistretta, A., Giorgianni, G., Platania, A., Gangi, S., et al., (2013). Health related quality of life in colorectal cancer patients: State of the art. *BMC Surgery, 13*(2), S15. https://doi.org/10.1186/1471-2482-13-s2-s15.

Michalczyk, K., Pawlik, J., Czekawy, I., Kozłowski, M., & Cymbaluk-Płoska, A., (2021). Complementary methods in cancer treatment-cure or curse? *International Journal of Environmental Research and Public Health, 18*, 356. https://doi.org/10.3390/ijerph18010356.

Mittal, A., Tabasum, S., & Singh, R. P., (2014). Berberine in combination with doxorubicin suppresses the growth of murine melanoma B16F10 cells in culture and xenograft. *Phytomedicine, 21*(3), 340–347.https://doi.org/10.1016/j.phymed.2013.09.002.

Nasr, I., McGrath, E. J., Harwood, C. A., Botting, J., Buckley, P., Budny, P. G., Fairbrother, P., et al., (2021). British association of dermatologists guidelines for the management of adults with basal cell carcinoma 2021. *British Journal of Dermatology*. https://doi.org/10.1111/bjd.20524.

Nicolas, D., Fabienne, D., & Véronique, P., (2014). Review: Vitamin E-based nanomedicines for anticancer drug delivery. *Journal of Controlled Release, 182*, 33–44.https://doi.org/10.1016/j.jconrel.2014.03.009.

Nuutinen, T., (2018). Medicinal properties of terpenes found in *Cannabis sativa* and *Humulus lupulus*. *European Journal of Medicinal Chemistry, 157*, 198–228. https://doi.org/10.1016/j.ejmech.2018.07.076.

Oh, C. C., Jin, A., & Koh, W. P., (2021). Trends of cutaneous basal cell carcinoma, squamous cell carcinoma, and melanoma among the Chinese, Malays, and Indians in Singapore from 1968–2016. *JAAD International, 4*, 39–45. https://doi.org/10.1016/j.jdin.2021.05.006.

Okhovat, J. P., Beaulieu, D., Tsao, H., Halpern, A. C., Michaud, D. S., Shaykevich, S., & Geller, A. C., (2018). The first 30 years of the American academy of dermatology skin cancer screening program: 1985–2014. *Journal of the American Academy of Dermatology, 79*(5), 884–891. https://doi.org/10.1016/j.jaad.2018.05.1242.

Olthof, M. R., Hollman, P. C. H., & Katan, M. B., (2001). Chlorogenic acid and caffeic acid are absorbed in humans. *The Journal of Nutrition, 131*(1), 66–71. https://doi.org/10.1093/jn/131.1.66.

Ong, Y. L. R., Sambrook, P., & Maddern, G., (2021). Oral squamous cell carcinoma resection and neck dissection mortality: A 10-year national audit study. *ANZ Journal of Surgery, 91*(1, 2), 145–151. https://doi.org/10.1111/ans.16463.

Ottino, P., & Duncan, J. R., (1997). Human study: Effect of vitamin E succinate on free radical formation, lipid peroxidation levels and cyclooxygenase activity in murine melanoma cells. *Nutrition. Research, 17*(4), 661–676. https://doi.org/10.1016/S0271-5317(97)00036-5.

Pal, H. C., Diamond, A. C., Strickland, L. R., Kappes, J. C., Katiyar, S. K., Elmets, C. A., Athar, M., & Afaq, F., (2016). Fisetin, a dietary flavonoid, augments the anti-invasive and anti-metastatic potential of sorafenib in melanoma. *Oncotarget, 7*(2), 1227–1241. https://dx.doi.org/10.18632%2Foncotarget.6237.

Pandey, L., Pasricha, R., Joseph, D., Ahuja, R., Yanthan, Y., Garg, P. K., & Gupta, M., (2021). Use of complementary and alternative medicine among patients with cancer in a sub-Himalayan state in India: An exploratory study. *Journal of Ayurveda and Integrative Medicine, 12*(1), 126–130. https://doi.org/10.1016/j.jaim.2021.01.001.

Patel, D., Shukla, S., & Gupta, S., (2007). Apigenin and cancer chemoprevention: Progress, potential and promise (review). *International Journal of Oncology, 30*(1), 233–245. http://dx.doi.org/10.3892/ijo.30.1.233.

Patra, V., GallaisSérézal, I., & Wolf, P., (2020). Potential of skin microbiome, pro- and/or pre-biotics to affect local cutaneous responses to UV exposure. *Nutrients, 12*, 1795. https://doi.org/10.3390/nu12061795.

Paunović, M. G., Matić, M. M., Ognjanović, B. I., & Saičić, Z. S., (2017). Antioxidative and haematoprotective activity of coenzyme Q10 and vitamin E against cadmium-induced oxidative stress in Wistar rats. *Toxicology and Industrial Health, 33*(10), 746–756. https://doi.org/10.1177/0748233717725480.

Pedrelli, V. F., Lauriola, M. M., & Pigatto, P. D., (2012). Clinical evaluation of photoprotective effect by a topical antioxidants' combination (tocopherols and tocotrienols). *Journal of the European Academy of Dermatology and Venereology, 26*(11), 1449–1453. https://doi.org/10.1111/j.1468-3083.2011.04219.x.

Pereira, L., (2018). Seaweeds as source of bioactive substances and skin care therapy-cosmeceuticals, algotheraphy, and thalassotherapy. *Cosmetics, 5*, 68. https://doi.org/10.3390/cosmetics5040068.

Piantelli, M., Rossi, C., Iezzi, M., La Sorda, R., Iacobelli, S., Alberti, S., & Natali, P. G., (2006). Flavonoids inhibit melanoma lung metastasis by impairing tumor cells endothelium interactions. *Journal of Cellular Physiology, 207*(1), 23–29. https://doi.org/10.1002/jcp.20510.

Piao, L., Mukherjee, S., Chang, Q., Xie, X., Li, H., Castellanos, M. R., Banerjee, P., et al., (2017). TriCurin, a novel formulation of curcumin, epicatechin gallate and resveratrol, inhibits the tumorigenicity of human papillomavirus-positive head and neck squamous cell carcinoma. *Oncotarget, 8*, 60025–60035. https://doi.org/10.18632/oncotarget.10620.

Ravindranath, M. H., Ramasamy, V., Moon, S., Ruiz, C., & Muthugounder, S., (2009). Differential growth suppression of human melanoma cells by tea (*Camellia sinensis*) epicatechins (ECG, EGC and EGCG). *Evidence-Based Complementary and Alternative Medicine, 6*(4), 523–530. https://doi.org/10.1093/ecam/nem140.

Ricci, S., Pinto, F., Auletta, A., Giordano, A., Giovane, A., Settembre, G., Boccellino, M., et al., (2019). The enigmatic role of matrix metalloproteinases in epithelial-to-mesenchymal transition of oral squamous cell carcinoma: Implications and nutraceutical aspects. *Journal of Cellular Biochemistry, 120*(5), 6813–6819. https://doi.org/10.1002/jcb.26905.

Ruiz-Nunez, B., Pruimboom, L., Dijck-Brouwer, D. J., & Muskiet, F. A., (2013). Lifestyle and nutritional imbalances associated with Western diseases: Causes and consequences of chronic systemic low-grade inflammation in an evolutionary context. *The Journal of Nutritional Biochemistry, 24*(7), 1183–1201. https://doi.org/10.1016/j.jnutbio.2013.02.009.

Sacco, A., Forgione, L., Carotenuto, M., De Luca, A., Ascierto, P. A., Botti, G., & Normanno, N., (2020). Circulating tumor DNA testing opens new perspectives in melanoma management. *Cancers, 12*, 2914. https://doi.org/10.3390/cancers12102914.

Sakkas, H., Bozidis, P., Touzios, C., Kolios, D., Athanasiou, G., Athanasopoulou, E., Gerou, I., & Gartzonika, C., (2020). Nutritional status and the influence of the vegan diet on the gut microbiota and human health. *Medicina, 56*, 88. https://doi.org/10.3390/medicina56020088.

Saxena, M., Saxena, J., & Pradhan, A., (2012). Flavonoids and phenolic acids as antioxidants in plants and human health. *International Journal of Pharmaceutical Sciences Review and Research, 16*, 130–134.

Serafino, A., Vallebona, P. S., Lazzarino, G., Tavazzi, B., Rasi, G., Pierimarchi, P., Andreola, F., et al., (2004). Differentiation of human melanoma cells induced by cyanidin-3-O-β-glucopyranoside. *The FASEB Journal, 18*(15), 1940–1942. https://doi.org/10.1096/fj.04-1925fje.

Sevli, O., (2021). A deep convolutional neural network-based pigmented skin lesion classification application and experts evaluation. *Neural Computing and Applications, 33*, 12039–12050. https://doi.org/10.1007/s00521-021-05929-4.

Siegel, R. L., Miller, K. D., Fuchs, H. E., & Jemal, A., (2021). Cancer statistics. *CA: A Cancer Journal for Clinicians, 71*(1), 7–33. https://doi.org/10.3322/caac.21654.

Singh, S. P., Alvi, S. B., Pemmaraju, D. B., Singh, A. D., Manda, S. V., Srivastava, R., & Rengan, A. K., (2018). NIR triggered liposome gold nanoparticles entrapping curcumin as in situ adjuvant for photothermal treatment of skin cancer. *International Journal of Biological Macromolecules, 110*, 375–382. https://doi.org/10.1016/j.ijbiomac.2017.11.163.

Singh, T., & Katiyar, S. K., (2011). Green tea catechins reduce the invasive potential of human melanoma cells by targeting COX-2, PGE2 receptors and epithelial-to-mesenchymal transition. *PLoS One, 6*(10), e25224. https://doi.org/10.1371/journal.pone.0025224.

Sous, D., Armstrong, A. E., Huang, J. T., Shah, S., Carlberg, V. M., & Coughlin, C. C., (2021). Cutaneous reactions to pediatric cancer treatment: Part I. Conventional chemotherapy. *Pediatric Dermatology, 38*(1), 8–17. https://doi.org/10.1111/pde.14418.

Sreedhar, A., Li, J., & Zhao, Y., (2018). Next-gen therapeutics for skin cancer: Nutraceuticals. *Nutrition and Cancer, 70*(5), 697–709. https://doi.org/10.1080/01635581.2018.1470651.

Srinivas, N., Malla, R. R., Kumar, K. S., & Sailesh, A. R., (2021). Environmental carcinogens and their impact on female-specific cancers. Malla, R. R., & Nagaraju, G. P., (eds.), *A Theranostic and Precision Medicine Approach for Female-Specific Cancers* (pp. 249–262). Academic Press. https://doi.org/10.1016/B978-0-12-822009-2.00015-7.

Staniforth, V., Chiu, L. T., & Yang, N. S., (2006). Caffeic acid suppresses UVB radiation-induced expression of interleukin-10 and activation of mitogen-activated protein kinases in mouse. *Carcinogenesis, 27*, 1803–1811.https://doi.org/10.1093/carcin/bgl006.

Strashilov, S., & Yordanov, A., (2021). Aetiology and pathogenesis of cutaneous melanoma: Current concepts and advances. *International Journal of Molecular Sciences, 22*(12), 6395. https://doi.org/10.3390/ijms22126395.

Strickland, L. R., Pal, H. C., Elmets, C. A., & Afaq, F., (2015). Targeting drivers of melanoma with synthetic small molecules and phytochemicals. *Cancer Letters, 359*(1), 20–35. https://doi.org/10.1016/j.canlet.2015.01.016.

Su, S., Cheng, J., Zhang, C., Akihisa, T., Xu, J., Zhu, W., Liu, W., et al., (2020). Melanogenesis-inhibitory activities of limonoids and tricyclic diterpenoids from *Azadirachtaindica*. *Bioorganic Chemistry, 100*, 103941. https://doi.org/10.1016/j.bioorg.2020.103941.

Todorova, K., & Mandinova, A., (2020). Novel approaches for managing aged skin and nonmelanoma skin cancer. *Advanced Drug Delivery Reviews, 153*, 18–27. https://doi.org/10.1016/j.addr.2020.06.004.

Uddin, A. N., Labuda, I., & Burns, F. J., (2012). A novel mechanism of filaggrin induction and sunburn prevention by β-damascenone in Skh-1 mice. *Toxicology and Applied Pharmacology, 265*(3), 335–341. https://doi.org/10.1016/j.taap.2012.08.035.

Vaid, M., Singh, T., & Katiyar, S. K., (2011). Grape seed proanthocyanidins inhibit melanoma cell invasiveness by reduction of PGE2 synthesis and reversal of epithelial-to-mesenchymal transition. *PLoS One, 6*(6), e21539. https://doi.org/10.1371/journal.pone.0021539.

Vainio, H., & Rautalahti, M., (1998). An international evaluation of the cancer preventive potential of carotenoids. *Cancer Epidemiology, Biomarkers & Prevention, 7*, 725–728.

Valiahdi, S. M., Iranshahi, M., & Sahebkar, A., (2013). Cytotoxic activities of phytochemicals from *Ferula* species. *DARU Journal of Pharmaceutical Sciences, 21*, 1–7.https://doi.org/10.1186/2008-2231-21-39.

Van, D. R. M., Huang, Z., Giovannucci, E., Rimm, E. B., Hunter, D. J., Colditz, G. A., Stampfer, M. J., & Willett, W. C., (2000). Diet and basal cell carcinoma of the skin in a prospective cohort of men. *The American Journal of Clinical Nutrition, 71*(1), 135–141. https://doi.org/10.1093/ajcn/71.1.135.

Vishwakarma, V., New, J., Kumar, D., Snyder, V., Arnold, L., Nissen, E., Hu, Q., et al., (2018). Potent antitumor effects of a combination of three nutraceutical compounds. *Scientific Reports, 8*(1), 12163. https://doi.org/10.1038/s41598-018-29683-1.

Wang, L., Zhang, Z., Ge, R., Zhang, J., Liu, W., Mou, K., Lv, S., & Mu, X., (2019). Gossypetin inhibits solar-UV induced cutaneous basal cell carcinoma through direct inhibiting PBK/TOPK protein kinase. *Anticancer Agents in Medicinal Chemistry, 19*(8), 1029–1036. https://doi.org/10.2174/1871520619666190301123131.

Wolff, T., Tal, E., & Miller, T., (2009). Screening for skin cancer: An update of the evidence for the U.S. preventive services task force. *Annals of Internal Medicine, 150*(3), 194–198. https://doi.org/10.7326/0003-4819-150-3-200902030-00009.

Yang, G., Fu, Y., Malakhova, M., Kurinov, I., Zhu, F., Yao, K., Li, H., et al., (2014). Caffeic acid directly targets ERK1/2 to attenuate solar UV-induced skin carcinogenesis. *Cancer Prevention Research, 7*(10), 1056–1066. https://doi.org/10.1158/1940-6207.capr-14-0141.

Zhang, X. M., Chen, J., Xia, Y. G., & Xu, Q., (2005). Apoptosis of murine melanoma B16-BL6 cells induced by quercetin targeting mitochondria, inhibiting expression of PKC-α and translocating PKC-δ. *Cancer Chemotherapy and Pharmacology, 55*, 251–262. https://doi.org/10.1007/s00280-004-0863-5.

INDEX

G

N

O

P

Q

R

S